Chronic Disease Management for Small Animals

Edited by

W. Dunbar Gram
University of Florida College of Veterinary Medicine
Florida, US

Rowan J. Milner
University of Florida College of Veterinary Medicine
Florida, US

Remo Lobetti
Bryanston Veterinary Hospital
Bryanston, Johannesburg
South Africa

WILEY Blackwell

The right of W. Dunbar Gram, Rowan J. Milner, and Remo Lobetti to be identified as the authors of the editorial material in this work has been asserted in accordance with law.

Registered Office(s)
John Wiley & Sons, Inc., 111 River Street, Hoboken, NJ 07030, USA

Editorial Office
111 River Street, Hoboken, NJ 07030, USA

For details of our global editorial offices, customer services, and more information about Wiley products visit us at www.wiley.com.

Wiley also publishes its books in a variety of electronic formats and by print-on-demand. Some content that appears in standard print versions of this book may not be available in other formats.

Library of Congress Cataloging-in-Publication Data

Names: Gram,W. Dunbar, editor. | Milner, Rowan J. editor. | Lobetti, Remo, editor.
Title: Chronic disease management for small animals / edited by W. Dunbar Gram, Rowan J. Milner, Remo Lobetti.
Description: Hoboken, NJ : Wiley, [2017] | Includes bibliographical references and index. |
Identifiers: LCCN 2017020145 (print) | LCCN 2017027035 (ebook) | ISBN 9781119201588 (pdf) |
   ISBN 9781119201052 (epub) | ISBN 9781119200895 (pbk.)
Subjects: | MESH: Dog Diseases–diagnosis | Cat Diseases–diagnosis | Dog Diseases–therapy | Cat Diseases–therapy |
   Chronic Disease–therapy
Classification: LCC SF991 (ebook) | LCC SF991 .C55 2017 (print) | NLM SF 991 | DDC 636.70896–dc23
LC record available at https://lccn.loc.gov/2017020145

Cover Design: Wiley
Cover Images: (center left, center right) courtesy of Mary Gardner;
(bottom & center middle) courtesy of Remo Lobetti

Set in 10/12pt Warnock by SPi Global, Pondicherry, India
Printed and bound in Singapore by Markono Print Media Pte Ltd

10 9 8 7 6 5 4 3 2 1

Contents

List of Contributors

Michele Berlanda PhD
Department of Animal Medicine,
Production and Health
University of Padova
Legnaro, Italy

Richard K. Burchell BSc (Hons), BVSc,
MMedVet (Med), DECVIM-CA
Massey University Veterinary
Teaching Hospital
Massey University
New Zealand

Iwan A. Burgener Dr.med.vet., Dr. habil, PhD,
DACVIM, DECVIM-CA
Small Animal Internal Medicine
VetMedUni Vienna, Vienna, Austria

Sheila Carrera-Justiz, DVM, DACVIM
(Neurology)
Department of Small Animal Clinical
Sciences, University of Florida,
Florida, US

Sylvie Daminet DACVIM,
DECVIM-CA, PhD
Department of Small Animal Medicine
and Clinical Biology
Faculty of Veterinary Medicine
Ghent University, Belgium

Mary Gardner, DVM
Lap of Love Veterinary Hospice,
6061 Grandview Ave, Yorba Linda
CA 92886

W. Dunbar Gram, DVM, DACVD, MRCVS
Department of Small Animal Clinical
Sciences, University of Florida College of
Veterinary Medicine, Florida, US

Kate Hill BVSc MANZCVS DACVIM PhD
School of Veterinary Science
The University of Queensland, Australia

Ninette Keller BVSc, BVSc (Hons), MMedVet
(Med), Grad Cert Tert Ed
Veterinary Specialist Services
Carrara, Gold Coast, Australia

Frank Kettner MMedVet, DECVIM-CA
Tygerberg Animal Hospital
Cape Town, South Africa

Liza S. Köster BVSc MMedVet (Med) DECVIM-CA
(Internal Medicine)
Small Animal Hospital, Glasgow University
Veterinary School, 464 Bearsden Road,
United Kingdom

Remo Lobetti BVSc (Hons) MMedVet (Med) PhD
DECVIM-CA (Internal Medicine)
Bryanston Veterinary Hospital
Bryanston, Johannesburg, South Africa

Joanne L. McLean BSc (Vet Biol) BVSc (Hons)
MMedVet (Med), DECVIM-CA
Bakenkop Animal Clinic Centurion,
South Africa

Dani McVety, DVM
Lap of Love Veterinary Hospice
Florida, US

Rowan J. Milner BVSc (Hons), MMedVet (Med), PhD, DECVIM-CA, DACVIM
University of Florida College of Veterinary Medicine,
Florida, US

Caryn E. Plummer, DVM, DACVO
Department of Small Animal Clinical Sciences, University of Florida, Florida, US

Tanya Schoeman BVSc (Hons) MMedVet (Med) DECVIM-CA
Cape Animal Medical Centre
Kenilworth, Cape Town

Gilad Segev DVM, DECVIM-CA
Koret School of Veterinary Medicine
Hebrew University of Jerusalem
Rehovot, Israel

Justin Shmalberg, DVM DACVN DACVSMR CVA CVCH CVFT
Board-certified in Small Animal Clinical Nutrition and in Sports Medicine & Rehabilitation, Integrative Medicine (Nutrition, Acupuncture, Rehabilitation, and Hyperbaric Oxygen Therapy) University of Florida College of Veterinary Medicine, Florida, US

Simon Swift, MA, VetMB, CertSAC, DECVIM-CA (Cardiology) MRCVS
Department of Small Animal Clinical Sciences, University of Florida, Florida, US

Penny Watson MA VetMD CertVR DSAM DECVIM-CA
Senior Lecturer in Small Animal Medicine
Department of Veterinary Medicine
Madingley Road
Cambridge, United Kingdom

Eric Zini PD, PhD, DECVIM-CA (Internal Medicine)
Clinic for Small Animal
Internal Medicine
Vetsuisse Faculty
University of Zurich
Zurich, Switzerland
Department of Animal Medicine,
Production and Health
University of Padova
Legnaro, Italy
Istituto Veterinario di Novara
Granozzo con Monticello, Italy

Preface

The goal of this first edition of *Chronic Disease Management for Small Animals* is to provide a textbook aimed at the management of chronic diseases in dogs and cats. The format of the book is concise so veterinarians quickly can find answers to questions relating to chronic diseases. This book is not intended to be another internal medicine textbook, but rather serve to catch a reader's attention and to educate regarding compassionate therapies for chronic diseases.

Virtually all a veterinarian's professional education is focused on acquiring and assimilating knowledge to properly diagnose and cure diseases. With experience, we realize that a significant part of our day is devoted to managing chronic conditions, for which there is no cure. This reality can be a challenge not only for the veterinarian but also for the owner/caregiver. The steps required to make a correct diagnosis often require less financial and emotional commitment than long-term therapy and management. Client education and "shared decision making" are critical components of

successful therapy with the goal of improving both the patient's and the client's quality of life.

This book is aimed at both the recent graduate and seasoned practitioner. The recent graduate, with some level of comfort in the diagnosis and treatment of diseases, soon discovers that chronic and incurable conditions often require a different approach than what was taught in veterinary school. For the seasoned practitioner who has achieved success in the management of chronic diseases, the benefit of the book is an up-to-date reference guide.

The book is divided into three parts. Part One on Communication and Caregiving, is aimed at the impact chronic disease has on the quality of life for both the patient and the owner/caregiver. Part Two, which forms the bulk of the book, deals with chronic diseases outlining diagnostics, therapeutics, quality-of-life and end-of-life decisions. Part Three focuses on hospice care and end of life. It covers client and patient needs, quality of life, cultural sensitivities, dying naturally, euthanasia, and death.

Acknowledgments

Together, we would like to recognize and thank the individuals (both animal and human) as well as their caregivers who have taught us much about the management of chronic disease. They and their primary care veterinarians were our inspiration. The editors and project managers at Wiley, including Erica Judisch, were instrumental in bringing this book to fruition and we thank them for their expertise. Lastly, we are grateful for our families who continually encourage and support us and our careers.

Part One

Communication and Caregiving

1

Communication, Caregiving, and Chronic Disease

Dani McVety

Introduction

Disease is often conceptualized as a temporary state and recovery as close as a single dose of medication, a round of antibiotics, or a few days of rest. Sometimes the "quick fix" doesn't resolve the issue. Instead, we are left with the realization that sickness and death do not happen because medicine fails. Sickness and death happen because breakdown is the natural aging of biology.

Veterinary medical schools are designed to prepare their graduates for the practice of medicine. How prepared they are is directly related to how those institutions define that practice. Is it merely the ability to apply diagnostics and treatment protocols, surgical preparedness, and so forth? Or does the practice of veterinary medicine include something more: the ability to define and seek an optimal outcome when there is no quick fix or any fix at all?

Veterinarians need to graduate with the knowledge, experience, and resources clients need and expect to properly handle these situations. Veterinarians must learn and apply other nonmedical skills if they expect their medical knowledge to be put to good use, particularly in situations of chronic disease management. These nonmedical skills include displaying empathy and active listening. So what is the importance of learning these skills and methods that go beyond veterinary medical science? Simply put, these tools are needed when treating patients with chronic diseases.

Empathy, active listening, and other nonmedical skills form the solid rock upon which the veterinarian stands when implementing medical knowledge to the highest potential allowed by the client. Only by establishing rapport and trust with clients will veterinarians help them expend their financial, emotional, time, and physical resources to make the investment necessary to improve the health, well-being, and quality of life of their pet.

Managing chronic disease brings a great deal of change for both the patient and the family. This change can happen both quickly, in the form of a terminal diagnosis, and/or subtly, in the form of symptomatic changes evolving over a period of time. Establishing this solid trust-based relationship is particularly important. Therefore, how a veterinarian establishes a relationship with a client, then delivers the news of change, and finally manages the emotions surrounding the change may determine whether medical treatment is facilitated for the well-being of the pet. Because veterinarians have the obligation to deliver the best medical care to patients, which hinges almost entirely on the veterinarian–client relationship, they must develop and utilize the skill sets necessary to communicate with, find common ground with, and persuade their clients.

Chronic Disease Management for Small Animals, First Edition. Edited by W. Dunbar Gram, Rowan J. Milner and Remo Lobetti.
© 2018 John Wiley & Sons, Inc. Published 2018 by John Wiley & Sons, Inc.

Box 1.1

It would be interesting to investigate how veterinarians may be impacted in situations where the client could not serve as legal proxy.

In veterinary medicine, our clients served as proxy for their pet's wishes in almost every interaction they have with a veterinarian. As veterinarians, we have two parties to serve; the owner/client and the patient. (Shelter medicine is the only exception to this rule, as treatment of animals in a shelter setting rarely include an owner.) In human medicine, the client and the patient are generally one person. Even in pediatric medicine, the parent is the guardian of the child, not the owner of the child. The parent generally has the levity to make decisions, but if that decision is not in the best interests of the child (as reasonably determined in a court of law), then the parent will lose the ability to make decisions for that child. In fact, it took a groundbreaking case in 1984 (*In re Guardianship of Barry*, 445 So.2d 365 (Fla. 2d DCA 1984)) to determine that a parent *can* serve as proxy for their dying infant child's wishes, allowing the removal of life support in this case.

And particularly in cases involving chronic disease, we remove "life support" frequently in many different ways. Legally, clients are owners of the patient and our communication and established rapport with that owner is imperative if we are to gain the trust such that our medical knowledge will be put to use for the betterment of the pet and/or the treatment of a disease.

This first chapter will explore how veterinarians can properly implement techniques to communicate the ideas learned in medical school to the client to improve the treatment and/or supportive care for the betterment of the chronically/terminally ill or aging pet. We will then discuss various specific skills that will aid the veterinarian in setting up the conversation appropriately, ensuring all parties are on the same page, learning how to adjust one's communication under certain difficult situations, and, finally, having the conversation about potentially ending a pet's life to mitigate pain and suffering.

Overview

You are more likely get back on a horse if your dismount is smooth rather than if you are bucked off. The trauma of a difficult dismount may hinder your desire to return to the saddle; pet ownership is similar. When clients have a peaceful end-of-life experience with their pet, they will heal more quickly, return to pet ownership more quickly, and more readily be back in your clinic. The clients that feel that the loss of their pet is "so traumatic, there's just no way I'll ever get another dog" are usually the ones that we want to have adopt another animal! Those are the clients that truly care for their pets, providing good medical care and giving animals safe and loving homes.

This end-of-life experience applies to more than the actual euthanasia process. The experience begins much sooner, when a chronic or terminal condition arises, even if that condition is simply "old age." The presence of an undesirable situation leaves the client feeling cornered. Emotions are heightened. There is more sensitivity to a veterinarian's communication. Each may contribute to the client's difficulty in making a decision on a treatment plan. Therefore, how veterinarians respond and adjust their communication in this tense situation will impact whether treatment plans are accepted, productive, and helpful to the pet and client.

In this chapter, we will first explore the mentality of clients by understanding the emotional impact of chronic disease. We will explore how to establish relationships with clients, how they respond to stress, how to best approach clients, and finally how to adjust your verbal and nonverbal communication to reach maximal effect and avoid conflict.

Impact of Chronic Disease on Quality of Life for Both the Patient and Caregiver

Veterinary medicine aims to recognize and effectively manage pain in a way that decreases suffering and increases the patient's quality of life for those pets with chronic conditions. In assessing and determining quality of life, the term "quality" has many meanings. Essentially, "quality" signifies a "general characteristic or overall impression one has of something" (Welmelsfelder 2007). Veterinary professionals recognize quality as a separate entity from quantity, as the concept "more is better" is not necessarily true. Therefore, to optimize an ill patient's quality of life, the veterinarian might encourage treatments that favor the patient's perception of welfare rather than longevity.

Illustration of the above concept is seen through the treatment options for a pet diagnosed with cancer. The characteristic methods of cancer treatment are typically surgery, chemotherapy, and/or radiation. Upon evaluating the type of cancer, how quickly it grows or spreads, and its location, a veterinarian must weigh the effects of treatment to the patient's quality of life. This information is then shared with the caregiver, and together, they make an informed decision based on the client's ability to pay for, provide, and emotionally handle the care associated with extended treatment.

For instance, when deciding whether to perform surgery, the veterinarian should determine whether the costs to the animal outweigh the benefits. If the removal of a large tumor also requires removing a vital organ, thus resulting in the loss of an essential bodily function, the costs largely overtake the benefits. If the patient must live in anguish to increase lifespan, it is best to choose an alternative route that allows instead for comfort and contentment. However, if the treatment offers longer life expectancy in addition to a positive prognosis with only acute adverse effects, it is worth

further exploring. Often, those associated acute conditions can be remedied with medication or simple lifestyle changes, generating a wise investment in exchange for long-term well-being.

To understand how chronic diseases impact a companion animal, there must first be a clear understanding of what quality of life is and how it is assessed. We can expand on the previous definition of the term "quality" by defining "quality of life" as "the total well-being of an individual animal" (August et al. 2009). Although definitions of the term vary, most can agree that quality of life encompasses the physical, social, and emotional components of the animal's life (August et al. 2009) in the current daily environment.

Although veterinary medicine has made vast improvements in assessing quality of life, it wasn't until the past decade that it has been extensively studied and measured in companion animal medicine (Lavan 2013). Due to its complex nature and modernism, no accepted standards or protocols currently exist (August et al. 2009); however, various quality-of-life surveys have been developed and are tailored toward many of the individual chronic diseases. Overall, these questionnaires evaluate a combination of physical versus nonphysical factors, including needs satisfaction, sense of control, social relationships, physical functioning, hygiene, mental status, and management of stress (see Figure 1.1). The principal aim of the surveys is to broadly assess and evaluate over time the states and changes of comfort or discomfort (Lavan 2013).

Due to the common element of self-reporting in determining quality of life, which is obviously not possible for animals, research has been done to support and establish signs, symptoms, mannerisms, and other qualitative measures people can use to gauge this. Although many hope for a more scientific approach to quality for an animal, its primary reliance remains on human perception and interpretation (Welmelsfelder 2007). Hence, studies show that the skill to communicate with a companion animal is age-old and does

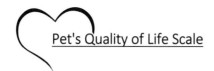

Pet's Quality of Life Scale

When evaluating the quality of life of your pet, personalized patient <u>and</u> family information is important when reaching an educated, informed, and supported choice that fits not only your pet's medical condition but also your wishes and expectations. In short, *quality of life* applies not only to the pet; it also applies to you!

Score each subsection on a scale of 0–2:

0 = agree with statement (describes my pet)
1 = some changes seen
2 = disagree with statement (does not describe my pet)

Social Functions

___ Desire to be with the family has not changed

___ Interacts normally with family or other pets (i.e., no increased aggression or other changes)

Physical Health

___ No changes in breathing or panting patterns

___ No outward signs of pain (excessive panting, pacing, and whining are most commonly seen)

___ No pacing around the house

___ My pet's overall condition has not changed recently

Mental Health

___ Enjoys normal play activities

___ Still dislikes the same thing (i.e., still hates the mailman = 0, or doesn't bark at the mailman anymore = 2)

___ No outward signs of stress or anxiety

___ Does not seem confused or apathetic

___ Nighttime activity is normal, no changes seen

Natural Functions

___ Appetite has stayed the same

___ Drinking has stayed the same

___ Normal urination habits

___ Normal bowel movement habits

___ Ability to ambulate (walk around) has stayed the same

Results:

0–8 Quality of life is most likely adequate. No medical intervention required yet, but guidance from your veterinarian may help you identify signs to look for in the future.

9–16 Quality of life is questionable and medical intervention is suggested. Your pet would certainly benefit from veterinary oversight and guidance to evaluate the disease process he/she is experiencing.

17–36 Quality of life is a definite concern. Changes will likely become more progressive and more severe in the near future. Veterinary guidance will help you better understand the end stages of your pet's disease process in order to make a more informed decision of whether to continue hospice care or elect peaceful euthanasia.

www.LapofLove.com | 1-855-933-5683

Figure 1.1 Quality of life scales.

Family's Concerns

Score each section on a scale of 0–2:

0 = I am not concerned at this time.
1 = There is some concern.
2 = I am concerned about this.

I am concerned about the following things:

___ Pet suffering

___ Pet dying alone

___ Not knowing the right time to euthanize

___ Concern for other household animals

___ Desire to perform nursing care for your pet

___ Ability to perform nursing care for your pet

___ Coping with loss

___ Concern for other members of the family (i.e. children)

Results:

0–4   Your concerns are minimal at this time. You have either accepted the inevitable loss of your pet and understand what lies ahead, or have not yet given it much thought. If you have not considered these things, now is the time to begin evaluating your own concerns and limitations

5–9   Your concerns are mounting. Begin your search for information by educating yourself on your pet's condition; it's the best way to ensure you are prepared for the emotional changes ahead

10–16   Although you may not place much value on your own quality of life, your concerns about the changes in your pet are valid. Now is the time to prepare yourself and to build a support system around you. Veterinary guidance will help you prepare for the medical changes in your pet while counselors and other health professionals can begin helping you with anticipatory grief

Discuss these questions below, and the entire Quality of Life Scale, with your veterinarian.

Below are some open-ended questions that assist gauge your family's time, emotional, and (when appropriate, financial) budgets:
1. Have you ever been through the loss of a pet before? If so, what was your experience (good or bad, and why)?
2. What do you *hope* the life expectancy of your pet will be? What do you *think* it will be?
3. What is the ideal situation you wish for your pet's end of life experience? (at home, pass away in her sleep, etc.)

Suggestions on using this quality of life scale:
1. Complete the scale at different times of the day, note circadian fluctuations in well-being. (We find most pets tend to do worse at night and better during the day.)
2. Request multiple members of the family complete the scale; compare observations.
3. Take periodic photos of your pet to help you remember their physical appearance.

Resources:
1. AAHA/AAFP Pain Management Guidelines for Dogs and Cats, **www.aahanet.org/Library/PainMgmt.aspx**
2. Online hospice journal and quality of life scale: www.PetHospiceJournal.com

www.LapofLove.com | 1-855-933-5683

Figure 1.1 Continued

not need scientific validation to prove its worth (Welmelsfelder 2007).

The best approach to assessing animal quality of life is through a combination of interpretation of behavior and physical traits by both the caregiver and the veterinarian over time. The animal's owner has the day-to-day first-hand experience of understanding changes in mannerisms and personality. Owners also typically administer treatment at home and are the first to notice their pet's reaction, such as side effects to medications or response to a procedure or therapy. Correspondingly, veterinarians play the vital role of determining and communicating the options and effects of various treatments. Healthcare providers offer the knowledge of species- and breed-specific behavioral repertoires as well as extensive experience in observing and acting with different species in various contexts (Welmelsfelder 2007). This proficiency allows them to accurately judge and share with the caregiver the meaning of their pet's body language (Welmelsfelder 2007).

Ideally, quality-of-life surveys could be conducted and discussed with a veterinarian throughout the lifespan of the animal, regardless of health status. By regularly using a quality of life survey for both healthy and chronically ailing patients, the caregiver and the veterinarian can document changes over time, have a familiarity with quality-of-life assessments, and, most importantly, enable the ability to discern minor quality-of-life changes caused by aging, chronic conditions, and/or disability.

For animals suffering from chronic diseases, even the subtlest changes over time can offer a significant impact to their quality of life and may indicate the need for additional or more formal approaches to treatment. Depending on the specific ailments, many patients suffering from chronic diseases experience changes in their levels of "anxiety," "fear," "restlessness," "sociability," and "playfulness," which are witnessed and reported by the owner (Welmelsfelder 2007). In these quality-of-life assessments, it is important to distinguish between the physi-

cal and mental parameters. For instance, if an owner of an arthritic animal expresses that his/her pet is "slower during walks," a determination should be made on whether this is because of pain, a mental state, or weakness associated with aging, a physical parameter (Yeates and Main 2009). If the determination is "pain," adjustments should be made for alleviation.

Similarly, this "body language" established by the physical movement of the animal associated with corresponding psychological qualities displays the verifiable impression of chronic diseases on quality of life. Among countless examples, here are just a few:

1) Consider a sudden onset of blindness, affecting access to food and water (physical parameters), in addition to discerning whether the blindness leads to fear, distress, decreasing the animal's companionship with others, or inability to "explore" during walks (physiological parameters).

2) Diabetes mellitus is another common chronic condition among cats and dogs. If well managed and treated, a diabetic pet can enjoy the same quality of life as any other pet. However, if uncontrolled or mistreated, diabetes can cause increased water consumption and urination, weight loss, dehydration, weakness, seizures, and possibly death. These quality-of-life ailments are evident through the pet's body language, such as lethargy, smelling like urine, or acting depressed.

3) As common as osteoarthritis is, it might be hard to spot at first considering that the pet's behavioral changes could be subtle. Arthritis doesn't necessarily mean a poor quality of life for a pet; it is simply joint inflammation caused by an increase in stiffness and immobility. If this inflammation can be controlled, the pet may enjoy a relatively good quality of life. Changes like medications, therapies, and household adjustments can be made to control these painful symptoms. Pets display these symptoms of pain by avoiding once enjoyable activities, acting

depressed, moving less, decreasing their hygiene (unable to keep clean due to immobility), and/or changing their eating habits. Anti-inflammatory drugs, holistic therapies, acupuncture, herbal supplements, and household alterations, such as keeping food and water at a comfortable height, adding nonskid runners to avoid slips, and extra warmth at night, can help to regulate the symptoms and provide for a happier life.

As indicated in the examples above, chronic diseases can have a significant bearing on a companion animal's quality of life. However, with careful selection and administration, therapies and treatments can help to assure good quality of life. Side effects must be considered so the measures executed will denote visible changes in quality of life or will otherwise provide a positive prognosis for long-term quality despite acute ailments.

While organ systems and treatment issues vary by illness, they all share the commonality of requiring daily attention from a caregiver to perform routine tasks for monitoring and management. Research has highlighted the enormous devotion owners have to their pets and the efforts and expenses they are willing to incur to provide optimal healthcare for them (Kelly 2014). There is an undeniable overlap in comparing the management of a pet's discomfort to that of a human; for both, the caregiver often administers a scheduled regimen of medication, monitors for signs of adverse reactions, and is prepared to transport the patient for emergency treatment if needed. The stakes are high if the conditions are not treated properly, as common results are brain damage or death. Among many examples, this is the case with diabetes management and allergic reactions to medications. This ambiance creates an immense amount of pressure and highly stressful conditions for the caregiver. As a result of the pressures associated with providing care, a caregiver is likely to experience substantial adjustment problems, higher levels of psychological distress,

deprived health, and reduced well-being; thus referred to as "caregiver burden" (Kelly 2014; Christiansen et al. 2013).

The pressure is better understood when compiling research that supports the notion of viewing a pet in much the same way as a child. A survey conducted by the American Veterinary Medical Association (AVMA) found that of 47,842 US households, nearly half (49.7%) of the respondents owning at least one pet "considered their pets to be family members" (Kelly 2014). Furthermore, similar to the human caregiving model, women are typically the primary caregivers of pets; AVMA's national study showed that 74.5% of pet owners with primary responsibility for their pets were female (Kelly 2014). Based on this, a conclusion can be made that caregivers of pets, especially mothers, endure the same form of quality of life reduction as do human caregivers.

The most common challenges reported by caregivers are the time it takes to provide extra care, changes in the use of the home to tailor the pet's needs, and restrictions relating to work, a social life, and finances (Christiansen et al. 2013). Many individuals described these changes as "time-consuming," "tough," "concerning," and "annoying" while also being "sad" and "frustrated" with the decline in the human–animal relationship. It is common to hear owners speak of "loss," "guilt," and "emotional distress" when caring for a chronically ill patient, as they are trying to weigh treatment options to euthanasia. Overall, caregivers tend to agree with veterinary professionals that the quality of life of their pet is more important than longevity. In fact, in a recent study, 86% of owners of dogs being treated for cancer were willing to exchange their dog's survival time for an improved or stable quality of life.

As advances in veterinary medicine continue, managing the quality of life for both the chronically ill patient and the caregiver is becoming increasingly possible. Palliative care providers offer guidance to families faced with caring for a pet; they aid in creating plans for living well based on the animal's needs and assist in treatment options to provide optimal quality of life for their patients (August *et al.* 2009). They also help to develop and administer the caregivers' goals while providing emotional and spiritual support. By establishing and following the treatment options provided by a veterinary professional and confiding in this professional, both the pet and the caregiver can enhance their shared quality of life, maximize their time spent together, and make important decisions when the pet's life can no longer be prolonged due to an unacceptable quality of life.

Part 1: Know Yourself—Set the Stage for Collaborative Decision Making, Active Listening, and Caregiving

> *It's not what you look at that matters, it's what you see.*
> —Henry David Thoreau

Trust is the foundation for collaborative decision making toward a common goal. The veterinary–client–patient relationship is based on that one shared goal: the well-being of the pet. The client may bring a dog into the emergency room at 2:00 a.m. after seeing a tapeworm in the feces while being completely oblivious to the swollen lymph nodes and coughing that has "just recently started, but I'm not too worried about it." Treatment of the tapeworm, or at least some dedicated time discussing the plan for treatment, is essential to establish trust with this client before an in-depth discussion on oncology ensues. Otherwise, the client will feel like you did not treat the most immediate and pressing issue (what the client sees with his/her own eyes) and instead chose a more expensive and deadly route.

In the example above, both the client and the veterinarian are "right." Both have the pet's best interests at heart. But the important thing is to get on the same page first to

maximize a positive outcome. The satisfaction of both parties with the outcome is pliable, mendable, and will change over time based on the knowledge at hand, but without establishing trust and rapport first, the client may not trust an expensive oncology workup after the original concern was simply a tapeworm.

Under the right circumstances, significant rapport can be built in a short amount of time. Experts estimate that it takes anywhere from a few seconds to 2–3 minutes for an immediate "good gut feeling" about someone to be established. In the author's opinion, it takes 1–2 seconds for clients (especially a stressed pet parent) to decide if they "like you" or not, 1–2 minutes for clients to decide if they trust you, and about 15 minutes for significant rapport to be established, even if you don't have all the answers. Simple things such as eye contact, smiling, open-ended questions, facing the patient, and even physically touching the person will leave the client feeling like the appointment lasted twice as long as it actually did.

Box 1.2
Physicians that had never been sued (no-claims) were compared with ones that had been sued two or more times. No-claims primary care physicians used more statements of orientation (educating patients about what to expect and the flow of a visit), laughed and used humor more, and tended to use more facilitation (soliciting patients' opinions, checking understanding, and encouraging feedback). Additionally, no-claims primary care physicians spent an average of 3.3 minutes longer in routine visits (Levinson *et al.* 1997).

Setting the stage for this type of trusting relationship to be established and to use the tools discussed later in this chapter starts with the veterinarian even before entering the exam room. When dealing with clients, particularly in a stressful or sad situation, such as chronic disease management, there are three rules that should always be followed:

1) Maintain self-control by actively listening and controlling your reactions.
2) Detach from the outcome; expect that you will not "win" every discussion.
3) Identify the shared value system between you and the client; remain focused on the common goal(s).

Self-Control

It is the veterinarian's role to be and appear to be in complete control when those around him/her are not. Control indicates confidence, and confidence earns trust. When setting the stage for good, constructive, collaborative decision making, self-control is the most important and powerful tool the veterinarian has. This is, of course, much easier said than done. The basis of this rule is to remain in compassionate control of the appointment flow, allowing the client to feel secure and well guided throughout the interaction with the veterinarian. It also requires active listening with little to no negative emotional reaction to the client's words. It requires you to put yourself in the position of the client and listen to his/her story from that viewpoint, not yours.

Imagine that a client is having the worst day of his/her life. Perhaps a spouse was just diagnosed with a terminal illness or the client lost his/her job. The client may need to focus this discontent and, quite naturally, you may become the target. To mitigate against this, first build a constant stream of empathy for the situation. Still, the client may begin to complain about a mistake he/she felt you made. Instantly reacting in an emotional, hostile, or defensive manner will scar the relationship immediately. Instead, continue to actively listen: let the client vent his/her frustration. Often such hostility is simply grief over a condition the client wishes to be different. Instead, remain poised and concerned but confident. Focus

on a solution or on better explaining the proposed course of care. If it's appropriate, there will always be time to share your side of the story later. It is far better to be kind than to be right.

Tips for maintaining self-control in the exam room:

1) Remember it's not about your feelings.
2) Remember the outcome is not happening to you.
3) Control fear and anger.
4) Use "emotional labeling" ("I can tell you are upset/angry/hurt").

Detaching from the Outcome

Detaching from the outcome is simply about understanding that you will not always "win" a disagreement with a client. Some clients are too entangled in their grief to fully listen or understand your suggestions. They may appear to be "picking a fight" with you from the very beginning. Being attached to the outcome of the disagreement (e.g., pushing the client to approve your treatment plan) too early may set the stage for resentment, particularly in clients with personalities that need time to establish a relationship with you and process information. Actively listening and requesting clarification and feedback from these clients will help them feel that you are not pushing an agenda on them but rather that you are there to support their pet in the same way that they are.

Shared Value Systems

Remaining focused on the shared value systems that both the veterinarian and the client have reminds both parties of the purpose of the interaction. Phrases like "we are both in this for the same reason, we both want Max to feel better" will remind them that everyone wants the same thing. Particularly when emotions rise or there is a moment of impasse, this is an important tool to use.

Maintaining self-control, detaching from the outcome, and focusing on shared value systems will leave the client feeling nonjudgmentally validated. People do not want to be judged in any thought or opinion that they have or in any action that they take. It doesn't mean you agree with someone. Validation is taking the time to listen to what their needs, wants, dreams, and aspirations are. You may not always understand, but simply by your listening, the client will feel validated and the stage for collaborative decision making will be set.

Part 2: Verbal Communication

Structure allows for flexibility in a conversation. It may sound counterintuitive, but when you have a structured conversation in place for any type of medicine; general practice, emergency, specialty medicine, and even geriatric medicine, that structure will allow you to walk a family through a conversation confidently and competently and therefore provide space to adjust yourself to their wishes and concerns more easily. Do not be afraid of the conversational structure provided here or sounding too rehearsed; when used properly, the flow patterns can ensure the veterinarian remains in compassionate control of the situation, exuding the confidence and competence clients desperately want and need at a difficult time.

As we move through this discussion, remember that veterinary medicine these days is more like pediatrics than the "horse mechanics" we were generations ago. Pets are family now. They have moved from the barnyard to inside the home to our bedroom ... and even under our sheets! A survey conducted by the AVMA (AVMA 2012) found that of 63.2% of people surveyed considered their pets to be family members. Another 35.8% considered their pets to be pets or companions, and only the remaining 1% considered their pets to be property.

The Use of Pet Pronouns

The words we choose to use when describing pets must be reflective of the importance they hold in the family. Sure, some people may view their pet as "just a dog," but those people will be only slightly offended by your endearing use of the word "baby," as compared to the owner who refers to herself as "Charlie's mom," who will be much more offended by the use of the pronoun "it"!

Through many discussions with thousands of veterinary professionals, it is the author's conclusion that about half of the veterinary team is willing to say the word "baby" when referring to a client's pet. Of course, that doesn't mean we all prefer this term. Many of us are not completely comfortable with its use, but adopt it based on the reaction from pet parents ("pet parent" is also a phrase gaining traction in our industry). These words can be used in a clinic to give a much more family oriented feel. But once the pet's name is known, there is no greater word than the name given to him/her by his/her owners.

Along these same lines, we have adopted the use of "pet parent" in our practice but still generally use the word "owner" when referring to the case among colleagues. Although "pet parent" may not seem preferable at first, the upside of a clinic conveying "we understand the importance of the pet in the family" is much more beneficial than risking the downside of appearing "cold" or "rude." It's rare that someone is genuinely offended by the use of these overly "fluffy" words, even if it's not his/her first choice either. But with 84% of pet owners referring to themselves as "mom" or "dad," this doesn't seem too far off the mark (JAVMA 2000).

Tone of Voice

Cats and dogs both use different vocal tones at different times of stress, attraction, play seeking, or almost any other behavior. Humans also deepen their voice while making their speech sound "more pleasant" when talking to someone they find attractive. A recent study illustrated this point (Hughes, Farley, and Rhodes 2010):

> We examined how individuals may change their voices when speaking to attractive versus unattractive individuals, and if it were possible for others to perceive these vocal changes. In addition, we examined if any concurrent physiological effects occurred when speaking with individuals who varied in physical attractiveness. We found that both sexes used a lower-pitched voice and showed a higher level of physiological arousal when speaking to the more attractive, opposite-sex target. Furthermore, independent raters evaluated the voice samples directed toward the attractive target (versus the unattractive target) as sounding more pleasant when the two voice samples from the same person presented had a reasonably perceptually noticeable difference in pitch.

The idea of using a lower-pitched voice to influence others in a multitude of ways has been known for quite some time. Margaret Thatcher was known to have too "shrill" a voice at the beginning of her career; so much so that she was not allowed on party broadcasts. But before her election in 1979, she worked with a speech coach to help lower her pitch and develop her infamously calm, authoritative tone. Her biographer Charles Moore later wrote, "Soon the hectoring tones of the housewife gave way to softer notes and a smoothness that seldom cracked except under extreme provocation on the floor of the House of Commons" (Gardner 2014).

Aside from lowering the vocal tone, a common mistake is the use of "upspeak." A frequent mistake in women (though men can do this as well!), the offender ends every sentence on a higher note than the rest of the speech. Doing this makes everything that's said sound like a question and, most importantly, gives up the confidence we wish to convey to our clients. Some professionals feel this kind of tone is very "California/Valley Girl," with the perception that this speech pattern makes its users appear young, immature, and overall uncertain. Instead of ending a statement on a high note (literally, not figuratively), try ending it on a consistent or even lower pitch (NOT softer) to convey a strong sense of confidence.

Salutations

We've all been there, the typical "hi, how are you" followed by the "great, how are you?" and then, it's really bad, one more "I'm great, how are you"...and then you're lost. When responding to the customary "how are you?" find and use (and reuse!) a phrase that you really love: "loving life and living the dream!" or "this is the best day of my life" or "it couldn't be better, I get to play with animals all day!" Any of these will leave the client feeling happy (hopefully) and, at minimum, spark a curiosity in him/her that may lead to an interesting conversation.

Sounding Persuasive

Though there are hundreds of tips on sounding persuasive, we have chosen our top three: talk moderately fast, use just enough pitch, and use powerful pauses.

1) Rate of speech: Speaking at a regular rate, perhaps even moderately fast, has been shown to be positively correlated with perceived intelligence. "Interviewers who spoke moderately fast, at a rate of about 3.5 words per second, were much more successful at getting people to agree than either interviewers who talked very fast or very slowly," said Jose Benki, a research investigator at the University of Michigan Institute for Social Research (Swanbrow 2011). Throw in a bit of humor, and you have a recipe for winning someone over!

2) Pitch variation: Some researchers have shown that the more active the pitch and variation, the more energetic and engaging a person may appear. This isn't always the case, however: "We found only a

marginal effect of variation in pitch by interviewers on success rates. It could be that variation in pitch could be helpful for some interviewers but for others, too much pitch variation sounds artificial, like people are trying too hard. So it back-fires and puts people off," said Benki (Swanbrow 2011).

3) Powerful pauses: "When people are speaking, they naturally pause about 4 or 5 times a minute," according to Benki. "These pauses might be silent, or filled, but that rate seems to sound the most natural in this context. If interviewers made no pauses at all, they had the lowest success rates getting people to agree to do the survey. We think that's because they sound too scripted. People who pause too much are seen as disfluent. But it was interesting that even the most disfluent interviewers had higher success rates than those who were perfectly fluent (and did not use pauses)."

Particularly in a high-paced, knowledge-based profession like veterinary medicine, you are best to make your verbal deliveries with mini-mal variation, focusing instead on tone, include natural…steady…frequent…pauses!

Sounding Honest

In Alex Pentland's book *Honest Signals: How They Shape Our World*, the author points out a couple of things to keep your eye on (Pentland 2010):

1) Speech mimicry and behavioral mimicry: Are they using the same words you use? Speaking at a similar speed and tone? Are they sitting the way you sit? Is a subtle, unconscious game of follow-the-leader going on? This is a sign the other person feels emotionally in sync with you. It can be faked but that's rare and difficult to pull off consistently across a conversation.

2) Consistency of emphasis and timing: This is a sign of focus and control. Someone who is less consistent is less sure of them-selves and more open to influence.

Win Them Over Again

If all else fails, what are two things you can do to win someone over? Robert Cialdini, author of the must-read book *Influence*, provides these important tips (Cialdini 1993):

1) Give honest compliments: It may not be easy, especially if the person has been dis-tancing him-/herself from you for a while. But if you're objective, the other person probably has some qualities you admire. If you take positive action and compliment people, it may well break the ice and make them re-evaluate their perceptions of you.

2) Ask for their advice: Cialdini notes this strategy—which involves asking for pro-fessional advice, book suggestions, and so forth—comes from Founding Father Ben Franklin, a master of politics and relation-ship building. "Now you've engaged the rule of commitment and consistency," says Cialdini, in which others look at their actions (giving you advice or a book) and draw a conclusion from it (they must actually like you), a surprisingly common phenomenon in psychology. "And sud-denly," says Cialdini, "you have the basis of an interaction, because now when you return it, you can return it with a book you think he or she might like."

Verbal communication is, indeed, extremely important in the communication we have with clients. The delivery, consistency, and accompanying nonverbal cues give the client the feeling that we are either listening and engaged or detached and uninterested. We have a choice, and with proper education, we can be in a better position to choose the best route for our patient, our client, and our team. Table 1.1 gives examples of average and ideal ways to express ourselves.

Part 3: Nonverbal Communication

A veterinary clinic's curb appeal does not stop at the clinic door. It extends all the way into the exam room and, most importantly,

Table 1.1 Examples of Average and Ideal expressions.

Average	Ideal
So let's get going. (moving appointment along)	I certainly feel he's ready and I have so much information to share with you, I want to make sure we cover it all.
	I'm going to step out and let my team know we need a bit more time.
I need to go. (appointment is taking too long)	I have another family to help, but Fluffy is top priority right now.
You will know when it's time.	We will work together to know when it's the best time.
You are doing the right thing.	We are doing the best thing.
Don't worry about him.	He is in good hands.
There's nothing more you can do.	You have done an amazing job.
He is out of pain.	He feels so much better now.

to the entire team! Every person our clients interact with will receive a "snap judgment" from his/her first impression. How long does this take? For years the general rule has been 7 seconds, but a few years ago a group of psychologists found that it takes about one-tenth of a second to form an impression of a stranger, simply from his/her face (Willis and Todorov 2006). They also found that longer exposure to the stranger does not significantly alter the impression; it only boosts confidence in the initial judgment.

What does this mean to a veterinary team? It means that we have a very, very small amount of time to make a positive impression on our clients. This positive impression is not only essential from a business standpoint (you want them to come back!) but also from a medical one. Our clients need to trust us; they need to believe that we care about their pet the same way they do. Without the belief and trust that the client and the veterinarian have the same desired outcome, trust and rapport will not be established, and the

client may not accept the treatment plan that the veterinary professional team has offered. Which is, after all, the reason we are in business: to care for, treat, heal, and support animals.

Of course, the importance of body language or nonverbal communication is not a new concept. The "7-38-55 Rule" was first developed in 1971 by University of California, Los Angeles psychology professor Albert Mehrabian (Mehrabian 2009): 55% of what we convey when we speak comes from our body language, 38% from our tone of voice, and a mere 7% from the words we choose. This study has been widely misinterpreted by stating "97% of what we convey is nonverbal" instead of garnering a greater understanding of vocal (tone, cadence, etc.) and body language cues, which are inappropriately combined to come up with the "97%."

Mehrabian more clearly states the following on his website:

> Total Liking = 7% Verbal Liking + 38% Vocal Liking + 55% Facial Liking. Please note that this and other equations regarding relative importance of verbal and nonverbal messages were derived from experiments dealing with communications of feelings and attitudes (i.e., like–dislike). Unless a communicator is talking about their feelings or attitudes, these equations are not applicable.

Although this landmark study is riddled with criticism and misinterpretation, it remains an important and highly cited illustration of the value of nonverbal communication. Many other studies have arisen since, each with a new methodology and with the continued conclusion that nonverbal cues are 3–4 times more influential than verbal cues.

Before we dive into the real content, it's important to understand that reading body language is not the same as mind reading. This is the difference between "observation" and "evaluation." Reading someone's nonverbal cues is about observation; we want to find natural tendencies in someone's physical behavior (called their "baseline"), then look for deviations from their baseline, and, finally, ask open-ended questions to find the root cause of the change.

For example, you may walk into a room and find two people seated; both have their arms crossed, while one has both feet flat on the floor and the other has her legs crossed at the knee. You might assume that the closed-off body postures mean they are both are upset, and perhaps the female is even more upset because her legs are crossed as well. This may be true, but probably not. Jumping to conclusions so quickly and, for example, immediately putting your guard up or responding with your own closed-off body language may start you off on a bad foot (no pun intended) by eliciting defensive behavior from these clients. In this example, crossed arms might be this gentleman's natural baseline, and the female may simply be cold!

Remember, reading body language is about observing someone's baseline, finding where there are deviations from that baseline, and using powerful questions to find the underlying cause of the deviation.

The Basics

The basics of body language are pretty simple. Across species lines, animals (human and nonhuman) use adaptations to increase or decrease their physical presence. A bear stands on his back legs to appear taller, cobras expand their hood when they are threatened, and the mantis lifts her front limbs while displaying a conspicuous eyespot to scare or distract a predator.

Humans present similar nonverbal "tells" by puffing their chest and standing taller when an attractive woman walks by or throwing both hands up in the air after accomplishing a huge milestone (even humans who have been blind since birth exhibit these behaviors).

The opposite is true as well; a dog cowers in the back of a cage or tucks his tail, an embarrassed child covers her face. We tend to minimize our physical presence when we want to disappear!

Each unique area of our body displays our emotions differently. The face is the most important when it comes to first impressions, and the feet most important when you want to know whether a negotiation is being tipped in your favor.

Personal Curb Appeal

When you want to make the most positive impression possible on a client, there are four main areas to consider: initial facial expressions, the introduction to the client, nonverbal cues (aka nonverbals) while speaking, and physical appearance. Each of these areas has been proven to influence the impression someone has on another person.

Facial Expressions

Judgments based on facial appearance or expression play a very powerful role in how we get treated (Mehrabian 2009). In fact, in a court of law, it's been shown that "mature faces" receive harsher judicial outcomes than those with a "baby face," and having a face that is thought to be "competent" (as opposed to trustworthy or likable) may be highly predictive of whether a person gets elected to public office (Zebrowitz and McDonald 1991). Also, like it or not, attractive people are more favorably viewed in general, leading to overall better outcomes in life, in addition to being thought of as more trustworthy (Subhani 2012).

What is a good way to use your facial expressions to improve your curb appeal? Smile. Yes, simply smile. Of course, we have all been subjected to the "fake smile" versus the "genuine smile"! This distinction has been researched for quite some time; so much so that a genuine smile is now described with the name "Duchenne smile" after the French physician Guillaume Duchenne, who studied the physiology of facial expressions in the nineteenth century (Harker and Keltner 2001).

The *Journal of Personality and Social Psychology* described the difference from the anatomical perspective (Harker and Keltner 2001):

1) The Duchenne smile involves both voluntary and involuntary contraction from two muscles: the zygomatic major (raising the corners of the mouth) and the orbicularis oculi (raising the cheeks and producing crow's feet around the eyes).
2) A fake smile involves the contraction of just the zygomatic major since we cannot voluntarily contract the orbicularis oculi muscle.

Interestingly, the fake smile is controlled by the motor cortex, while more complicated emotion-related expressions, like the Duchenne smile, are controlled by the limbic system.

Yes, our clients can tell the difference! A genuine, warm, sincere expression of happiness that conveys a welcoming greeting is related to emotion, while the cheesy grin is simply a forced muscle action. So make sure your greeter (whomever that might be) smiles because he/she is happy to be there, not because he/she is forced to!

The Nonverbals of Introduction
Upon being greeted with the warm, genuine smile, the customary introduction ensues. Even if this is a long-standing client, there is still a formal greeting ritual we all engage in. The first 7 seconds may be too long for a first impression, but it's the perfect amount of time for a good introduction.

In our current Western society, the handshake occurs first and, as long as it's a good one, is the universally accepted sign of professionalism, politeness, and confidence. A good handshake is an art! Whether you're the veterinarian or the support staff, make sure you initiate the handshake before the client does to show a confident welcome. Remember, clients are coming into your "home" (the clinic), and you want them to feel that you genuinely appreciate their presence. Make hand contact palm to palm, web

to web (the "web" is the flap of skin between your thumb and pointer finger), while keeping the angle of your hand either perpendicular to the ground or palm facing slightly up. Palm down in a handshake indicates power. Don't squeeze too tightly, nor too loosely, and maintain consistent tension as you say your greeting. Also, make sure to shake everyone's hand in the pet's family, not just the primary owner—even the children. (What a way to inspire a new generation of veterinarians!)

While shaking the client's hand, maintain good eye contact and introduce yourself, even if you believe he/she knows your name (but not with close friends, of course!). Clients may have forgotten your name since their last visit, and setting your clients up for success by knowing your name helps build their confidence.

Because the introduction is about 7 seconds long, make sure it's meaningful. Step in front of the receptionist's desk to shake the client's hand, use a two-handed handshake (both of your hands around their one hand), lean gently forward to show appreciation for the client coming in, and/or bend down to pet his/her dog (cats may not appreciate this, though!).

Nonverbals to Gain Rapport
After you've made an amazing first impression, followed by a confident introduction, it's time to complete the circle so that the client builds the trust, rapport, satisfaction, and connection with the entire veterinary team. These skills all enforce the concepts of active listening, engaged interaction, and supporting the client's concerns.

These concepts are broken into three anatomical areas: the top, middle, and lower body regions.

Body Language in the Top Third
Eye contact is incredibly important! But how much is too much? At what point does it start to become creepy? One study on the Royal Society Open Science website (Binetti *et al*. 2016) found that, when asked to stare at a

video of an actor staring back at them, participants had a "preferred gaze duration" of 3.3 seconds (give or take 0.7 seconds). The authors also found that the rate of pupillary dilation (an automatic reflex) was a good indicator of how long people wanted to gaze; the longer their preferred gaze, the faster their pupils expanded. (Don't get too attached to this difference, however. The change was so subtle that it was only seen with eye-tracking software, which would be awkward to follow in real life!)

Make your eye contact consistent by looking only inside the imaginary triangle between the two points about 1 inch above each eye and the tip of the nose; going farther down to the mouth or chin is more indicative of a social or amorous relationship.

Aside from the eyes, do not bite, tense, purse, or conceal your lips. Janine Driver, renowned body language expert, says, "when we don't like what we see or hear, our lips disappear" (Lyintamer 2014). This is evidenced by turning both lips into our mouth, similar to spreading lip balm once it's been applied.

When nodding your head, a gentle, 1 second nod implies active listening, whereas faster head nods may tell your listener "hurry up, I don't have time for this." Make your nods slow and small with a closed mouth (which indicates you are listening).

Hands and arms are the second component of this category. Many of us will find ourselves wringing our hands or picking at our fingernails at any given moment. This may increase when we are nervous and evolve from a normal, baseline behavior into what is considered "pacifying" behavior. This is a normal reaction to nervousness or discomfort. (Again, we don't know WHY someone may be nervous or uncomfortable, but we can simply make the observation, then follow up with a powerful question.)

On the deeper meaning of hand positions, Adam Kendon, author of *Gesture: Visible Action as Utterance*, says (Kendon 2004):

Gestures of the Open Hand Prone or "palm down" family are used in contexts

where something is being denied, negated, interrupted or stopped, whether explicitly or by implication. Open hand Supine (or "palm up") family gestures, on the other hand, are used in contexts where the speaker is offering, giving or showing something or requesting the reception of something.

When auditing the body language of your own hands and arms, use open, offering palms when escorting a client to an exam room, offering to take their coat, or asking if there's "anything else you need?"

Body Language in the Middle Third

Where someone's torso is facing may be one of the most important indications of where they want (or don't want!) to be. The "belly button rule" dates back to the 1930s. Since then, numerous scientists and body language experts have reinforced the theory. Most notably, psychology professor Mehrabian has said, "the belly button rule is the most important indicator of reading a person's intention."

During an introduction, face your belly button toward them. This indicates genuine interest and engagement. While you're writing in the patient's chart as the client actively describes his/her pet's history (or anything else he/she feels is important to you), you may turn your shoulders slightly away in recording notes, as long as your belly button remains mostly pointed toward the person talking.

Body Language in the Lower Third

Many experts feel that it's easier to read someone's feelings by looking at his/her feet than any other part of the body. In fact, this concept especially applies to interactions when one party is attempting to "convince" another, which can be the case when a veterinarian (or anyone else on the team) is presenting an estimate to a client. Studies have actually shown that crossed legs can have a devastating effect on a negotiation.

In *How to Read a Person Like a Book*, authors Gerard Nierenberg and Henry H. Calero reported that the number of times settlements were reached increased greatly when both negotiators had uncrossed their legs. In fact, they found that out of 2,000 videotaped negotiation transactions, not one resulted in a settlement when even one of the negotiators had his/her legs crossed (Nierenberg and Calero 1971).

So what is "good" body language in this lower part of the body? Because building a rapport with clients is our main goal, you want to be perceived as interested and actively listening. Uncross your legs, both feet flat on the ground, sit on the edge (but not too far forward) of the seat, and lean slightly forward. (This is a great stance to take when writing the clinical history while listening to the client.) For the best effect possible, don't jiggle your feet, wrap your toes around the edge of the chair, or cross your legs or your ankles. And if you see the client doing any of these unwanted behaviors, it might be a good time to audit your own body language or other communication styles (tone or phrasing) to compensate for the potential misalignment. Of course the client might simply be cold!

Physical Appearance

You may not be into fashion or up on the latest trends, but that's not what having a "nice" appearance is all about. Being well dressed has everything to do with appearing put together, not being a mannequin for the latest crop top or fringe boots. Just as our clients will judge the veterinarian's surgical skills by the neat row of sutures, they will also judge our entire team's knowledge, professionalism, compassion, and overall trustworthiness by the way we choose to dress ourselves that morning.

We've all heard the saying "dress for the job you want" or "clothes make the man." Well, those sayings have real research, and lots of it, to back them up! In 1955, a group of researchers had a man cross a city street against traffic (Lefkowitz, Blake, and Mouton 1955). When this man was dressed in a suit, 3.5 times as many people followed him as when he was wearing a "work shirt and trou-

sers." Regardless of background demographics, a business suit is universally seen as a form of authority.

Taking this one step further, not only is being well dressed seen as a reason for others to follow you but also a reason for others to do what you ask them to do. In another study (Bickman 1974), an experimenter would stop someone on the street, point to a person about 50 feet away (this person far away was an accomplice), and say, "You see that guy over there by the parking meter? He's over parked but doesn't have any change. Give him a dime!" The experimenter would then leave. When dressed in a uniform (anything relating to authority), most people complied with the instruction to give the other person money. When dressed in regular clothes, however, compliance was less than 50%!

But how does this translate into the exam room? What about the white coat hypertension we hear so much about? It appears this may be an overreaction, making it the exception, not the norm. In a written survey in 2005, patients were asked to review pictures of physicians in four different dress styles, then answer questions relating to their preference as well as their willingness to discuss sensitive issues (Rehman *et al.* 2005):

On all questions regarding physician dress style preferences, respondents significantly favored the professional attire with white coat (76.3%, P < .0001), followed by surgical scrubs (10.2%), business dress (8.8%), and casual dress (4.7%). Their trust and confidence was significantly associated with their preference for professional dress (P < .0001). Respondents also reported that they were significantly more willing to share their social, sexual, and psychological problems with the physician who is professionally dressed (P < .0001). The importance of physician's appearance was ranked similarly between male and female respondents (P = .54); however, female physicians' dress appeared to be significantly more important to respondents than male physicians' dress (P < .001).

The conclusion from this study was obvious: "Respondents overwhelmingly favor physicians in professional attire with a white coat. Wearing professional dress (i.e., a white coat with more formal attire) while providing patient care by physicians may favorably influence trust and confidence-building in the medical encounter."

More recently, in 2015 a comprehensive international review of studies on physician attire was published on the British Medical Journal Open website, adding to the previous study's findings (Petrilli *et al.* 2015),. The authors confirmed the idea that, yes, most people prefer their doctor to be dressed formally, and they also stressed that how you feel about your doctor's attire can depend greatly on your age and/or culture. For example, in general, Europeans and Asians of any age, and Americans over age 50, trusted a formally dressed doctor more, while Americans in Generations X and Y tended to accept less-dressy physicians more willingly. Doctors in other roles, however, such as surgery or emergency, appear more insulated from this effect, and patients are much more willing to see their doctor in scrubs.

Even if you are not the veterinarian, pick your attire carefully. What you choose to put on your body says more to the client about your professionalism and trustworthiness than you may think!

Conclusion

Curb appeal does not stop at the clinic's entrance. And fortunately for veterinary professionals, those clinic doors are human sized, not small doggy doors (until pets earn a monetary income, this will be the case)! We have to interact with, connect with, and, ultimately, win the trust of our clients if our professional knowledge is to be put to good use. Without that rapport with our clients, something every person of the veterinary team is responsible for upholding, our treatment plans may not be accepted and/or compliance may not be achieved. Only through immediate, consistent, and appropriate maintenance of this bond will the patients receive the best possible medical care and our clients be happy to see us again!

References

August K, Cooney K, Hendrix L, Mader B, Pierce J, Shanan, A. 2009, Animal hospice and palliative care guidelines. International Association of Animal Hospice and Palliative Care (IAAHPC). 2009: 1–51.

AVMA. U.S. pet ownership and demographics sourcebook. 2012.

Bickman L. The social power of a uniform. Journal of Applied Social Psychology. 1974; 4: 47–61.

Binetti N, Harrison C, Coutrot A, Johnston A, Mareschal I. Pupil dilation as an index of preferred mutual gaze duration. Royal Society Open Science. 2016.

Christiansen SB, Kristensen AT, Sandoe P, Lassen J. Looking after chronically ill dogs: impacts on the caregiver's life. Anthrozoos. 2013; 25(4): 519–533.

Cialdini R. Influence. HarperCollins. 1993.

Gardner B. From shrill housewife to Downing Street: the changing voice of Margaret Thatcher. Daily Telegraph, November 25, 2014. Online at: http://www.telegraph.co.uk/news/politics/11251919/From-shrill-housewife-to-Downing-Street-the-changing-voice-of-Margaret-Thatcher.html.

Harker L, Keltner D. Expressions of positive emotion in women's college yearbook pictures and their relationship to personality and life outcomes across adulthood. Journal of Personality and Social Psychology. 2001; 80(1): 112–124.

Hughes SM, Farley SD, Rhodes BC. Vocal and physiological changes in response to the physical attractiveness of conversational partners. Journal of Nonverbal Behavior. 2010; 34(3): 155–167.

JAVMA. Survey says: owners taking good care of their pets. Online at: https://www.avma.org/News/JAVMANews/Pages/s020100d.aspx. 2000.

Kelly MA. Managing a pet's chronic illness. PhD diss., University of Illinois Chicago. 2014.

Kendon A. Gesture: visible action as utterance. Cambridge University Press. 2004.

Lavan RP. Development and validation of a survey for quality of life assessment. Veterinary Journal. 2013; 197: 578–582.

Lefkowitz M, Blake RR, Mouton JS. Status factors in pedestrian violation of traffic signals. Journal of Abnormal Social Psychology. 1955; 51: 704–706.

Levinson W1, Roter DL, Mullooly JP, Dull VT, Frankel RM. Physician-patient communication. The relationship with malpractice claims among primary care physicians and surgeons. Journal of the American Medical Association. 1997; 277(7): 553–559.

Lyintamer, NBC's Today show invites back comedic communications consultant and top keynote speaker Janine Driver. Online at: http://www.lyintamer.com/lt-blogs/85-nbc-s-today-show-invites-back-comedic-communications-consultant-and-top-keynote-speaker-janine-driver. 2014.

Mehrabian A. Silent messages – a wealth of information about nonverbal communication (body language). Self-published. 2009.

Nierenberg G, Calero HH. How to read a person like a book. Simon and Schuster. 1971.

Pentland A. Honest signals: how they shape our world. MIT Press. 2010.

Petrilli CM, Mack M, Petrilli JJ, Hickner A, Saint S, Chopra, V. Understanding the role of physician attire on patient perceptions: a systematic review of the literature: targeting attire to improve likelihood of rapport (TAILOR) investigators. British Medical Journal Open. 2015.

Rehman SU, Nietert PJ, Cope DW, Kilpatrick AO. What to wear today? Effect of doctor's attire on the trust and confidence of patients. American Journal of Medicine. 2005; 118(11): 1279–1286.

Subhani MI. Physical attractiveness or referrals: which matters the most? Submitted to International Journal of Accounting and Finance. 2012.

Swanbrow D. Persuasive speech: the way we, um, talk sways our listeners. Michigan News May 11, 2011. Online at: http://ns.umich.edu/new/releases/8404-persuasive-speech-the-way-we-um-talk-sways-our-listeners.

Welmelsfelder F. How animals communicate quality of life: the qualitative assessment of behavior. Animal Welfare. 2007; 15: 25–31.

Willis J, Todorov A. First impressions: making up your mind after a 100-ms exposure to a face. Psychological Science. 2006; 17(7): 592–598.

Yeates Y, Main D. Assessment of companion animal quality of life in veterinary practice and research. Journal of Small Animal Practice. 2009; 50: 274–281.

Zebrowitz LA, McDonald SM. The impact of litigants' baby-facedness and attractiveness on adjudications in small claims courts. Law & Human Behavior. 1991; 15: 603.

Part Two

Syndromes and Clinical Signs of Chronic Disease

2

Pruritus, Atopic Dermatitis, and Pyoderma

W. Dunbar Gram

Introduction

Dermatitis, cutaneous infections, and pruritus consistently are some of the most common reasons caregivers bring pets to veterinarians. They often have an underlying allergic primary disease process. These symptoms may be chronic or recurrent; often presenting during the first as well as the last year of life. While a single etiology may be present, it is common that multiple diseases and factors are concurrent contributing issues. These factors may vary from episode to episode, season to season, year to year and with the general health of the patient. Canine atopic dermatitis is "A genetically-predisposed inflammatory and pruritic allergic skin disease with characteristic clinical features associated with IgE antibodies most commonly directed to environmental allergens" (Halliwell 2006). A somewhat similar disease occurs in cats and is referred to as "Feline Atopic Syndrome" (Foster 2014).

A chronic, life impacting but nonlethal disease can be difficult for a caregiver to accept and challenging for the veterinarian–client relationship. In these situations, empathetic client communication, client engagement, and client education are essential for both the short- and long-term well-being of the patient (Knesl, Hart and Fine 2016). It is important for the veterinarian to "meet the client/caregiver where they are," within their comfort zone, walk alongside them, and get to know their motivation, fears, goals, and limitations. Once the client is comfortable with the relationship, the veterinarian and the caregiver can better work together for the benefit of the patient. The relationship is often dynamic. Motivations, fears, goals, limitations, medical knowledge, and therapeutic options may change with time, particularly with a chronic disease. Both parties should be adaptable and mutually respectful of each other's importance regarding the health of the patient.

The "good and the bad" aspects of chronic dermatological disease are inherent. Seldom does a dermatology patient face an acute life-threatening situation with all the emotional and financial aspects that accompany them. Yet, very few dermatologic diseases are curable, and consequently chronic management is necessary. Additionally, symptoms may wax and wane independently of therapeutic intervention, leading to the incorrect assumption that a therapeutic intervention is beneficial and should be continued. Most therapies are purely palliative and have potential side effects as well as contraindications. Allergen specific immunotherapy (ASIT) is the only specific therapy for atopy (Mueller 2014). It can reverse an integral part of the underlying pathogenesis and in some cases effect a virtual cure for canine atopic dermatitis (DeBoer 2014).

Chronic Disease Management for Small Animals, First Edition. Edited by W. Dunbar Gram, Rowan J. Milner and Remo Lobetti.
© 2018 John Wiley & Sons, Inc. Published 2018 by John Wiley & Sons, Inc.

Summation of effect and threshold pruritus theory can be used to help explain how various factors contribute to the clinical signs (Tater 2012). In this explanation, the threshold at which clinical signs are noted can be represented by a horizontal line. Under that horizontal line are vertical bars stacked upon each other, like building blocks. Once the stacked bars are taller than the line, the threshold is breached. At this point, clinical signs become evident. In some cases, a single factor may be large enough to reach the threshold and in other cases, several factors may be needed. Some veterinarians may use gestures instead of lines or bars to make this point to clients. In this situation, one hand or forearm represents the threshold and the other hand is far beneath the threshold. With the mention of each potential contributing factor, the lower hand incrementally is raised closer to, and eventually exceeds, the threshold.

In a verbal analogy of this concept, the threshold is the top of a drinking glass and the goal is to avoid having water overflow out of the glass. If a glass is filled to the brim (but not overflowing) with water, a single small pebble placed in the water will lead to the glass being too full and water then spilling out. In order to prevent this spillage, the obvious approach would be to prevent a pebble from falling into the glass. While this approach may seem appropriate for the flea-allergic dog where the flea represents the pebble, the scenario is potentially more much more complex. For instance, if the glass was not entirely filled to the brim it could accommodate one or more pebbles without spilling. This translates into the clinical situation in which a dog with a combination of environmental allergies and mild flea allergy may not be able to tolerate any flea bites during the height of pollen season (cup filled to the brim with water). The same patient potentially could tolerate a flea bite or two during a time of year when the pollen count is low (when the cup is not as full).

Diagnosis

Although "management of chronic disease" is the focus of this book, curable dermatological diseases should be considered in the list of differential diagnosis during the initial evaluation and upon follow-up visits for a patient with pruritus. No widely accepted single clinical classification of chronic pruritus exists (Metz, Grundmann, and Stander 2011). In an effort to provide concise information and offer alternative categorization of potential differential diagnoses, a brief review follows.

Traditional lists of differential diagnoses are helpful to ensure that common causes are not overlooked. The author has promulgated the "PAIN 4 ME" mnemonic to assist with recall of differential diagnosis and emphasize the importance of certain etiologies from a dermatology perspective. Each of these diseases may directly or indirectly cause a patient to become pruritic. They are grouped together by broad etiological categories including a reminder within the "number 4" category. The reminder emphasizes that lists are inherently incomplete. Clients and patients may benefit from referral to a specialist who can then build upon the previous efforts by the care-giving team.

Differential Diagnosis Grouped by Broad Categories of Etiologic Agents

- P parasitic (demodex, flea, scabies, other mites)
- A allergic (flea, environmental, food, contact)
- I immune mediated
- N neoplastic
- 4 four or more potential other causes or forward the client/patient to a specialist
- M microbial (bacterial, yeast, dermatophyte)
- E endocrine

Although this grouping can be an effective means of remembering potential etiologies, the reality of clinical practice may lead to them being categorized differently. From one point of view, common diseases (e.g., flea allergies, environmental allergies, and infections) should be considered first. Another important consideration relates to how quickly a disease may be confirmed and controlled. Practical issues such as the cost of diagnostics and therapeutics are often the cornerstone of collaborative decision making between a veterinarian and client. Discussions regarding cost should include both short-term as well as long-term costs, particularly with chronic disease processes. The cost of chronic allergen specific immunotherapy is typically less expensive and associated with fewer side effects than chronic palliative antipruritic therapy.

It can be helpful during client discussions to group etiologies according to the following list in conjunction with a discussion of cost. Additionally, more than one etiologic agent is often present at the same time.

Alternative Categorization of Potential Etiologies

- *Common:* Bacterial and yeast infections, flea-induced pruritus, atopic dermatitis
- *Confirmable during exam:* Bacterial and yeast infections, flea infestation, demodex, scabies (although possible to confirm, fewer than 50% of patients will have a positive skin scrape)
- *Controllable quickly:* Scabies, bacterial and yeast infections (but likely to recur due to underlying etiology). Some cases of food allergy and flea bite pruritus
- *Curable:* Scabies (not always intensely pruritic), dermatophytoisis (variably pruritic), demodicosis (variably pruritic)

Some common diseases, such as infections (bacteria or yeast) are quickly identifiable but may be only part of the problem as they are secondary to an underlying primary disease. Management of the pruritic patient often requires the veterinarian and caregiver to remain constantly vigilant for bacterial infections, yeast infections, ectoparasites as well as other factors. For the pruritic patient, treatment of common, confirmable, and/or quickly controllable diseases is often pursued while utilizing palliative antipruritic therapy. Many patients may have more than one disease or factor contributing to pruritus at the same time making this approach a time- and cost-effective option. Once the contributing factors and diseases have been cured or controlled, the palliative antipruritc medical therapy and potential costs side effects can be reassessed. The medication may be discontinued or tapered. Table 2.1 lists some of the primary, secondary, and coexisting diseases that may be pruritic.

Superficial bacterial pyoderma and yeast infections can be identified during an office visit and successfully treated within 3 to 4 weeks. If the infections remain after systemic antimicrobials, additional diagnostics or therapeutics should be considered. For bacterial infections, a bacterial culture and sensitivity is appropriate. If topical therapy has not been utilized, it may be reconsidered. For yeast infections, a different systemic antifungal agent should be considered along with topical therapeutic options (Lewis 2016). While most infections technically are curable, the improvement is often temporary because they are virtually always secondary to an underlying primary disease process. For patients in which the infection is the final factor leading to the pruritic threshold being reached, the treatment of secondary infection, without controlling the underlying primary etiology, may be temporarily successful in controlling pruritus but not result in long-term control of the underlying disease. Endocrine diseases are seldom pruritic, but from a dermatology perspective, recurrent pyoderma can be the only presenting complaint with hypothyroidism and hyperadrenocorticism. With these patients, the pruritus is not usually as severe and typically totally resolves with appropriate infection control. This scenario emphasizes the need for follow-up appointments and cytologies towards the end of the course of antimicrobial therapy. Clients may be reluctant to follow

Table 2.1 Primary, secondary, and coexisting diseases that may be pruritic. (Many patients have more than one concurrently.)

Differential diagnosis	Long-term therapy	Length of time until control
Bacterial infection	Manage underlying disease	3–4 or more weeks
Yeast infection	Manage underlying disease	2–4 or more weeks
Scabies	Not necessary	2–4 weeks
Demodicosis	Seldom necessary	2–4 months or more
Food allergy	Avoidance of allergen	2 months
Flea bite pruritus	Avoidance through flea control	1–6 months depending upon environmental flea burden and patient hypersensitivity
Atopy	Allergen specific immunotherapy Avoidance of allergen if possible Various adjunctive medical therapy	3–12 months Variable Variable: hours to weeks

up with their veterinarian when their pet is clinically normal. When antibiotics are initially prescribed, a client-focused discussion pointing out that repeated use of antibiotics has been reported to be a factor in the development of multi-drug resistant infections helps emphasize the importance of identifying and treating the underlying condition. Treatment of the underlying condition does not simply mean treating pruritus because many antipruritic medications (steroids, oclacitinib, ciclosporin) may be contraindicated with bacterial infections and demodicosis (Lewis 2016; Miller, Griffin, and Campbell 2013). Dermatophyte infections are much less common in dogs compared to cats, but certain strains of dermatophytes can be quite pruritic. A dermatophyte culture should be considered in virtually all patients with dermatologic abnormalities.

Scabies is a relatively rare diagnosis and can be difficult to confirm. Nevertheless, it is extremely important because it is a curable cause of pruritus and can affect both allergic and not allergic patients. Empirical therapy is often necessary to rule out this contagious parasite that can also cause allergic reactions. Some individuals develop a hypersensitivity to scabies mites. This hypersensitivity reaction could in part account for the observation that pruritus may not be observed in all dogs from a household with a scabies positive pet (Lewis 2016; Miller *et al.* 2013). Some scabicidal agents also provide other benefits, such as flea control and heartworm prevention. These can be excellent choices as part of a complex parasite control plan.

Demodicosis is a relatively common, quickly confirmable diagnosis that in many cases can be successfully treated within a few months. It should be on the differential diagnosis list initially and at virtually each reevaluation of the same patient (cats and dogs) (Lewis 2016; Miller *et al.* 2013). In dogs, this is particularly true if drugs, such as steroids or oclacitinib, are being utilized for control of pruritus. The author has been referred many patients with undiagnosed demodicosis who were previously well controlled atopic patients receiving long-term medical therapy for pruritus. These patients can be challenging to manage because they require therapy for the demodicosis as well as a workup for the underlying reason that led to the long-term use of antipruritic drugs.

Atopic dermatitis is a common cause of pruritus but a definitive diagnosis can be elusive (Lewis 2016; Miller *et al.* 2013; Jackson and Mueller 2012; Favrot *et al.* 2010; Deboer and Hillier 2001). The presence of a positive allergy test does not confirm the diagnosis, it must be correlated with the history, clinical signs, and response the therapy. The diagnosis should never be made without a thorough workup and exclusion of other causes. Importantly, confirmation of atopic dermatitis does not mean that it is the ONLY factor contributing to the current clinical signs. Atopic dermatitis may simply be a coexisting diagnosis that is actually well controlled at the time the patient presents with pruritus caused by another diagnosis. For example, an atopic patient is at least equally as likely to contract an infectious parasitic disease (e.g., scabies) as a non-atopic patient. Due to the pruritic patient's past history and previous workup (including lack of response to scabicidal therapy), one might assume that a current episode of pruritus is associated with an allergy flare due to a change in seasons (allergen load). The patient may actually be itching due to scabies recently acquired from another dog. More common than sarcoptes mites, an undetected low level of flea exposure is often the cause for an exacerbation of pruritus in an atopic patient.

A 2010 clinical practice guideline by the International Task Force on Canine Atopic Dermatitis published a succinct table of Favrot's Criteria for canine atopic dermatitis (see Table 2.2) (Favrot *et al.* 2010).

Adverse reaction to food is a relatively rare, but potentially totally controllable cause of pruritus in some patients. Other symptoms, such as gastrointestinal, may also be noted. The reader is referred elsewhere for a more in-depth discussion of the differences between food allergy and adverse reaction to food. Within 2 months of initiating a strict (no treats or flavored oral medications) dietary trial, symptoms should abate with either disease, eliminating the need for long-term medical therapy. In many patients, concurrent atopic dermatitis and/or flea induced pruritus may be a factor. Secondary infections are common. The clinical signs of food allergy can be indistinguishable from the clinical signs of environmental allergy (Carlotti 2014), yet the latter can be much

Table 2.2 Favrot's 2010 criteria for canine atopic dermatitis.

1. Onset of signs under 3 years of age
2. Dog living mostly indoors
3. Glucocorticoid-responsive pruritus
4. Pruritus sine materia at onset (i.e. alesional pruritus)
5. Affected front feet
6. Affected ear pinnae
7. Nonaffected ear margins
8. Nonaffected dorso-lumbar area

A combination of five satisfied criteria has a sensitivity of 85% and a specificity of 79% to differentiate dogs with AD from dogs with chronic or recurrent pruritus without AD. Adding a sixth fulfilled parameter increases the specificity to 89% but decreases the sensitivity to 58%.

Source: Favrot *et al.* 2010.

more complicated to manage (Lewis 2016; Miller *et al.* 2013).

Flea-induced pruritus is a commonly overlooked but manageable cause of pruritus. This is especially true when the typical distribution pattern of flea allergy is not present. This terminology is used in an attempt to emphasize the importance of strict flea control, even when fleas seem unlikely as a contributing factor. For many atopic pets, the mechanical stimuli of a flea bites alone can trigger pruritus without true flea allergy being present (summation of effect and threshold.) These atopic pets as well as flea allergic pets can itch due to flea bites in households without any perceived flea infestation (lack of typical flea allergy distribution pattern). This problem can be difficult for many pet owners and even veterinarians to understand and accept. In these situations, the adult flea numbers are so low that they are not seen on pets or humans in the environment. For basic flea control needs of a non-allergic pet, a single product is often sufficient. For an allergic (atopic or flea allergic) pet, a trial 2–4 month or more period of a "Double Down" flea control program may be advisable (see Box 2.1). This protocol typically uses two different products with different active

---

Box 2.1

"Double Down" Flea Control Benefits

- For the pruritic patient on a hypoallergenic dietary trial, some flea control products can also provide heartworm prevention during a hypoallergenic dietary trial. The use of an unflavored oral product or topical product is necessary in order to provide continuous heartworm prevention during the workup of a pruritic patient. Some situations and client preferences lead to diagnostics and therapy for flea bite associated dermatitis, food allergy and scabies concurrently during a 2–4 month period of time.
- Some flea control products also have scabicidal attributes. Scabies is one of the very few truly curable pruritic diseases and should not be overlooked as a potential diagnosis at the initial assessment or even during follow up visits of a patient that has been diagnosed with other diseases such as atopic dermatitis.
- A few weeks after administration of a flea product, the often-increasing length required for a flea to die becomes important. It may allow undetected flea bites to add to the summation effect with pruritus inducing factors. The resulting increase in pruritus may be noted in the days to weeks preceding the routine repeat application of the single product.

---

ingredients and benefits. One product is used at the beginning of the month and another product is used in the middle of the month (Gram and Short 2015). It is important to know the active ingredients of products in order to avoid using different brand names but similar active ingredients.

"Double Down" protocol for flea control can be helpful in various pruritic scenarios. For the flea allergic pet, the "Double Down" protocol helps overcome pruritus associated with a reduced speed of kill seen with most flea control products. For virtually all flea control products, the speed of kill is typically faster for the first few weeks after a product is utilized compared to the time period before repeat applications. During the regulatory approval process/efficacy trials, the percentage of fleas killed is often measured 48 hours after product administration. While this is adequate for flea control in a non-allergic patient, clinically it can be a problem for flea allergic pets. The not-yet-dead fleas may feed several times over a period of many hours before they die. Caregivers often report an increase in pruritus in the days to weeks immediately preceding the due date for repeat administration of a flea product without fleas or flea feces being noted. Many

studies report the percentage of fleas killed 28 days after product application whereas many months are actually 31 days long. The label instructions on some products may not allow more frequent application. Client compliance and delay in product use further exacerbates the slower residual speed of kill issue for the allergic patient. The use of a different product at different times of the month overcomes this issue. It also allows the use of products with different attributes in addition to flea control that may be useful during the workup of a pruritic patient, such as scabicidal activity or topical heartworm prevention during a hypoallergenic dietary trial.

Pruritus Diagnosis Summary

Neither intradermal allergy test nor serum allergy test should be used as a screening test for pruritic patients suspected of having atopic dermatitis (Lewis 2016; Miller *et al.* 2013; Deboer and Hillier 2001). There is no substitute for a veterinarian's clinical judgment coupled with a physical examination and complete history (see Box 2.2). With that information, the list of differential diagnoses can be narrowed down provided the diagnoses are presenting with their typical characteristics.

Box 2.2

Pruritus Diagnosis Summary (These considerations should not be overlooked during initial and reevaluation appointments).

- Obtain a thorough history and perform complete physical examination in order to narrow down the list of potential differential diagnoses.
- Remember to rule out curable disease and contagious diseases such as dermatophytosis and scabies. A history of negative findings does not mean that these could not be a new problem.
- Ensure that a patient does not have a confirmable or controllable primary disease or secondary factor. Evaluate for parasitic and microbial diseases by performing appropriate cytologies and skin scrapes for dermodicosis, which previously may have been or difficult to confirm.
- Consider food allergy: relatively rare but controllable without medication. Client receptivity and compliance can pose a challenge when performing a strict hypoallergenic dietary trial consisting of novel or hydrolyzed proteins and avoidance of treats and flavored oral medications (such as heartworm and flea control products).
- Consider empirical ectoparasite therapy for scabies and fleas utilizing "Double Down" flea control, even if parasites are not confirmed on examination.
- Consider antipruritic therapy in order to provide comfort for the patient and the caregiver while working to identify and control the primary disease. Educate the caregiver regarding risks and benefits of both short-term and long-term therapy as well as the costs.
- If the work up and treatment for other diseases is negative and medical therapy is necessary for more than 3 months out of the year, consider intradermal allergy testing or serology based allergy testing from a reputable laboratory.

Specialists often see patients with common diseases and an atypical presentation. Within three months of a multifaceted diagnostic and therapeutic approach, most etiological agents can be controlled or ruled out as potential contributing or coexisting factors. In some situations, ruling out one single differential diagnosis at a time is appropriate. In many situations, however, more than one factor is present concurrently. Following a thorough assessment of a patient's history, physical examination findings, successful treatment of secondary infections, careful modification of a parasite control plan, and a stringent dietary change for several months, the likely diagnosis of atopic dermatitis may be made by exclusion of other causes. Demonstration of IgE antibodies via intradermal allergy testing or serum testing is covered in depth by many other publications. They are not pathognomonic for the diagnosis of atopy. These adjunctive tests should only be used, after a well-orchestrated clinical workup. Tests are performed in order to identify important allergens to be avoided or included in allergen specific immunotherapy. Currently available types of "allergy testing" should not be performed as a screening test for atopic dermatitis. Many clinically normal animals will actually test positive (Lewis 2016; Miller *et al*. 2013; Jackson and Mueller 2012). Allergen specific immunotherapy is an often overlooked and effective means of providing long-term management of a pruritic patient with atopic dermatitis.

Management

The caregiving client is a critical component of the management of chronic disease. Academic evidence-based reviews are a key factor in determining therapeutic options to discuss with a client. It is however important not to overlook the potential benefit of over the counter (OTC) products, such as fatty acids and antihistamines. Because they may not have been subjected to the rigorous process of governmental regulatory approval, funding for high quality clinical trials may be relatively lacking. It is not uncommon for the resulting evidence-based assessment to read something akin to "insufficient evidence for or against the use of these products." The option of utilizing readily available and often less expensive OTC products can be clinically useful and help integrate clients into the decision-making process. This optional therapeutic approach may not be appropriate in all situations. For most cases with pruritus, it gives the client time to adjust to the reality of chronic caregiving and to be included as a critical component of the long-term decision-making team. The severity and distribution of the pruritus will influence therapeutic options. Generalized lesions will likely be treated differently than localized lesions and acute flare episodes may be treated differently than chronic disease (Favrot *et al.* 2010).

A veterinarian's compassionate discussion of therapeutic costs and options, including OTC products, can result in reaffirmation of the importance of shared decision making with regards to the management of chronic disease. With this type of healthy relationship, should the OTC products not provide adequate relief; the client may then feel more comfortable scheduling a follow up with their veterinarian. In some cases, after educating a client who has chosen nonprescription therapy, I have written a proposed course of optional prescription drug therapy to be initiated in the very near future. Instructions also include the need to schedule a follow up visit 1 to 3 weeks after starting the new course of prescription therapy. This patient care/client situation is obviously complex and not appropriate in all situations but can extremely helpful on a number of levels and sincerely appreciated by many clients. As an example, in this era of antibiotic stewardship, I have used this option for the treatment of pyoderma. Clients are given the option of topical nonprescription/non-antibiotic therapy or systemic prescription antibiotic therapy.

Should they choose topical therapy, I inform them that I am happy with that decision, and it would be best if I could reevaluate in one month in order to ascertain the response to therapy. If clients have costs or scheduling concerns, another option may be possible. A note is made in the pet's record, "Within the next 3 weeks, if no improvement is seen, the client may ask for the antibiotics that were discussed during the evaluation today". I then further emphasize the importance of keeping following up assessments with an office visit, 2 to 3 weeks after starting and while still using the antibiotic. A similar approach is sometimes used for palliative pruritus relief in the atopic patient and with drugs such as steroids or oclacitanib. In this situation, client education is centered on long-term control as well as potential acute etiological flare factors such as parasites, food reactions, and infections. If an infection is not present, I may offer various topical options or OTC antihistamines but make a note in the record that should adequate relief not occur within a few days, various options are available. The client may schedule a reevaluation or request a prescription product that is already noted in the record. Additionally, the record has instructions regarding when to schedule a reassessment office visit and further discuss options for chronic management.

The multitude of factors contributing to pruritus in the atopic patient can be complex and a multimodal approach to therapy is common. Palliative therapy is appropriate in the short term while working up a patient, addressing contributing factors and treating the underlying disease process. The American College of Veterinary Dermatology (ACVD) task force on canine atopic dermatitis states the following general principles of therapy: "The treatment of canine atopic dermatitis is multifaceted and consists of a combination of actions that include the use of allergen avoidance, anti-inflammatory agents, allergen-specific immunotherapy and antimicrobial drugs (Table 2.3). The importance and order of these treatment steps vary from patient to

Table 2.3 Pruritus therapies.

Diagnosis	Chronic therapy recommendations
Flea-bite-induced pruritus	If the only diagnosis is flea bite pruritus, stringent flea control is the long term treatment of choice. Palliative antipruritic therapy may be necessary for a few months until flea control can be achieved or during exacerbations.
Food-induced pruritus	If the only diagnosis is food allergy, a strictly followed hypoallergenic diet is the long-term treatment of choice. Palliative antipruritic therapy may not always be helpful for food allergy/adverse reactions to food.
Atopy-induced pruritus	If the only diagnosis is atopic dermatitis, allergen specific immunotherapy (ASIT) is the long-term treatment of choice for patients. Palliative adjunct antipruritic therapy may be necessary either temporarily or for longer duration. For patients with symptoms present for less than 3 months out of the year and not anticipated to suffer from progression of their disease, palliative antipruritic therapy may be the only therapy necessary. Atopic dermatitis is often a progressive disease and medical therapeutic options may need to be changed periodically. For patients, particularly those of predisposed breeds in many geographic areas, allergy testing and ASIT may be considered before 18 months of age.

patient" (Olivry and Sousa 2001). More recently, the recognition of a defect in the epidermal barrier function in atopic patients has led to a renewed emphasis regarding skin, coat care, and shampoo therapy (Favrot *et al.* 2010; Santoro *et al.* 2015). For more information regarding acute and rescue palliative therapy the reader is referred to the section later in this chapter.

A systematic evidenced-based review in 2010 evaluating interventions for the management of atopic dermatitis in dogs found six interventions to demonstrate some evidence of efficacy to decrease pruritus and/or skin lesions. These included topical tacrolimus, topical triamcinolone, oral ciclosporin, oral glucocorticoids, subcutaneous recombinant gamma interferon, and subcutaneous allergen specific immunotherapy. Importantly, one study showed a particular essential fatty acid supplement to reduce prednisolone use (Olivry *et al.* 2010). This review was published before the commercial availability of oclacitanib, which is effective and indicated for control of pruritus associated with allergic dermatitis and control of atopic dermatitis in dogs at least 12 months of age (Apoquel product information 2016).

For a variety of reasons, many veterinarians utilize oral prednisone/prednisolone, oral oclacitanib or oral ciclosporin when faced with the reality of managing chronic pruritus due to atopic dermatitis. While all three of these medications have proven to be quite useful for this purpose, each has its own nuances. As previously discussed, antihistamines and fatty acids should not be overlooked as potential adjunctive therapy. They may help reduce the use of these prescription medications while reducing costs and concerns about potential side effects. All of these may be useful while waiting for allergen specific immunotherapy to become effective or as adjunctive chronic therapy.

Prednisone has been used for many decades as a very cost-effective means of controlling pruritus (and inflammation). Most veterinary practitioners are well acquainted with their efficacy and side effects. Depending on dosage, they may have different attributes. The prednisone/prednisolone dosages below are those generally utilized for dogs. Individual patient variation is common and patients should be monitored (Miller *et al.* 2013).

- *Immunosuppressive:* 2.2–4.0 mg/kg/q24h or divided BID for 4–10 days, then tapered to every 48 hours
- *Anti-inflammatory:* 1.1–2.2 mg/kg/q24h or divided BID for 2–6 days, then tapered to every 48 hours
- *Antipruritic:* 0.5 mg/kg/q 48 h
- *Replacement:* 0.2–0.3 mg/kg/q24h

Most atopic patients, without a pyoderma, respond well to a single SQ dexamethasone SP injection (see acute/rescue therapies later in this chapter), followed the next day by the initiation of oral prednisone approximating the daily replacement dosage of 0.2–0.3 mg/kg but actually administered every 48 hours. Over time, this results in a dosage that is cumulatively 50% of the physiological replacement dose. With every 48-hour administration, the effect on the hypothalamic-pituitary-adrenal axis should be minimal. This regimen is not effective in all cases, particularly those that are more symptomatic. It is tailored to the individual patient, who should be monitored periodically. More severely affected patients may temporarily require a higher dose of oral prednisone after a dexamethasone injection. This protocol has also been utilized concurrently in the short to intermediate term with each of the other therapies discussed later. The careful use of a cost-effective medication such as prednisone is an important consideration for many clients.

Oclacitanib (Apoquel®), a synthetic Janus Kinase (JAK) inhibitor, has recently become widely available. Like steroids, it is fast acting. The veterinary package insert states the following indications: "Control of pruritus associated with allergic dermatitis and control of atopic dermatitis in dogs at least 12 months of age." The dosage is 0.4–0.6 mg/kg twice daily for up to 14 days and then administered once daily for maintenance therapy. The package insert precautions state that "Dogs receiving Apoquel® should be monitored for the development of infections, including demodicosis and neoplasia." In order to help prevent long-term twice a day dosing by clients, many veterinary dermatologists start dosing with only a once a day schedule.

Ciclosporin Modified (*Atopica*® and generic equivalents in "modified" form so as be microemulsified for better absorption) is a cyclic polypeptide, immune modulating agent that has been commercially available for dogs for many years and somewhat more recently for cats. Unlike prednisone and oclacitanib, it is not fast acting and may require 3–6 weeks or more of therapy to determine its efficacy. The package insert states the following indications for dogs: "for the control of atopic dermatitis in dogs weighing at least 4 pounds body weight" and over 6 months of age. In cats, it is indicated: "for the control of feline allergic dermatitis as manifested by excoriations (including facial and neck), military dermatitis, eosinophilic plaques, and self-induced alopecia in cats at least 6 months of age and at least 3lbs (1.4 kg) in body weight." The dosage in dogs is 3.3–6.7 mg/kg/day as a single daily dose for 30 days (Atopica product information 2016) and then it may be tapered in some patients. This is done by decreasing the frequency of dosing to every other day or 2–3 times a week. For cats, it is available in liquid form and the dose is 3.2 mg/lb/day (7 mg/kg/day) as a single daily dose for a minimum of 4 to 6 weeks or until resolution of clinical signs, and then tapered in a manner similar to the protocol for dogs. Ciclosporin should be used with caution with drugs that affect the P-450 enzyme system, such as ketoconazole. Vomiting and/or diarrhea are the most commonly observed adverse reactions. Hypertrichosis, gingival hyperplasia, and papillomas are rare but well recognized in association with ciclosporine use. The feline product insert "Warnings" states: "Atopica for cats is a systemic immunosuppressant that may increase the susceptibility to infection and the development of neoplasia." In dogs, the label contraindications states: "Atopica is contraindicated for use in dogs with a history of neoplasia."

Allergen-specific immunotherapy (ASIT) was subjected to a systematic review that confirmed the safety and efficacy of subcutaneous ASIT in reducing the signs of atopic dermatitis (Favrot *et al.* 2010). After that publication, sublingual allergen specific immunotherapy (SLIT) has also been widely adopted. The general consensus among dermatologists who also utilize ASIT is that SLIT is effective and safe. Importantly, the

2010 clinical practice guidelines from the International Task Force on Canine Atopic Dermatitis states that "ASIT is the only intervention that has the potential to prevent the development of signs and alter the long-term course of the disease." For patients who have symptoms which do not respond to symptomatic medical therapy or experience unacceptable side effects, even for relatively short periods of time, ASIT is indicated (Favrot *et al.* 2010).

A primary care veterinarian may refer a patient for allergy testing and ASIT or SLIT. This is common because immunotherapy is not as straight forward to utilize as pharmacological therapy. Consequently, clients can become discouraged and unfortunately discontinue therapy before allowing adequate time to provide observable benefit, which can take as long as 12 months. The protocol including dose, frequency, and duration of therapy is typically tailored to the patient and client's needs and a complex decision process. While waiting for the immunotherapy to become effective, judicious use of concurrent medical therapy in a gradually tapering manner can help control a patient's symptoms while serving to continually educate the caregiver about short and long-term goals. In some patients, the overall degree of pruritus may not obviously change, but eventually all medical therapy can be discontinued and an adequate level of comfort achieved without the use of drugs. Many practitioners utilize ASIT and SLIT with good results. If good results are not obtained, clients may then inappropriately believe that changes in testing modality and/or immunotherapy protocol are not indicated. This complicated situation is best discussed with a caregiver before allergy testing in conjunction with the option of referral to a veterinarian with specialty training in this complex modality.

The use of safe, cost-effective, and easily followed regimens for acute pruritus relief coupled with education allows the primary care practitioner, referral specialist, and client to work together towards a collaborative long-term plan aimed at controlling chronic pruritus and recurrent pyoderma due to atopic dermatitis.

Acute and Rescue Palliative Therapy

Most pruritic patients are also inflamed. In situations where topical therapy is not enough, judicious systemic short-term glucocorticoid use can be an extremely effective tool to control an acute flare up of pruritus associated with atopic dermatitis that is not complicated by significant secondary infection. For 25 years, this author has utilized a dexamethasone dosage similar to that used when performing a high dose dexamethasone suppression test in order to provide acute relief from pruritus and inflammation. This dosage is widely considered safe and appropriate as a diagnostic tool even in a difficult to control diabetic patient in order to rule out Cushing's disease. Virtually all atopic patients without secondary infections should experience a significant reduction in pruritus lasting 1–4 days. If temporary relief is not noted, the tentative diagnosis of an acute atopic dermatitis exacerbation as the sole factor should be reevaluated and other causes of pruritus reconsidered. A similar improvement can also be achieved with oral glucocorticoids but side effects such as polyuria, polydypsia and polyphagia are more likely and client compliance issues can complicate the assessment and plan. Oclacitanib can also be utilized to provide quick relief of pruritus. It is the author's clinical impression that the use of anti-inflammatory dosages as opposed to "antipruritic doses" of glucocorticoids as a "crisis buster" is more likely to result in breaking the cycle of itch and inflammation and in decreasing the chronic need for prescription products. After the inflammation/itch cycle has been broken and the inciting factor(s) removed, three scenarios may occur. First, no further therapy may be necessary until the next time an inciting factor leads to the pururitic threshold being reached. Second, mild concurrent atopy may then be adequately controlled by OTC products such as antihistamines and fatty acids. These products are more likely to be beneficial when used chronically to prevent flare ups than during an acute episode. Their consistent chronic used may decrease the need for long-term use of prescription products and rescue therapy. Third, pruritus will return and be symptomatic enough that prescription antipruritic therapy will be necessary. It is often a judgment call related to historical and physical examination findings that lead the veterinary practitioner and caregiver to suspect that this will be the case and that intermediate term prescription management will be necessary. See earlier discussion regarding chronic management.

Common "Crisis Buster" drugs with a quick onset of activity for acute somewhat generalized pruritus associated with atopic dermatitis:

- Dexamethsone injection (anti-inflammatory/antipruritic dose)
- Oral prednisone, prednisolone or methylprednisolone (anti-inflammatory/antipruritic dose)
- Oral prednisolone/prednisone (antipruritic dose)
- Oral oclacitanib

Oral medications do offer patients and clients (who previously have been educated about reasons for acute exacerbations and therapeutic options) short-term "crisis buster" pruritus control without an acute care evaluation by their veterinarian. Many clients appreciate options for acute relief at the same time they are being educated about the potential side effects of long-term medical therapy. This balance of easy to follow symptom relief and client education emphasizes the need to identify and change the course of the underlying disease process.

In these situations, empathetic client communication, client engagement, and client education are essential for the both the short- and long-term well-being of the patient (Knesl *et al.* 2016).

My standard dexamethasone SP dose is 1 mg/10 pounds SQ or IV. This is equivalent to 0.75 mg Dexamethsone/10 pounds. Using generally accepted steroid strength conversion values (5 mg pred/0.75 mg dexamethasone), this converts to prednisone at a dose of 1.1 mg Pred/kg. As stated elsewhere, the anti-inflammatory dose of pred is 1.0–1.5 mg/kg/day, for 7 to 10 days. The anti-inflammatory dose is approximately 2 to 3 times the antipruritic dose. However, most pruritic patients are also inflamed. In these cases, I simply give one injection of dexamethasone SQ to "break the inflammatory cycle" and often do not need any more steroids while utilizing other medications. If more steroids are needed, I will then start oral prednisone 1 day later, at a standard antipruritic dose of 0.5 mg/kg every 2 to 3 days and taper further over time. If the inflammation is severe, I will use a higher dose. For convenience sake, I often simply have the clients start the pred pills the day after the injection. For practical reasons, I typically administer the dexamethsone subcutaneously, but will consider intravenously (IV) if necessary. I use the IV route if the client is uncertain regarding the response to steroids in the past. In this situation, we call the client 24 hours later to document the response. Clinically, this technique works well in patients who have been well controlled with immunotherapy and/or other forms of medical therapy, but have suffered an exacerbation. Compared to dogs, cats seem to require about twice the dose of oral GC to achieve the same effects. Prednisolone should be used instead of prednisone in this species.

I emphasize the words *simply* and *convenience* because the patient's primary caregiver (the client) is often burdened with many other tasks. I feel this approach is both medically appropriate and helps prevent caregiver burnout as well as many financial concerns. Many clients may become emotionally and financially exhausted when overburdened with caring for an allergic pet. The doses discussed were arrived at by comparing them to what would be necessary if prednisone were utilized, but trying to avoid the mineralocorticoid side effects. I justify the use of injectable dexamethasone SP by comparing the dose used in a high dose dexamethasone suppression test. The same drug at a similar dose is used for a diagnostic test in a difficult to control diabetic dog who is also a Cushings suspect (high dose dexamethasone suppression test).

Quality of Life for Patient and Caregiver

A patient affected with chronic dermatologic disease offers the potential to "make or break" the relationship between a client and veterinarian. Multiple visits, treatment costs, and potential medication side effects all offer the potential for the caregiver/client to become frustrated. Although a few dermatological diseases are curable, many are not.

Ignoring the underlying disease and repeated use of antibiotics to treat secondary bacterial skin infections, is associated with an increased risk of a patient developing a methicillin resistant staphylococcal infection. Many incurable diseases, such as flea allergy and food allergy, may be managed without long-term antipruritic medications. Short-term careful use of palliative antipruritic medications help keep the patient and client comfortable while working to identify the primary etiology or eliminate the allergen causing the problem. These medications should not be substitutes for identifying and addressing the underlying disease process. When long-term medications are necessary, follow-up patient visits and client education including the option of referral to a specialist are important factors in the care of the patient and relationship between the client and veterinarian.

References

Apoquel product information Veterinary product and label information veterinary package insert. https://www.zoetisus.com/apoquel-pet-owner/pdfs/apoquel_pi.pdf, (accessed July 17, 2016).

Atopica product information Veterinary product and label information veterinary package insert. http://us.atopica.com/en/easset_upload_file971_94950_e.pdf (accessed 17 July, 2016).

Carlotti DN. Cutaneous manifestations of food hypersensitivity. In: C Noli, A Foster, and W Rosencrantz, Eds. Veterinary allergy. John Wiley & Sons, Ltd, 2014: 109.

DeBoer DJ. Guidelines for symptomatic medical treatment of canine atopic dermatitis. In: C Noli, A Foster and W Rosencrantz, Eds. Veterinary allergy. John Wiley & Sons, Ltd. 2014: 95.

DeBoer DJ, Hillier A. ACVD Task force on canine atopic dermatitis (XV): Fundamental concepts in clinical diagnosis. Veterinary Immunology and Immunopathology. 2001; 81(3–4): 227–231.

Favrot C, Steffan J, Seewald W, et al. A prospective study on the clinical features of chronic canine atopic dermatitis and its diagnosis. Veterinary Dermatology. 2010; 21: 23–30.

Foster A. Feline allergy. In: C Noli, A Foster, and W Rosencrantz, Eds. Veterinary allergy. John Wiley &Sons, Ltd. 2014: 201.

Gram D, Short J. Fleas and ticks in small animals. Grupo Asís Biomedia. 2015.

Halliwell R. Revised nomenclature of veterinary allergy. Veterinary Immunology and Immunopathology. 2006; 114(3–4): 207–208.

Jackson HA, Mueller RS. Atopic dermatitis and adverse food reactions. In: HA Jackson and R Marsella, Eds. BSAVA manual of canine and feline dermatology. British Small Animal Veterinary Association. 2012: 130–140.

Knesl O, Hart BL, Fine AH. Opportunities for incorporating the human-animal bond in companion animal practice. Journal of the American Veterinary Medical Association. 2016; 249(1): 42–44.

Lewis DT. Dermatologic disorders. In: M Schaer and F Gaschen, Eds. Clinical medicine of the dog and cat, 3rd edn. CRC Press. 2016: 767–817.

Metz M, Grundmann S, Stander S. Pruritus: an overview of current concepts. Veterinary Dermatology. 2011; 22(2): 121–131.

Miller WH, Griffin CE, Campbell KL. Eds. Muller and Kirk's small animal dermatology, 7th ed, Elsevier Mosby. 2013.

Mueller RS. Allergen-specific immunotherapy. In: C Noli, A Foster, and W Rosencrantz, Eds. Veterinary allergy. John Wiley &Sons, Ltd. 2014: 85.

Olivry T, Foster AP, Mueller RS, et al. Interventions for atopic dermatitis in dogs: a systematic review of randomized controlled trials. Veterinary Dermatology. 2010; 21(1): 4–22.

Olivry T, Sousa C. The ACVD task force on canine atopic dermatitis (XIX): general principles of therapy. Veterinary Immunology and Immunopathology. 2001; 81(3–4): 311–316.

Santoro D, Marsella R, Pucheu-Haston C, et al. Review: Pa (2001) thogenesis of canine atopic dermatitis: skin barrier, and host-micro-organism interaction. Veterinary Dermatology. 2015; 26(2): 84–e25.

Tater KC. An approach to pruritus. In: HA Jackson and R Marsella, Eds. BSAVA manual of canine and feline dermatology. British Small Animal Veterinary Association. 2012: 37–45.

3

Managing Mobility: An Integrative Approach (Orthopedic and Neurologic Impairments of Mobility)

Justin Shmalberg

Introduction

Mobility impairment affects the majority of aging dogs and cats. Younger animals may experience an insidious onset due to trauma, congenital malformation, or environmental conditions. Osteoarthritis, intervertebral disc disease, muscle strain, and related musculoskeletal disorders are generally chronic and variably treatable, but in all cases affect caretakers who are concerned about their pet's quality of life and chronic management. Caretakers expect their pets to be mobile, interactive, and pain-free when ambulating, and a deviation from this expectation can emotionally impact owners and influence treatment decisions. The ability to normalize or manage an animal's declined mobility is paramount to maintaining a pet's quality of life in addition to the well-being of the owner.

Diagnosis

Impaired mobility arises from a number of conditions, each with unique treatment approaches. Mobility impairment should be defined in comparison to an individual animal's baseline, which is generally before injury and often at its optimum immediately after the end of growth and development. Therefore,

impairment in mobility may be characterized by one or more of the following:

1) A reduction in the amount of time an animal can ambulate. An example would include paresis secondary to intervertebral disc disease.
2) A change in the quality or character of movement, e.g. animals with proprioceptive deficits, muscle strains, or compensatory weight shifting secondary to osteoarthritis.
3) An inability to rise from a lying or seated position. Osteoarthritis and intervertebral disc disease may require short- or long-term assistance, through the use of direct manipulation, slings, and special harnesses.
4) Painful movement. Pain should be considered impaired mobility even when visual changes in locomotion are not present. Chronic muscle or articular pathology may, in early stages, produce discomfort without obvious gait abnormalities.

The diagnostic approach for disorders of movement should be methodical and comprehensive. Animals with relatively clear primary diagnoses may have secondary or compensatory changes that promote or induce other injuries. The vast majority of mobility changes will have a neurologic or musculoskeletal origin, and as such, the history and physical examination should be

Chronic Disease Management for Small Animals, First Edition. Edited by W. Dunbar Gram, Rowan J. Milner and Remo Lobetti.
© 2018 John Wiley & Sons, Inc. Published 2018 by John Wiley & Sons, Inc.

comprehensive and include an assessment of neurologic function, soft tissue pain, joint function, and orthopedic integrity.

History and Physical Examination

Owners should be asked to describe the ways in which their pet's mobility has changed and whether there was an acute inciting incident or if it developed slowly without a definitive origin. It should be determined whether clinical signs are variable, and if so, what the potential triggers may be. This includes whether increased activity results in increased impairment and whether the condition is better after resting or with activity. Paretic and muscle disorders often benefit from periods of rest due to increased tissue fatigue, whereas osteoarthritic disorders frequently improve as the animal ambulates throughout the day. Urinary and fecal habits should be evaluated for functional impairment which may impact quality of life, owner outlook, or the incidence of urogenital infections.

Special consideration should be given to cats, which as a species may be less overt with clinical signs of mobility disorders. Screening questions can include whether the cat is still able to jump to the same height, whether they continue to be found in similar areas throughout a house rather or if they are more sedentary in a particular area. A general assessment of activity can be solicited from the owner – if such information cannot be provided, an accelerometer may be used to monitor activity and to compare to published averages. A period of weight gain in the absence of dietary change may indirectly suggest reduced voluntary activity.

A comprehensive rehabilitation exam benefits all dogs with changes in their ability to ambulate. This examination should include the elements in the following subsections.

Comprehensive Physical Examination with a Systems Approach

Aging animals in particular may present with concurrent medical conditions. An ophthalmic examination allows for screening for changes that may impact vision, assessment of the integument may provide information about nutritional status and the presence of any chronic dermatoses, assessment of dentition allows for the recognition of conditions causing oral pain, cardiothoracic abnormalities may reveal disorders expected to reduce stamina (heart disease, chronic bronchitis), abdominal palpation could reveal concurrent neoplasia or gastrointestinal disorders, body condition should be assessed given the obvious impacts of adiposity on joint and spinal loading, and the urogenital system externally examined as dogs with impaired mobility are predisposed to urinary tract infections and perineal dermatitis.

Neurologic Examination

Animals are frequently misdiagnosed with orthopedic issues when the primary pathology is neurological and vice versa. Consequently, an abbreviated neurological examination can quickly and simply screen for common neurogenic causes on a differential diagnosis list.

The neurologic examination should minimally include the following:

1) Assessment of a patient's affect and behavior. Altered mentation and behaviors are suggestive of forebrain disease. Aging animals should be evaluated for cognitive dysfunction.
2) Assessment of critical cranial nerves which could influence mobility. This includes menace detection (cranial nerves II and VII), pupillary light reflex (II, III), palpebral reflex (V, VII), assessment of facial symmetry (VII), and a gag reflex (IX, X). Any head tilt should be closely evaluated for central or peripheral vestibular causes.
3) An evaluation of an animal's stance can suggest different neurologic lesions. A wide-based stance is characteristic of proprioceptive ataxia, a narrow stance may be due to paresis, and decreased weight bearing could be either pain or root signature.

4) Proprioception should be evaluated in all patients. This should be done with adequate support of an animal because allowing a pet to bear weight on the dorsal surface of its paw may test sensory rather than proprioceptive fibers. Proprioceptive fibers, located primarily in the outer tracts of the spinal cord are often first affected by many compressive myelopathies. Hopping and wheel-barrowing provide additional tests of proprioception.

5) Withdrawal reflexes should also be assessed in all patients. A weak or absent withdrawal reflex is suggestive of a disorder affecting either the peripheral nerves (neuropathy) or a central lesion within the area of the reflex arc (C6-T2 for forelimbs, L4-S2 in the hindlimbs).

6) Additional reflexes may be tested to further localize pathology. These are described in greater detail elsewhere, but it is important to note that the forelimb reflexes are less reliable in normal patients than are those of the hindlimb. The patellar reflex examines the cranial portion of the reflex arc whereas the gastrocnemius and cranial tibial reflexes assess the caudal portion.

7) Examination of anal tone is advised in all older animals with impaired mobility. A rectal examination, apart from being a component of a comprehensive physical examination, can provide assessment of the lumbosacral space, disorders of which may be characterized by pain, neurologic deficits, and/or abnormal micturition or defecation.

Orthopedic Examination
The orthopedic examination should be systematic in order to best evaluate potential pathology. A system whereby the examiner moves from head to tail, and from ventral to dorsal, appears to enhance the ability to detect lesions. This procedure can be done as follows:

1) Cervical range of motion should be evaluated. Both neurologic (intervertebral disc disease, cervical spondylomyelopathy) and orthopedic diseases (arthritis) may cause resistance to range of motion.

2) The forelimb should be evaluated by starting with the digits and moving proximally. Digital osteoarthritis and sesamoiditis are frequently overlooked as a source of mobility impairment. The carpus should be evaluated for laxity as well as crepitus. The elbow should be evaluated in extension and the presence of any effusion determined. Long bones should be palpated, especially in large breed dogs at risk of osteosarcoma. The shoulder joint is supported by soft tissues and as such the range of motion in the shoulder should be evaluated in all directions. Retired canine athletes may be at increased risk of medial shoulder instability, characterized by an increased abduction angle. Delayed cranial reach of the shoulder may be due to infraspinatus pain and contracture. The biceps should be evaluated for tenosynovitis – the area of the bicipital bursa and the insertion should both be evaluated. The scapula itself should be moveable based on its muscular attachment. Reduced flexion of any joint may be suggestive of osteoarthritis.

3) The thoracolumbar spine should be evaluated for pain from the spinal column or from the surrounding epaxial musculature. The presence of kyphosis may suggest underlying pain in this area, and both kyphosis and lordosis may result in altered carriage of the limbs and changes in stride length and quality.

4) The hindlimb is evaluated in a similar fashion as the forelimb, with digits and sesamoids being evaluated first. The tarsus should be examined for reduced range of motion. Long bones should be palpated, especially the proximal tibia and distal femur in large dogs. Stifle range of motion should be assessed and compared to the contralateral side. Medial buttress should be assessed. The thickness of the patellar tendon should be palpated, and the presence of effusion caudal to this tendon noted. Cranial drawer and tibial

thrust testing should be completed, and drawer should be evaluated in flexion to assess for chronic partial tears. The hip can be examined dynamically by placing a hand over the hip during gaiting and passively by an assessment of extension.

5) Pelvic symmetry should be evaluated and lumbosacral and tail palpation performed.

Soft Tissue Assessment

The examination of soft tissue and fascia is commonly overlooked in a patient with mobility impairment. However, some soft tissue pathology may be the primary source of pain or alterations in gait, and most animals with chronic orthopedic or neurologic pain will display secondary discomfort, spasm, or strain in adjacent soft tissue structures. A skilled soft tissue assessment takes a commitment to the assessment of various muscles and ligaments in normal patients on routine physical examination. Careful monitoring of a patient's demeanor or behavior during muscle manipulation can provide feedback on potential discomfort in a certain area. The following represents a list of major muscle groups that warrant examination.

1) *Brachiocephalicus*: This muscle of the neck can become a source of discomfort due to strain from forelimb lameness, contralateral hindlimb lameness, or primary cervical pathology. Many dogs affected by these conditions will display significant pain on palpation.

2) *Infraspinatus and supraspinatus:* These muscles may produce primary shoulder pathology and instability when injured, but may also be a source of discomfort with forelimb pathology or in overweight animals.

3) *Triceps:* The triceps should be evaluated in animals with elbow pathology. The long head of the triceps appears particularly predisposed to sensitivity.

4) *Epaxial muscles:* Sensitivity in the epaxial muscles can be both a primary and secondary finding. Concurrent evaluation of the patient's neurologic status is critical.

5) *Iliopsoas:* The combined psoas major and iliacus muscles are a common cause of mobility impairment in canine athletes but may also be a secondary source of pain in animals with hip or stifle disorders. The muscle can be assessed by lateral palpation of the lumbar vertebrae and by palpation of the muscle when the hindlimb is extended and internally rotated. Abduction may also trigger discomfort when the coxofemoral joint is extended.

6) *Sartorius:* This muscle lies cranially to the quadriceps and is frequently sore and contracted in patients with cranial cruciate insufficiency or coxofemoral disease.

7) *Pectineus:* The pectineus functions as an adductor of the hindlimb and is located on the medial surface of the proximal hindlimb coursing from the iliopubic eminence to the femur. The muscle is a frequent cause of discomfort in animals affected by hip dysplasia and/or arthritis.

8) *Calcaneal tendon complex:* Stifle flexors joining the calcaneal tendon are predisposed to injury with significant load bearing. More commonly, however, pain may cause persistent activation of the muscles including the gracilis, biceps femoris, and semitendinosus.

Differential Diagnoses

A comprehensive physical examination permits broad categorization of a patient's symptoms and allows the practitioner to better localize the anatomic site of mobility impairment if not apparent during visual gait assessment.

Neurologic findings should prompt consideration of a select group of common differential diagnoses, and mobility impairment will most commonly be a result of pathology in the spinal column. Spinal dysfunction may generally be graded using five categories:

1) Spinal pain only
2) Ambulatory paresis

3) Nonambulatory paresis
4) Plegia with pain sensation
5) Plegia without deep pain sensation

Intervertebral disc disease is the most commonly encountered chronic neurologic impairment affecting mobility. Large breed dogs will typically present with chronic lesions of lower severity and some present exclusively with proprioceptive deficits. Conversely, Dachshunds and other chondro-dystrophic breeds may present with either chronic or acute disc protrusions. Many such dogs have other sites of disc protrusion, and therefore may require chronic management even after acute decompressive surgery.

Congenital malformations should be considered in young animals with ataxia or other neurologic signs. Large breed dogs with cervical spondylomyelopathy may respond well to integrative treatments when signs are mild to moderate. Small-breed dogs with caudal occipital malformation and other congenital malformations respond variably to integrative interventions.

Acute vascular events and trauma to the spine may cause significant and sudden presentation of neurologic symptoms. Fibrocartilaginous embolism is a frequent cause of asymmetrical hindlimb plegia which generally has an excellent rate of recovery. Similarly, noncompressive traumatic lesions to the spinal column typically result in lesion improvement. However, both may cause chronic mobility impairment when recovery is incomplete.

Neoplastic lesions may present as progressive chronic conditions, and the presence of asymetrical muscle mass with a root signature in an older dog should prompt this differential diagnosis.

Osteoarthritis is the most common cause of impaired mobility in animals, and more than half of all small animals living to life expectancy will have evidence of the condition. Radiographic diagnosis is generally definitive, but the presence of reduced range of motion and significant crepitus are strong indicators of this chronic inflammatory con-dition. Young animals with developmental orthopedic disease, especially of the elbows, often present with early-onset arthritis which can significantly impact an animal's lifelong comfort level and in some cases may result in euthanasia before life expectancy is reached. Osteoarthritis can affect any joint, including the articular facets. Degenerative joint disease should be distinguished from traumatic arthritis, infectious arthritis, and immune-mediated polyarthropathies. In areas where rickettsial diseases are common, screening should be performed.

Developmental orthopedic diseases including hip dysplasia and elbow dysplasia (characterized by ununited anconeal process, fragmented medial coronoid process, osteo-chondrosis dissecans, and/or elbow incon-gruity) are important causes of lameness in young animals and predispose to degenerative joint disease. Early prophylactic integrative interventions may reduce the onset of clinical signs. Gait abnormalities are frequently observed by the owners, and examination may reveal the presence of incongruity, pain, and effusion.

Active dogs and performance animals may present with chronic orthopedic injuries resultant from a single episode of trauma. These include digital fractures, especially in racing Greyhounds, carpal or tarsal chip fractures, or avulsion injuries. Radiographs or computed tomography, when available, are generally adequate to distinguish degenerative joint disease from chronic conditions amendable to surgical intervention.

Older dogs should be carefully evaluated for early neoplastic lesions causing mild lameness or subtle changes in mobility. Osteosarcoma, for example, has been identified due to the presence of increased temperature over the distal radius of a Great Dane during a rehabilitative examination for hindlimb lameness. Such examples illustrate the importance of a comprehensive examination.

Soft tissue pathology may be identified in either an orthopedic examination or in a dedicated soft tissue assessment.

The characterization of such lesions remains controversial. The human literature refers to myofascial trigger points as hyperirritable areas within a taut band of muscle. The molecular mechanisms of such phenomena are unclear, however, it is thought that such palpable areas represent non-neurologic activation of muscle fibers which then induce secondary inhibition of the muscle and weakness. These areas are characterized by an aversive response on palpation, and are frequently addressed with local manipulative therapies.

Muscle strains are more commonly recognized by practitioners than trigger points and typically result from eccentric loading, that is stretching of a muscle during activation. The established grading system in veterinary medicine is as follows:

Grade 1: mild: myositis and bruising but minimal disruption of architecture
Grade 2: moderate: myositis and partial tearing of fascia and/or muscle
Grade 3: severe: tearing of the fascial sheath, disruption of fibers, hematoma

Muscles responsible for significant loading, such as the biceps, gracilis, iliopsoas are most commonly affected. The grading system is of less utility for chronic lesions. Chronic repetitive strain results in a combination of Stage 1-like inflammation and local trigger points with secondary muscle inactivation.

Chronic tendonitis occurs in several areas in the dog, and is most common in active animals or those with previous surgical intervention. Patellar tendonitis, for example, is a possible complication of osteotomies for cruciate ligament insufficiencies. Biceps tenosynovitis with or without calcification is encountered in some dogs. Other areas of potential tendonitis are less common; for example, the tendon of the abductor pollicus longus (dewclaw) may be subject to repetitive strain. Tendon strains are described similarly as to those affecting muscle:

Grade I: minor stretching or tearing
Grade II: partial tear with functional preservation

Grade III: near complete or complete tear with secondary instability and functional compromise.

Sprains describe acute ligamentous injury, and are therefore separate from strains. If severe, surgical intervention is typically required to restore stability.

Infectious and neoplastic causes of myositis are far less common than primary pathology resultant from repetitive strain or acute eccentric loading. The practitioner must carefully assess examination findings to determine whether soft tissue pathology is primary or compensatory to another inciting cause, such as osteoarthritis or paresis.

Diagnostic Challenges

Endocrine disorders may affect muscle, tendons, ligaments, and peripheral nerves. For example, hypothyroidism in some cases induces a peripheral neuropathy in dogs and selective atrophy of muscle fibers. Hyperthyroidism is associated with general weakness in cats without definitive histologic lesions. Hyperadrenocorticism induces changes in muscle condition, such as necrosis and atrophy of faster twitch muscle fibers, as well as in fibroblast maturation.

Metabolic disorders and electrolyte disturbances cause weakness, fatigue, and other symptoms which must be separated from primary causes of impaired mobility. Patients with potassium abnormalities, diabetes, hypertension, and others must be examined in the context of the patient's entire medical history and symptoms. When metabolic conditions are identified, concurrent management is indicated.

Mobility declines with age and caretakers may be financially unprepared or unwilling to invest in the cost of diagnostic evaluations for suspected non-surgical lesions. Such owners should be counseled on the general disadvantages of empiric treatment. However, many treatment modalities can be elected without specific knowledge of the precise lesion localization because of systemic treatment effects. Radiographs are likely the most accessible and cost-effective of tests for orthopedic localization. Other considerations include computed tomography (CT), with its advantage of being multi-dimensional and more time and cost effective for the assessment of multiple joints. CT rarely provides adequate resolution for neu-rologic lesions, except in the case of a miner-alized disc protrusion. Alternatives include MRI, at a significant owner investment, or for muscle and tendon injuries, diagnostic ultrasound. The latter requires a linear high frequency probe and a trained operator.

Novel Diagnostics

A variety of new diagnostic resources are available. Gait analysis is increasingly com-mon in rehabilitative practice and allows for generation of patient-specific data on the rel-ative weight distribution between limbs. The advantage over force plates are that entire gait cycle parameters can be analyzed instead of simply one leg at a time. Standing force ana-lyzers may provide information about inac-tive weight distribution, but similar information may be obtained from looking carefully at the amount of central pad contact in a dog's comfortable standing position. Kinematic data uses analysis of video footage to determine joint angles during motion. Similar work has been done using walking fluoroscopy. Thermal cameras are available that purportedly detect cutaneous tempera-tures, elevations of which may be suggestive of tissue inflammation. These technologies are typically reserved for those cases in which a definitive localization cannot be made dur-ing the comprehensive evaluation or are reserved for confirmation of clinical suspi-cions. Overreliance on technology in the diagnosis risks missing pathology which may be identified on a thorough examination.

Comorbidities

Obesity must be prioritized in any patient with impaired mobility, and the concurrent management of obesity is discussed later. Obesity results in increased mechanical load-ing in patients with impaired mobility. The hor-monal effects of adiposity, such as on adipokine balance, may actually worsen osteoarthritis and other conditions by causing a chronic inflam-matory state. Dogs fed to maintain lean body mass have a lower risk of arthritis, and when arthritis does occur, a reduced severity of clini-cal signs. Moreover, overweight dogs live an estimated two fewer years than lean dogs.

The presence of any other systemic disease may increase a patient's fatigue and decrease adaptability to impaired mobility. Consequently, animals should receive a comprehensive health screen before treatment of mobility is initiated.

Prognosis

Most chronic mobility disorders are incura-ble. Surgical interventions may improve an acute deterioration in the case of interverte-bral disc disease or severe hip dysplasia. More commonly, however, patients develop impairment of other joints, other discs, or have progression of non-surgical osteoar-thritis. The goals of most interventions are to preserve existing function, to maintain or improve muscle mass, to maintain existing neurologic function, and to provide general comfort through a multimodal approach.

A New Integrative Approach

Normal functional mobility relies on a complex synergy between multiple body systems and tissues. The approaches designed to preserve such function should be equally multimodal. A multifaceted approach of weight management, drug therapy, nutritional management, dietary supplements, surgery, and exercise has long been advocated for osteoarthritis. A similar individualized patient approach should be elected for all mobility disorders and can be divided into the following categories:

1) *Controlled exercise:* Exercise should be low-impact, high-resistance in order to preserve muscle mass without overloading

joints. Hydrotherapy may be especially helpful for severe cases of altered ambulation.

2) *Pain control:* A combination of therapeutic modalities should be used to address pain. These may include acupuncture, pharmaceutical drugs, nutraceuticals, soft tissue therapies, and photobiomodulation.

3) *Nutrition:* Nutritional requirements change as an animal's condition or diagnosis changes. A dog with significant paresis and intolerance to exercise may require caloric reduction. However, the amount of protein per calories should be elevated to maintain lean body mass.

4) *Tissue stimulation:* Endogenous reparative process may be engaged with a variety of modalities, such as platelet therapies, shockwave, acupuncture, electrostimulation, stem cells, and others. The suitability of such modalities is tissue- and condition-dependent. Treatment of issues following secondary compensation is critical.

5) *Weight management:* Obesity must be avoided in all animals with compromised mobility.

Therapeutics

Acute Management and Stabilization

Acutely nonambulatory patients are often best managed with hospitalization. The emotional distress of the owner and the need to prevent further declines generally makes this the best approach. Moreover, advanced imaging may be required and if so, referral to a specialty practice for the short term may be indicated. The most common causes of acute impairment will be neurologic in origin and surgical intervention may be indicated depending on the presenting signs. There is no evidence to support the use of steroids in acute spinal trauma, and their use in humans may increase complication rates. Therefore, pain control, if necessary, and non-steroidal anti-inflammatory drugs (NSAIDs) may be preferred. Orthopedic causes of impaired

mobility will be managed similarly, and drug therapy is discussed in greater detail in the following section.

Chronic Therapeutic Options

If owners confront a condition that is likely to be progressive, it is important to have early and extensive conversations regarding their goals, treatment philosophies, financial or logistical limitations, as well as the point at which they feel that mobility could impair their animal's quality of life. The latter is difficult to raise when an animal's condition is stable and mild, but such documented conversations serve as important reference points for future decisions about care and end-of-life.

Therapeutic interventions are best offered and administered in a stepwise fashion in order to better assess a patient's response to a particular intervention, especially given that the chronic management of most patients will be multimodal. Owners are overwhelmed by the diversity of options and the relative merits if presented at an initial evaluation.

Pharmacologic Interventions

Mobility disorders without an inflammatory component or pain generally fail to respond to pharmacologic interventions. In some cases of severe muscle atrophy, the use of anabolic steroids has been proposed to build muscle mass. However, physiotherapy and elevated dietary protein are preferred strategies to help to maintain lean body condition.

If a patient has reduced mobility due to an inflammatory condition such as osteoarthritis, the following drugs may be of benefit.

- *Prednisone (0.5–1 mg/kg/day), prednisolone (same dose, cats) or equivalent steroid:* Animals which respond should be tapered to the lowest effect dose. Many dogs can demonstrate a response at 0.25 mg/kg every other day, which is consistent with 'physiologic' dosing but which appears to still ameliorate clinical signs in some patients. Steroids are not recommended by the author as a first-line in the management of intervertebral disc disease.

- *Carprofen (2.2 mg/kg BID) or equivalent non-steroidal anti-inflammatory drug in dogs:* Carprofen remains the most well-studied of all the NSAIDs in dogs and is effective in the management of mobility reductions secondary to degenerative joint disease. Many geriatric dogs benefit from lower doses at the same frequency, especially in combination with analgesics when appropriate.
- *NSAID use in cats:* A number of NSAIDs are now labeled for use in cats, but their use should still be approached with caution and with the dose titrated to the lowest effective dose. Meloxicam and robenacoxib are labeled for use in cats, but only short-term. The American Association of Feline Practitioners maintains guidelines for the use of NSAIDs in cats which should be reviewed prior to their use.

Pain may have primary or secondary effects on mobility, and in either case should be treated aggressively. Adjunctive agents are often necessary even when administering a glucocorticoid or NSAID. The following therapeutic options are available.

- *Tramadol:* 5 mg/kg q6–12 h dogs, 2 mg/kg q12–24 h cats. Tramadol is extremely well tolerated in both species with minimal risk of a meaningful overdose. The dose appears to be highly variable and must be adjusted to the patient.
- *Amantadine:* 3–5 mg/kg q12–24 h. This drug works on the NMDA receptor but without the dissociative effects associated with ketamine. It has been shown to be well-tolerated in dogs, especially in combination with an NSAID. Experience in cats is limited, and once daily dosing at the low end of the dose range is prudent.
- *Buprenorphine:* 5–20 ug/kg q8h sublingually (cats). This opioid can be used chronically as needed but may be difficult to administer to some cats and has the disadvantage of needing to be dosed more frequently than other options.
- *Gabapentin:* 5–10 mg/kg q12h starting dose. Gabapentin has been suggested for chronic and neuropathic pain although its efficacy has been variable depending on the condition for which it was administered. It is recommended an adjunctive agent for that reason.
- *Amitriptyline:* 0.25–2 mg/kg q12–24 h. This tricyclic antidepressant may have effects on chronic pain through central mediation of pain. Caution should be used with other tricyclic drugs, selective serotonin reuptake inhibitors (SSRIs), and monoamine oxidase inhibitors (MAOIs).
- *Fentanyl patch:* 2–5ug/kg/h, to a maximum of a 100 ug/h patch for large dogs, rounded to the nearest size patch and 25 ug/h for cats. Fentanyl patches provide analgesic support for at least 72 hours, but potentially for up to a week in some patients. Onset may be delayed 4–24 hours after application, and animals should be monitored so as to not remove or ingest the patch.
- *Topical lidocaine patches:* Patches are cut to size and deliver drug to the area deep to the patch. Effects will be limited to the site of contact and by duration of drug delivery, which is about 12–24 hours.

Intra-articular Injections

Degenerative joint disease may be managed with a combination of local and systemic therapies. Intra-articular injections are a valuable adjunct if isolated joints are a significant source of lameness or pain. Elbow arthritis particularly benefits from this approach. The following therapeutics can be adminstered intra-articularly.

1) *Triamcinolone:* A glucocorticoid with documented efficacy at reducing inflammation. The recommended dose is not well established, but doses of 3 mg for small joints or feline injections have been recommended. Doses of 6 mg for larger canine joints are often used. If multiple

joints are to be injected, a total dose not to exceed 1 mg/kg has been used by the author. Systemic absorption will occur, and there will be some suppression of the adrenocortical axis but side effects are typically mild. Theoretical contraindications on cartilage growth exist, but some literature suggests that the inflammatory environment of the joint is more hostile to cartilage repair than is a glucocorticoid injection. Animals typically respond within 5–7 days, and effects may be sustained for 1–2 months.

2) *Morphine:* Intra-articular (IA) morphine has been shown to have postoperative analgesic effects in animals and sustained effects in human osteoarthritic patients. Doses of 0.1–0.5 mg/kg have been reported, with the author dosing on the high end. The duration of IA morphine is unknown, but is likely effective at least for several days. Given the uncertainty about dosing, the author typically mixes with another IA agent.

3) *Local anesthetic:* Bupivicaine or mepivacaine (0.5% solution) can be administered concurrently with other agents to reduce postinjection discomfort resultant from the capsular distension associated with an IA injection. Doses of 0.5 mg/kg have been used postoperatively for analgesia, but the volume may be determined by the practical volume limits if other agents are given.

4) *Regenerative therapies:* Platelets and stem cells are discussed in greater detail later but are equipped to provide growth factors and stimulate tissue repair. It remains unclear as to whether IA stem cell injections cause differentiation of cells into chondrocytes or if the stem cells have other indirect effects on reducing joint inflammation and inducing tissue repair.

5) *Prolotherapy:* Prolotherapy, or the injection of irritants, in the joint remains uncommon in veterinary medicine but it has attracted significant attention in human medicine. IA concentrated dextrose solutions produced equivalent effects to IA steroids in some human studies. However, a study of osteoarthritic dogs found no benefit to IA injections of 5 mL of 25% dextrose.

Nutrition and Supplements

Dogs and cats with impaired mobility require evaluation of dietary intake. The three major considerations are as follows:

1) Caloric intake. If animals are less active than expected, caloric expenditure is likely to decrease. Most pet dogs require no more than $95 \times$ (ideal body weight in kg)$^{0.75}$ kcal per day. Paralyzed humans display a reduction in caloric intake of about 1/3 although this may be mediated by a reduction in muscle mass. Pet foods vary widely in caloric content and therefore owners should be given specific instructions on what and how to feed. These recommendations are consistent with current AAHA guidelines that all patients receive a nutritional recommendation.

2) Protein content. Most dogs with impaired mobility should be fed diets with elevated amounts of protein. Higher protein diets are shown to preserve lean body mass in aging animals and those with reduced activity. A diet with more than 75 grams of protein per 1000 calories fed should be administered. The protein content of a diet can be determined from the guaranteed analysis with the following formula:
   a) Add 1.5% to the minimum protein content listed on the bag.
   b) Divide the value by the caloric density of the food (kcal/kg) divided by 10,000.
   c) For example, consider a diet with 21.5% min. protein and 4,000 kcal/kg. An estimate of the number of protein grams per 1000 calories would be 57.5. This was calculated as follows: $((21.5 + 1.5)/(4000/10,000))$.

3) Omega 3 fatty acids. In patients with inflammatory conditions, the omega 3 fatty acids EPA (eicosapentaenoic acid) and DHA (docosahexaenoic acid) produce less inflammatory prostaglandins

and leukotrienes than omega 6 fatty acids. EPA and DHA are found in fish oils, algal oils, and krill oil. The dose of fish oil recommended is 1–3 mg of combined EPA and DHA for every calorie fed. A 40 pound dog consuming 1000 calories per day should be given 1,000–3,000 mg of EPA and DHA per day. Most standard 1 gram fish oil capsules contain 300 mg of combined EPA and DHA and therefore this patient would need between 3 and 10 capsules daily (assuming that the dietary concentration is low). Some therapeutic diets or fish-based commercial diets will meet this requirement with the diet alone.

Table 3.1 is a suggested macronutrient profile (expressed as grams per 1000 kcal) for dogs of normal body condition with mobility impairment.

Therapeutic diets should be critically evaluated as to whether they meet therapeutic goals for nutritional intake. Consider the comparison of diets labeled for degenerative joint disease shown in Table 3.2.

Dietary supplements may be of value in patients with altered mobility secondary to osteoarthritis. Table 3.3 is an abbreviated list of available therapeutic options.

Supplements may influence lean body mass, oxidative balance, and other possible biologic processes, and therefore be effective for both orthopedic and neurologic causes of mobility impairment (Table 3.4).

Weight Management

Calorie restriction must be initiated in overweight animals to achieve a slow rate of weight loss of 0.5% to 2% weekly. Higher rates may be associated with a greater risk of lean body mass loss. Diets high in protein appear superior to those with moderate amounts of protein, and the energy density of the diet is often decreased by: limiting the fat content (fat is more than two times more energy dense than protein and carbohydrate), increasing the moisture content, or by adding dietary fiber.

Table 3.5 shows the macronutrient composition in grams per 1000 calories recommended for weight-loss diets in animals with mobility challenges.

The caloric intake required for weight loss can be estimated in animals by reducing food intake by 1/3 from the known current weight-stable calorie intake. If an animal is actively gaining weight on a fixed number of calories it is more difficult to determine the amount of restriction required. Moreover, the diet history is often unknown or unclear because owners may be unaware of how much they are feeding

Table 3.1 Suggested macronutrient profile (grams per 1000 kcal) for dogs of normal body condition with mobility impairment.

Protein	Fat	Carbohydrate	EPA + DHA
75	>35	<100	>1

Table 3.2 Diets labeled for degenerative joint disease.

Nutrient (/1000 KCAL)	Diet A	Diet B	Diet C	Diet D
Protein (g)	51	79	66	76
Fat (g)	41	33	32	34
EPA + DHA (g)	1.26 (EPA)	NR	1.45	NR
Glucosamine (mg)	NR	340	237	137 (min)
Chondroitin (mg)	NR	NR	26	13
Caloric density (kcal/cup)	356	408	324	296

NR = not reported.

Table 3.3 Therapeutic supplements.

Supplement	Action and Dosing
Glucosamine and Chondroitin	• Glucosamine is a precursor to glycosaminoglycans in cartilage, such as chondroitin and hyaluronic acid • Oral absorption of these products has been demonstrated in dogs; however, clinical effects have been mixed • If given, owners should be prepared to administer for at least 2 months before making a determination about clinical utility • Dose: >25 mg/kg glucosamine daily and >15 mg/kg chondroitin daily • Injectable products such as Adequan provide the same precursors but without the uncertainty of oral absorption. The oral doses listed above is equivalent to the injectable dose assuming normal absorption by a particular animal
Green-Lipped Mussel	• Contains omega-3 fatty acids, minerals, and other compounds • One study found that some owners perceive huge improvements in OA even when dogs are given placebo or GLM. Claims of instant improvement should be critically evaluated • Dose: 30 mg/kg daily but the dose is not well-established
Methylsulfonylmethane (MSM)	• Dietary sulfur compound with unclear mechanisms, but interestingly, dimethyl sulfoxide (DMSO) is metabolized in part to MSM • Limited evidence of efficacy is available • Dose: >10 mg/kg daily
Boswellic Acid	• An anti-inflammatory herbal compound derived from frankincense • Laboratory studies suggest an anti-inflammatory effect but there are few studies in veterinary medicine • Dose: 40 mg/kg daily of boswellia resin. Pure boswellic acid products can likely be administered in 1/3 the amount of resin based on currently available scientific analyses (i.e., 10–15 mg/kg boswellic acids daily)
Curcumin	• Derived from the spice turmeric • NF-kB and COX-2 inhibitor • Poor gastrointestinal absorption • Subjective, but not objective, improvement in dogs with osteoarthritis • Dose: 40–50 mg/kg twice daily of an extracted form. Conventional curcumin powder may have poor absorption at practical doses
Avocado/Soybean Unsaponifiables (ASU)	• Positive effects in the synovial fluid of dogs and favorable human clinical trials have been reported • Increased tissue factor beta and secondary increase in collagen • Possible inhibition of NO synthase and matrix metalloproteinases • Dose: 10 mg/kg daily
Elk Velvet Antler	• Positive changes were reported in forceplate analysis and lameness in a clinic trial • Effects may be due to large concentration of collagen or unique proteins • Adrenal lesions and death were reported in two dogs receiving the product, but these could not be definitively linked to the product • Dose: 15–25 mg/kg twice daily
Other Supplements	• A number of supplements are used by animal owners but which require further investigation. These include gelatin hydrolysate, hyperimmunized cow milk proteins, and undenatured type II collagen • Doses are poorly established in veterinary medicine

Table 3.4 Nutritional Supplements.

Supplement	Action and dose
Branched Chain Amino Acids	• Includes leucine, isoleucine, and valine; leucine has been shown to stimulate skeletal muscle protein synthesis in a number of species • Dosing branched chain amino acids is difficult without knowledge of dietary amino acid composition • Dose: unknown, but a high protein diet is likely greater able to achieve the requisite dose than pure branched chain amino acids in supplement form
L-carnitine	• Not technically an amino acid, but critical for transporting long-chain fatty acids across the mitochondrial membrane for energy production • May promote weight loss during caloric restriction • Dose: 30 mg/kg daily (dogs), 50 mg/kg daily (cats)
S-adenosylmethionine (SAM-e)	• Contributes to production of glutathione, the primary intracellular antioxidant • Some human studies suggest positive effects on osteoarthritis • Dose: 20 mg/kg (dogs), 50 mg/kg (cats), but clinical data in dogs and cats is limited
Vitamin C	• Supplementation has been shown to increase serum or plasma levels; in one study, it increased cartilage weight in experimental canine arthritis • Possible side effects: Greyhounds ran slower when given vitamin C, and diarrhea has been reported • Dose: most canine studies administered 1 g of supplemental vitamin C.
Vitamin E	• Primary antioxidant within the cell membrane • Positive effects reported in osteoarthritis but also has general antioxidant properties • May reduce spinal injury when given *before* injury. The effects after injury are not well described • Dose: 10–20 iu/kg daily but variable across studies
Alpha Lipoic Acid	• Antioxidant and co-factor for mitochondrial enzymes • Component of an antioxidant mixture shown to reduce severity of canine cognitive dysfunction • May reduce severity of peripheral neuropathy and osteoarthritis in human studies • Dose: 11 mg/kg daily: dogs only • This compound has much greater toxicity in cats than in other species and the maximum tolerable dose is < 30 mg/kg daily for cats

Table 3.5 Recommended macronutrient composition (grams per 1000 calories) for weight-loss diets in animals with mobility challenges.

Protein	Fat	Carbohydrate	EPA + DHA
>110	<40	<90	>1

or may be feeding supplemental foods (treats, leftovers, etc.) as a large portion of the diet.

Most overweight or obese cats require calorie restriction to about 150–200 calories per day. The amount to feed dogs is predicated on ideal body weight, which can be calculated for dogs using the validated 9 point scoring system, in which a 4 or 5 score out of 9 is normal. For each point over 5, the animal's body weight is 15% greater than ideal body weight (IBW). This may be expressed mathematically:

$$\text{Current Body Weight (kg)} = \text{IBW} \times (1 + (\# \text{ points over } 5 * 0.15))$$

Therefore, an animal with a current body weight of 50 kg and a body condition score of 8/9 would have an ideal body weight calculated as follows: 50 kg = IBW (1.45), or IBW = 35.5 kg.

Ideal body weight should be used in all canine weight loss formulas. The most commonly used formula is 70* (ideal body weight in kg)$^{0.75}$ kcal per day. In the example above, the obese dog would be estimated to require about 1020 calories per day. The actual amount should be adjusted to achieve 0.5–2% of body weight loss weekly. Animals that are significantly impaired in their mobility may require fewer calories, by as much as 1/3 less than the calculated equation.

Increased exercise alone is generally insufficient to achieve weight loss. As an example, a 35 kg obese dog with an ideal body weight of 25 kg fed 1000 calories daily would use only 6% more calories daily if walked a total of 3.2 miles. While underwater treadmill therapy has been shown to be a part of a successful weight loss protocol, the effect of hydrotherapy alone remains unclear. Studies of normal dogs walking in an underwater treadmill demonstrated only slightly increased energy expenditure as compared to walking at the same speed on a dry treadmill.

Physiotherapy

Physiotherapy techniques are underutilized in the management of mobility disorders in veterinary medicine. Affected patients require therapeutic exercises to maintain or increase function and to build strength (Table 3.6). Such techniques have been critically evaluated after orthopedic surgery, specifically for cruciate insufficiency, and suggest a reduction in the time to a return of function. The specific exercises recommended should be tailored to the patient and advanced as the animal displays functional improvement.

Therapeutic massage is often considered with physiotherapy. Massage has not been

Table 3.6 Therapeutic exercises.

Exercise	Technique	Function
Passive range of motion	Each joint should be isolated and held in maximal comfortable extension for 10 seconds, then in flexion for 10 seconds	Improvement and maintenance of connective and soft tissue range of motion, movement of synovial fluid, activation of stretch receptors
Weave poles	Animals are asked to move in a weaving fashion around a linear series of objects with the distance between objects adjusted to the patient's limitations	Facilitates weight-shifting, improves active range of motion, challenges proprioceptive fibers
Cavalettis	Animals are led over objects of a certain height so that they must step over the barrier	Proprioceptive retraining, induction of active flexion of elbow and stifle, gait retraining
Wobble board or balance ball	Pets are placed on an unsteady object (either two or all limbs) and supported while balancing	Activation of reciprocal musculature, proprioceptive retraining, strength building
Isometric exercises	A muscle or group of muscles is exercised without the muscle lengthening or shortening. For example, placement of the hindlimbs of a paretic dog and application of ventral pressure causes muscles to work to maintain standing conformation	Low-impact strength training, activation of many motor units, provision of neural feedback in the event of spinal injury
Ground treadmill	The pet is asked to walk on a treadmill with or without an incline or decline	Endurance training, ability to monitor gait more closely, decline: weight shifting to forelimbs, incline: weight shifting to hindlimbs

subjected to robust clinical trials in dogs or cats, but anecdotally these species relax during manipulation of muscle groups, especially when myofascial trigger points are identified. There are a variety of techniques utilized, but focal digital massage of affected trigger points is often adequate, with the pressure adjusted to an animal's comfort. Larger areas, such as the epaxial muscles, can be massaged with the forefingers or through the use of vibrating massagers, if tolerated by the patients. The principles by which massage may induce a therapeutic effect include increased lymphatic flow, modulation of local pain mediators such as substance P and prostaglandins, positive cortical responses, increased local circulation, reductions in muscle fasciculation, and reduction of tissue or fascial adhesions. Most animals that display improved mobility following massage have secondary compensatory changes in soft tissue structures as a result of a primary injury.

Hydrotherapy

Mobility impairments in small animals are often due to an inability to support weight normally during a full gait cycle. Therefore, animals may display improved ambulation when load-bearing is reduced. Animals recovering from intervertebral disc protrusions will often ambulate first when body weight is supported. Hydrotherapy remains one of the more common methods of achieving this effect in dogs and occasionally in cats. The principles of aquatic therapy relate to the effects of the water on buoyancy and resistance. Underwater treadmill therapy reduces concussive forces on joints and promotes increased joint flexion and full active

extension. It may also improve muscular conditioning due to the increased work required to move against the density of the water. It has been used for both weight loss protocols and for postoperative rehabilitation of dogs following cruciate repair. Hydrotherapy techniques include swimming and underwater treadmill therapy. Animals in an underwater treadmill tend to use their hindlimbs more reliably than when swimming. The underwater treadmill will result in increased joint loading as compared to swimming and this is related to the height of the water (Table 3.7).

Swimming is often used rather than underwater treadmill when trying to manipulate an active range of motion; hip, stifle, and hock flexion were all increased in a pool as compared to a ground treadmill. However, hip and stifle extension angles are reduced. Severely osteoarthritic dogs are typically exercised more comfortably in a pool because they are completely non-weight bearing.

Underwater treadmill may be better for proprioceptive training and dynamic balance than swimming since neither is required with complete buoyancy. Additional data are required to better inform the optimal time for starting hydrotherapy but many authors advocate early use after acute loss of mobility and early initiation of any program for chronic mobility impairment.

Laser Therapy

Several classes of therapeutic lasers are available to veterinarians and are marketed for pain, inflammation, and wound healing. The most common are class IIIb lasers with a power of 0.5 Watts, and class IV lasers which generally offer a variable power of 0.5–15 Watts. Laser is

Table 3.7 Weight loading as a result of water height.

Water height	Percent of weight loading	Function
Tarsal/carpal	91	Increase active range of motion
Stifle/elbow	85	Maximal strength conditioning
Hip/shoulder	38	Reduced concussive forces, increased stability

an acronym for *light amplification by stimulated emission of radiation*. Light in the visible red and infrared spectra (600–1000 nm) exerts the biologic effects of photobiomodulation, which include:

1) Increased adenosine triphosphate (ATP) production through activity on mitochondrial cytochrome C oxidase
2) Induction of cellular antioxidant production due to a sublethal increase of free oxygen radicals
3) Vasodilation as a result of nitric oxide release from proteins.

The effects of laser on mobility have been theorized as a reduction in inflammatory mediators in osteoarthritic joints and on a reduction of inflammation. A neuroregenerative effect has been proposed, and a single clinical veterinary study reported a significant reduction in the time of ambulation following decompressive hemilaminectomy in dogs.

Animals with impaired mobility will likely require frequent and chronic treatments, with twice daily administration not uncommon among laser therapy protocols. Ten treatment sessions are likely necessary over a one month period to fully evaluate the clinical utility in a patient. The area to be dosed is generally roughly measured to estimate numerical area in cm^2. Approximately 5 Joules of laser energy per cm^2 is required in the affected tissue to achieve the effects of photobiomodulation. The power of a laser in Watts is equivalent to the number of Joules delivered per second. Animals should ideally be shaved before administration because melanin in pigment, and the air in the interface between laser and patient, may significantly reduce laser penetration. The depth of the tissue also influences the amount of photons absorbed by intervening tissue, and dosing should be increased 50% for lesions greater than 1 cm in depth and 100% more for lesions greater than 2.5 cm in depth. Photons emitted from a laser are unlikely to penetrate bone in sufficient amounts to achieve clinical effects, which should be considered when treating spinal lesions.

As an example of laser dosing, a 40 kg labrador has a circumferential area of 150 cm^2 around the stifle. The stifle joint is located deep to overlying tissue, and consequently an increase of 50% is elected. A Class IV laser is set to 10 W of power. The desired dose is $(150\,cm^2 \times 5\,J/cm^2 \times 1.5\,J)$, or 1125 Joules. A 10 W laser will provide 10 J/sec and therefore the treatment time is just under two minutes. A Class IIIb laser with a power of 0.5 W would take 40 minutes to treat the same area.

Shockwave Therapy

Extracorporeal shockwave therapy utilizes high energy sound or pressure waves to transfer energy to biologic tissues. More specifically, energy causes cavitation and microstresses in tissues and cells with high impedance. The resulting stress in the tissue stimulates an acute response which may stimulate a compensatory endogenous reparative phase of healing. Additional analgesic effects may be provided through modulation of serotonin. The modality may have particular utility in animals with impaired mobility secondary to chronic tendinopathy; increased collagen deposition and increased neovascularization have been reported following the therapy. Clinical utility may also exist for osteoarthritic patients as benefits have been shown in clinical studies of dogs, likely mediated by a reduction in nitric oxide and preservation of chondrocytes. The modality requires access to a shockwave unit and trode, and dogs should be sedated for the procedure. Doses of between 400–800 shocks are used per site, and treatments may be repeated every 1–3 weeks for acute injuries affecting mobility and on a patient-specific regular schedule for chronic diseases like osteoarthritis. Clinical responses and dosing frequencies appear to be patient- and condition-dependent, and further research is needed to inform optimal treatment protocols.

Therapeutic Ultrasound

Therapeutic ultrasound provides energy in the form of sound, which is absorbed by tissues of high protein content such as skeletal muscle, thereby providing deep heating to target tissues. Short-term (<10 minutes) heating of 1.6–4.6 °C was reported in the caudal thigh muscles of dogs following ultrasound with powers of between 1 and 1.5 W/cm^2. This short-term thermal effect of ultrasound may facilitate improved stretching and is most beneficial when followed by range of motion exercises. As an example, calcaneal tendon extensibility and tarsal flexion increased for 5 minutes following ultrasound application in dogs. Repeated and frequent administration may produce faster rates of healing in tendons and in other tissues. A therapeutic ultrasound unit typically has several settings (Table 3.8) which must be selected by the user.

Acupuncture

Acupuncture remains a source of significant controversy in veterinary medicine largely due to debates surrounding the antiquity of acupuncture, and available evidence suggests that modern veterinary acupuncture is a recent invention. A dated systematic review found there was insufficient evidence to recommend acupuncture in small animal patients, and studies have been conflicting; most studies of osteoarthritis failed to document an immediate benefit although long-term studies have not been performed. However, several studies of intervertebral disc disease suggest a benefit on return or improvement of ambulation. Research has

documented a variety of mechanisms by which acupuncture may influence pain reception or neural stimulation:

- endogenous opioid release
- substance P modulation
- serotonin modulation
- myofascial release and reduction of local inflammatory mediators
- histamine release
- cannabinoid receptor modulation
- stimulation of neurovascular bundles, Golgi tendon apparatus, and/or free nerve endings
- synaptic plasticity

Acupuncture points may be selected based on traditional or scientific approaches. Typically, 32 gauge stainless steel needles are used in dogs and 34 gauge or "hand" needles in cats. Acupuncture may be simply performed by any practitioner by identification of myofascial trigger points and placement of a needle at that site. Needle insertion has been shown to relax local muscle tension and to reduce pain. The fascia can be activated by twisting the needle after insertion.

The acupuncture point nomenclature used by many veterinarians trained in the modality is rather confusing and is derived from the human point system. Various organs are associated with meridians in Chinese thought, and controversy exists as to if and how acupuncture meridians or channels can be explained. Irrespective, the naming system does provide the ability to communicate point location. Table 3.9 lists the common points used in the management of mobility.

Cyanocobalamin injections (vitamin B12) may be administered into acupuncture points, but an advantage over conventional needling has not been scientifically validated. Cobalamin has a wide margin of safety and physiologic and cellular deficiencies have been reported in various conditions. Cobalamin functions as a methyl donor and does have a more complex absorption pathway than all of the other B vitamins. Some local effects on allodynia have been reported in rats, but this has not been confirmed for

Table 3.8 Ultrasound settings.

Setting	Options
Power	0.1–3 W/cm^2 with lower power for tendons and higher power for large muscles
Frequency	1 MHz for deep tissues, 3.3 MHz for superficial (<2 cm)
Continuous or pulsed	Continuous commonly used for chronic lesions, pulsed (decreased duty cycle) for acute. Continuous for thermal effects.

Table 3.9 Acupuncture points used in the management of mobility.

Acupuncture point	Point location
Bladder Meridian	Located in the epaxial musculature at each intervertebral space starting caudal to the scapula and ending cranial to the sacrocaudal space
Stomach 36	Located in the proximal cranial tibial muscle
Pericardium 8 and Kidney 1	Located beneath the central metacarpal and metatarsal pad, respectively
Liu feng	Located in the interdigital spaces with the needle inserted between the metacarpo- or metatarsophalangeal joints
Bladder 40	Located in the popliteal fossa caudal to the stifle
LI 10	Located between the extensor carpi radialis and common digital extensor, just distal to the elbow joint

dogs or cats. The administration of large doses (>1 mL/10 pounds) may cause red discoloration of the urine.

Electrostimulation

Percutaneous electrical nerve stimulation is most commonly performed through the use of electroacupuncture. Specific battery-operated units are available for this purpose. Electroacupuncture has been shown in multiple species to augment therapeutic response by increasing release of endogenous opioids, with frequency-dependent effects.

- Low frequency (2 Hz) electroacupuncture releases μ-acting opioids
- High frequency stimulation (100 Hz) affects κ receptors
- Veterinary studies frequently employ a mixed low and high frequency treatment of at least 20-minute duration
- Release of β-endorphins lasts at least three hours posttreatment in dogs

The advantage of percutaneous stimulation is the ability to better affect deep tissues and neural inputs. Patients with paresis or plegia would be expected to have better response than with transcutaneous electrical stimulation due to the loss of conductivity in deep tissues secondary to inherent tissue resistance. Electrotherapy studies that documented an improvement in spinal mobility utilized various electroacupuncture treatment protocols.

Transcutaneous electrical nerve stimulation (TENS) utilizes conductive pads to activate sensory nerve fibers and to modulate pain. This is an option for owners to administer at home because stimulatory units are inexpensive and easy to use after initial settings are made. TENS is most likely to be of benefit in animals with pain secondary to osteoarthritis; TENS treatments set to a frequency of 70 Hz improved ground reaction forces in osteoarthritic dogs. The effects are thought to be mediated by similar neuromodulatory mechanisms as electroacupuncture.

Neuromuscular electrical stimulation is an option available on most commercial TENS units and can be employed in the treatment of muscle atrophy by recruiting motor fibers. Increased muscle mass was documented in dogs receiving this type of stimulation following surgical repair of a cranial cruciate ligament repair. TENS or Neuromuscular Electrical Stimulation (NMES) could be theorized to be more beneficial than electroacupuncture for the treatment of large areas given the greater current dispersal area over the pads as compared to needles. Table 3.10 lists the common TENS and NMES settings.

Hyperbaric Oxygen

Hyperbaric oxygen therapy may provide similar physiologic effects, but on a systemic basis, as laser photobiomodulation. Hyperbaric oxygen is known to induce the following:

1) ATP production by providing additional oxygen for phosphorylation

Table 3.10 Common TENS and NMES settings.

Common TENS Settings		Common NMES Settings	
Frequency	30–150 Hz	Frequency	25–50 Hz
Pulse duration	50–100 us	Pulse duration	100–400 us
		Ramp	2–4 s
		On/off	1:3 to 1:5

2) Compensatory increase in intracellular antioxidant production due to sublethal doses of free oxygen radicals
3) Posttreatment vasodilation due to nitric oxide release

Hyperbaric oxygen is well tolerated according to a veterinary retrospective on its use in dogs, but it does require access to a specialized pressure chamber. There is a paucity of clinical data on the utility of the treatment for disorders of mobility. However, research in humans and laboratory animals suggests that it may be effective for the management of postsurgical edema of tissues and of the spinal cord. Practices are increasingly employing the therapy for severe spinal cord injury, with treatment times of about an hour, pressures of about 2 atmospheres absolute (2 ATA), pure oxygen, and a frequency determined by condition severity. The reduction in spinal edema, if confirmed in dogs, would be of benefit from chronic non-surgical lesions in spinal cords, such as those associated with symptomatic cervical spondylomyelopathy. The increase in endogenous antioxidants may also be beneficial in osteoarthritis, and hyperbaric oxygen can be considered when an animal has severe degenerative joint disease in multiple joints, making laser therapy impractical.

Regenerative Medicine

Regenerative therapies rely on endogenous substances to release reparative growth and tissue factors and to reduce inflammation (Table 3.11). The primary regenerative techniques utilized in dogs and cats are platelet therapies and stem cell injections. Platelets can be harvested using anticoagulant and various commercial collection systems.

Table 3.11 Regenerative therapies.

Growth factor	Functions
PDGF-BB (and other isoforms)	Mitosis of fibroblasts, angiogenesis, expression of other growth factors
TGF-beta	Extracellular matrix and type 1 collagen synthesis, mesenchymal stem cell proliferation
bFGF	Angiogenesis and proliferation of mesodermal cells
VEGF	Angiogenesis and endothelial cell proliferation
EGF	Angiogenesis and cellular mitosis activation
IGF-1	Cell proliferation and survival, platelet signaling and activation, myoblast proliferation
CTGF	Angiogenesis and developmental chondrogenesis

Plasma containing lower concentrations of platelets may be harvested with the addition of 1 mL of ACD anticoagulant to 10 mL of collected blood and centrifugation. However, in-house processing should confirm the presence of platelets with a hemocytometer. Platelets exert clinical effects through the release of alpha granules which contain a number of growth factors. Clinical benefits are reported in patients with impaired mobility due to osteoarthritis, cranial cruciate ligament rupture, and chronic tendinopathy.

Autologous stem cells are typically processed from adipose tissue harvested via surgical collection of falciform ligament or subcutaneous fat. The cells are also known as mesenchymal or adipose-derived stem cells, and these cells can theoretically differentiate into adipocytes, chondrocytes, or osteoblasts. Canine clinical trials with osteoarthritis patients revealed modest and temporary reductions (<6 months) in clinical signs. Some data suggest that some remaining intact cartilage scaffolding is necessary for positive clinical effects. Given the current cost of stem cells, they are often reserved for when other options fail.

Veterinary Spinal Manipulation

Veterinary spinal manipulation therapy, also referred to as veterinary chiropractic, operates under the assumption that mobilization of joints can reduce physical pain, diminish inflammation, and thereby improve normal ambulatory function. The majority of the research in veterinary spinal manipulation has been performed in horses. Some authors theorize that chiropractic "adjustments" engage the myofascial planes and therefore produce similar effects as tissue massage, acupuncture, and other rehabilitation techniques. Some conventional practitioners and specialists have reservations about the modality especially in animals with intervertebral disc disease. Consequently, advanced training is recommended if this modality is to be used in the management of mobility impairment.

Homeopathy

Classical homeopathy remains controversial as a concept due to the underlying foundational principle that "like cures like" and that dilute quantities of a substance are more potent than more concentrated remedies. Most homeopathic agents induce the clinical signs they are designed to treat if given undiluted. As there is generally a lack of identifiable molecules of this parent compound, homeopathy is regarded as fairly safe. There are new products, however, that combine agents and use less dilute quantities of the classical substances. One such proprietary product, Zeel, was reported as being as efficacious as carprofen in a clinical trial in osteoarthritic dogs. Other products have not been subjected to critical appraisals in dogs and cats, although many are regarded as of low toxicity and risk.

Assistive Devices and Orthotics

Dogs with chronic mobility impairment may benefit from custom assistive devices which improve ambulation. Orthopedic conditions that may benefit include carpal or tarsal instability, cruciate ligament insufficiency, and medial shoulder instability. Retraining devices are available for patients with neurologic deficits, and custom wheelchairs may provide therapeutic benefits in some patients and provide a means of ambulation for nonambulatory animals.

Carpal and tarsal instability may be treated with moldable supportive wraps or in severe cases, custom orthotic solutions with a custom and adjustable hinge to limit hyperflexion or hyperextension. Mediolateral instability may also be addressed through the use of such devices. Custom orthotics typically reduce the risk for pressure sores, but they may still occur so an experienced fitter and molder should prepare the replicas for the company producing the devices. Orthotics have been designed to limit the cranial motion of the tibia in dogs when surgical repair of cruciate insufficiency is not feasible for any number of reasons. It is presently unclear whether these prevent tibial movement or instead if they provide sensory feedback or prevent internal rotation of the tibia. Some dogs do respond favorably, but those with meniscal injury will commonly display continued discomfort. Medial shoulder instability can be a source of mobility impairment, and animals can be managed with custom neoprene hobbles to prevent abduction. Most veterinary orthotic companies will address unique and challenging requests for patients with unique needs.

Dogs with proprioceptive deficits benefit from devices that prevent flexion of the carpus or extension of the tarsus. There are products, such as the Biko brace, which connect the distal limb to the torso with elastic material to prevent tarsal extension and secondary trauma to the dorsal aspect of the pes. Other devices include straps from the distal tibia to the metatarsals to hold the tarsus in flexion. These can be extremely effective at providing proprioceptive support for animals with deficits.

Wheelchairs no longer have the social stigma in animals due to their increased prevalence of use and owners' acknowledgements that dogs enjoy the ability to ambulate more normally with such assistive devices. Some severely paretic dogs benefit from a four-wheel or 'quad' cart to be able to move their limbs during rehabilitation. Dogs with a chronic inability of ambulate can use a cart for mental stimulation and to prevent the animal from being in a recumbent position for extended periods of time. Long-term cart or wheelchair use is best achieved with an adjustable device which has been customized to the particular patient. Ideally, the back should be in a normal anatomic alignment and care should be taken to avoid overloading the forelimbs with an improperly fitted cart. Contact areas, such as those around the harness or leg stirrups used to secure the patient to the cart, should be examined frequently for pressure sores or dermal irritation.

Assistive devices have a high rate of acceptance among owners when they are presented with videos of dogs in similar conditions. The customized solutions cost more than off-the-shelf solutions but are generally worth the investment given the improvements in mobility and the reduction in side effects from using an ill-fitting orthotic or cart.

Surgical Intervention/Salvage Procedures

Surgical intervention is appropriate in many of the acute impairments in mobility which occur, namely cruciate insufficiency and intervertebral disc disease. In some cases, however, the degree of severity of the clinical signs may warrant an attempt at conservative management. Dogs less than 13 kg can display positive functional outcomes without surgery when affected with cruciate insufficiency. Larger dogs too may benefit from a rehabilitative approach. In the event meniscal damage is suspected at the time of acute injury, or during chronic management, many such animals benefit from meniscal exploration and debridement. Animals with chronic intervertebral disc disease may be managed with a combination of integrative modalities, such as acupuncture, laser, hydrotherapy,

and physiotherapy. Comorbidities in many cases increase the risk of surgery in older patients. The options should always be presented to the owner at the time of evaluation, but there are an increasing number of therapies to try before surgery may prove necessary.

Non-responsive or severe conditions may benefit from surgical intervention. Surgery should be considered in the following conditions of impaired mobility.

- Grade 3–5 intervertebral disc disease
- Intervertebral disc disease with uncontrolled pain
- Severe hip osteoarthritis (femoral head and neck excision, total hip)
- Severe tarsal or carpal osteoarthritis (arthrodesis)
- Severe stifle or elbow osteoarthritis (arthrodesis, joint replacement)
- Medial patellar luxation with severe limitations in mobility
- Cranial cruciate ligament rupture +/– meniscal injury
- Juvenile hip dysplasia (Double pelvic osteotomy (DPO), Triple pelvic osteotomy (TPO), pubic symphysiodesis)
- Lumbosacral stenosis with severe or worsening clinical signs
- Significant cervical spondylomyelopathy (distraction-fusion)
- Amputation for significant disease of a single limb

Most of the surgeries performed for mobility impairment benefit from postoperative rehabilitation and many of the aforementioned modalities. Increasing evidence suggest that such interventions may improve outcome at a faster rate than normal activity or activity restriction.

Rescue Therapies

Animals with a sudden and unexpected deterioration are generally treated with an increased frequency of modalities listed earlier. In addition, the dose of anti-inflammatory drugs may be increased as well as the dose of analgesics.

Impacts of Interventions

The management of chronic impaired mobility requires frequent communication between the owner and attending veterinarian. In addition, the cost of medications, supplements, and treatments may be significant and lifelong in many cases. However, such modalities may extend an animal's life and improve comfort. Owners are increasingly willing to pursue such approaches to disease management. The increased care and attention provided to their pet may strengthen their bond so long as the level of care required does not rise to the level of creating fatigue. A time commitment by the owner is generally required for these chronic protocols, as the work cannot all be done by the veterinary team. Owners are frequently assigned tasks to extend the benefits of veterinary interventions, and failure to do so may impact the rate of recovery. Animals typically prove quite resilient in managing their deficits and most enjoy therapies designed to improve function. The ability to interact with other people, dogs, and environments may have benefits on outcome that are difficult to judge and to measure.

Owners should be counseled at the start of management that their pet's protocol will be individualized and that the early interventions will be used to assess response. Animals may worsen following an intervention, especially physiotherapy, and owners should be educated about the process. Owners must also accept that the optimal program for their pet is unknown at the outset of treatment and as such they will have to face a period of uncertainty. They are critical members of the wellness team and need to be actively engaged and given input on the process.

Expected Outcome and Possible Adverse Effects

The outcome for many nonsurgical interventions designed to improve mobility are unavailable in the scientific literature. The combination of modalities employed in most cases further complicates any definitive assessment of prognosis. However, when integrative interventions have been evaluated against inactivity or drug therapy alone, findings are generally positive. Moreover, adverse effects are typically limited to transient and reversible worsening of an animal's condition. The progressive individualization of protocols generally ameliorates such iatrogenic deteriorations over time. However, some animals will fail to respond to any and all suggested modalities. In these patients, difficult decisions about surgical interventions, if available, and quality of life will need to be discussed.

Quality of Life

Mild to moderate impairments in mobility may be of no functional significance to some animals and their owners. In these cases, the cost of treatment to maintain stability or to prevent secondary complications may be the primary factor an owner considers in assessing the treatment plan for their pet. Some owners may need to be shown videos of dogs in various states of immobility to better understand the functional limitations and behaviors of affected dogs. Patients who are not suffering from pain generally do not require constant inventory of the patient's clinical condition. The exception would be for animals with concurrent pain, in which case pain inventories can be utilized to track progress in controlling such signs, which are likely to be of great significance to animal and owner.

Severely impaired mobility without significant pain or discomfort is arguably one of the most difficult situations an owner may encounter if an animal's cognition is normal. The resiliency of pets produces a situation in which they may be emotionally unaffected by their altered mobility even when completely nonambulatory or paralyzed. Consequently, owners may significantly struggle with a decision on whether to continue treatment or to euthanize based upon their animal having a progressive decline, as compared to a sudden worsening of a terminal clinical condition. Therefore, owners often have time to consider all possibilities and to err on the side of waiting for an additional deterioration before confronting end-of-life or quality-of-life issues. Such declines may be gradual and the owner may not recognize deterioration, or when worsening of signs does occur the owner may recant previous statements about their endpoints of care. Frequent visits between the veterinarian and the owner may forge a strong enough bond whereby the veterinarian's assessment carries significant decision-making influence. Many veterinarians struggle with such responsibility and try not to

advocate in any potential benchmark in the animal's care. However, this subjective assessment of the veterinarian may be required by the owner and unfortunately quality of life assessments specifically targeting mobility have not yet been validated in dogs or in cats. There are however other scoring systems which may be adapted for this purpose.

Patient Assessment/Scoring Systems

The following scoring systems are applicable to mobility impairment when pain is present.

For osteoarthritis, Table 3.12 is an example of a subjective scoring system which is

Table 3.12 Clinical scoring system for assessing dogs with osteoarthritis.

Criterion	Clinical evaluation
Lameness	1) Walks normally 2) Slightly lame when walking 3) Moderately lame when walking 4) Severely lame when walking 5) Reluctant to rise and will not walk more than five paces
Joint mobility	1) Full range of motion 2) Mild limitation (10–20%) in range of motion; no crepitus 3) Mild limitation (10–20%) in range of motion; with crepitus 4) Moderate limitation (20–50%) in range of motion; ±crepitus 5) Severe limitation (>50%) in range of motion; ±crepitus
Pain on palpation	1) None 2) Mild signs; dog turns head in recognition 3) Moderate signs; dog pulls limb away 4) Severe signs; dog vocalises or becomes aggressive 5) Dog will not allow palpation
Weight-bearing	1) Equal on all limbs standing and walking 2) Normal standing; favours affected limb when walking 3) Partial weight-bearing standing and walking 4) Partial weight-bearing standing; non-weight-bearing walking 5) Non-weight-bearing standing and walking
Overall score of clinical condition	1) Not affected 2) Mildly affected 3) Moderately affected 4) Severely affected 5) Very severely affected

Source: McCarthy (2007). Reproduced with permission of Elsevier.

1. Fill in the oval next to the one number that best describes the pain at its worst in the last 7 days.

○ 0 ○ 1 ○ 2 ○ 3 ○ 4 ○ 5 ○ 6 ○ 7 ○ 8 ○ 9 ○ 10

No pain   Extreme pain

2. Fill in the oval next to the one number that best describes the pain at its least in the last 7 days.

○ 0 ○ 1 ○ 2 ○ 3 ○ 4 ○ 5 ○ 6 ○ 7 ○ 8 ○ 9 ○ 10

No pain   Extreme pain

3. Fill in the oval next to the one number that best describes the pain at its average in the last 7 days.

○ 0 ○ 1 ○ 2 ○ 3 ○ 4 ○ 5 ○ 6 ○ 7 ○ 8 ○ 9 ○ 10

No pain   Extreme pain

4. Fill in the oval next to the one number that best describes the pain at it is right now.

○ 0 ○ 1 ○ 2 ○ 3 ○ 4 ○ 5 ○ 6 ○ 7 ○ 8 ○ 9 ○ 10

No pain   Extreme pain

Description of function:

Fill in the oval next to the one number that best describes how during the last 7 days pain has interfered with your dog's.

5. General Activity:

○ 0 ○ 1 ○ 2 ○ 3 ○ 4 ○ 5 ○ 6 ○ 7 ○ 8 ○ 9 ○ 10

Does not interfere   Completely interferes

6. Enjoyment of life

○ 0 ○ 1 ○ 2 ○ 3 ○ 4 ○ 5 ○ 6 ○ 7 ○ 8 ○ 9 ○ 10

Does not interfere   Completely interferes

7. Ability to Rise to Standing From Lying Down

○ 0 ○ 1 ○ 2 ○ 3 ○ 4 ○ 5 ○ 6 ○ 7 ○ 8 ○ 9 ○ 10

Does not interfere   Completely interferes

8. Ability to Walk

○ 0 ○ 1 ○ 2 ○ 3 ○ 4 ○ 5 ○ 6 ○ 7 ○ 8 ○ 9 ○ 10

Does not interfere   Completely interferes

9. Ability to Run

○ 0 ○ 1 ○ 2 ○ 3 ○ 4 ○ 5 ○ 6 ○ 7 ○ 8 ○ 9 ○ 10

Does not interfere   Completely interferes

10. Ability to Climb Stairs, Curbs, Doorsteps, etc.

○ 0 ○ 1 ○ 2 ○ 3 ○ 4 ○ 5 ○ 6 ○ 7 ○ 8 ○ 9 ○ 10

Does not interfere   Completely interferes

Overall impression:

11. Fill in the oval next to the one number that best describes your dog's overall quality of life over the last 7 days.

○ Poor   ○ Fair   ○ Good   ○ Very Good   ○ Excellent

Figure 3.1 Canine brief pain inventory. *Source:* Courtesy of Dr. Dorothy Cimino Brown.

consistent with those often published in studies examining an intervention (McCarthy et al., 2007).

A more general canine brief pain inventory may be more applicable to other conditions (Figure 13.1, PennVet, 2013):

Feline pain inventories are unfortunately not yet validated, so clinicians are left with subjective assessments of activity and comfort, recognizing that feline pain manifests quite differently than canine pain.

When mobility impairment is not associated with pain, currently validated tools do not appear adequate to objectively assess an animal's progress. Consequently, a hybrid system may be necessary.

Figure 13.2 is an example of a questionnaire which could be used for patients with altered mobility but without significant pain. The survey has not, however, been subjected

to validation and as such should be used with caution and in combination with other assessment findings and tools.

End-of-Life Decisions

Owners who care for dogs with mobility impairments may develop caretaker fatigue but simultaneously be so dedicated to their pet that they are reluctant to consider euthanasia when an animal's condition deteriorates. Owners need specific guidance as to the pain status of their animal and the secondary complications and management that come with a further decline in mobility. Contextual information is also critical for most owners. For example, a 15-year-old greyhound with progressive paresis and fecal incontinence will encounter significantly

1. How would you rate your pet's current mobility?
   a. 1 = no mobility without complete assistance, 10 = normal mobility
2. How often does your pet need your assistance in any capacity due to his or her mobility?
   a. 1 = more than 10 times daily, 5 = five times daily, 10 = never
3. Describe the three activities during which you feel your animal derives the greatest enjoyment, and how your pet's mobility interferes with that activity
   a. Activity 1: 1 = unable to perform 10 = does not interfere at all
   b. Activity 2
   c. Activity 3
4. Please rate how your pet's mobility influences eating and drinking:
   a. 1 = completely interferes, 10 = causes no issues
5. Please rate how your pet's mobility affects control of urination?
   a. 1 = unable to urinate without assistance 5 = needs a moderate amount of assistance or has infrequent urinary accidents 10 = does not affect
6. Please rate how your pet's mobility affects control of defecation?
   a. 1 = unable to defecate without assistance 5 = needs a moderate amount of assistance or has infrequent defecation accidents 10 = does not affect
7. Describe the percentage of time you spend caring for your animal as opposed to interacting in a way which does not involve being a caretaker, providing food, assisting with mobility, etc.
   a. 1 = 100 % of time spent caring for my pet when we interact, 10 = only care necessary is providing water and food; all other time is normal activity
8. Please describe your outlook on your pet's condition
   a. 1 = extremely pessimistic 10 = extremely optimistic
9. Please rate your pet's quality of life given his or her current mobility
   a. Extremely poor b. poor c. acceptable d. good e. extremely good

Figure 3.2 Questionnaire for patients with altered mobility but without significant pain.

more challenges than a 3-year-old dachshund with grade 5 spinal dysfunction after intervertebral disc protrusion. The greyhound in this example likely has lesser functional capacity to accommodate for other comorbidities should they occur, and with their occurrence being far more likely as a function of aging. Owners may voluntarily raise the issue of euthanasia at the time of a deterioration but then indicate they are not ready for such a decision. In these cases, owners likely have reached a point whereby they subconsciously understand that their animal's quality of life may justify humane euthanasia. It is important for veterinarians to establish open communication with these clients during regular treatment assessments and to provide scoring systems if necessary for objective evaluation. Owners otherwise may delay the decision while their pet continues to worsen. Veterinarians with a long relationship with patients may also need to solicit outside opinions from colleagues to maintain objectivity. When the decision is reached that a patient is to be euthanized, the location, timing, and conditions of the euthanasia will all be important and care should be taken to accommodate owner's concerns and to create a supportive and comfortable environment in which the euthanasia occurs. Chapter 36 covers this issue in more detail.

References

McCarthy G, O'Donovan J, Jones B, McAllister H, Seed M, Mooney C. Randomised double-blind, positive-controlled trial to assess the efficacy of glucosamine/chondroitin sulfate for the treatment of dogs with osteoarthritis. The Veterinary Journal. 2007; 174: 54–61.

PennVet Canine Brief Pain Inventory (Canine BPI). 2013. Online at: http://www.vet.upenn.edu/research/clinical-trials/vcic/pennchart/cbpi-tool accessed 25 May 2017.

4

Chronic Diseases of the Eye and Adnexa

Caryn E. Plummer

Introduction

There are various ophthalmic conditions that can become chronic and require diligent therapy and monitoring. This chapter will discuss the most common chronic, incurable but manageable ophthalmic diseases such as dry eye and glaucoma, as well as some of the less commonly encountered "chronicopathies" of the eyes.

Chronic ocular and adnexal disease in the companion animal requires a uniquely dedicated owner if optimal outcomes are to be achieved. It is the responsibility of the veterinarian to educate clients in the need for diligent care and monitoring. Ocular pain is a profound impediment to life quality and this fact is consistently under-recognized by both the pet-owning public and the veterinary community.

Adnexa

Chronic Blepharitis

Blepharitis, or inflammation of the eyelids, typically presents with clinical signs that vary based on etiology, chronicity, and degree of self-trauma but generally exhibits some degree of eyelid swelling, hyperemia, alopecia, crusting, and secondary keratitis and conjunctivitis (Peña and Leiva 2008)

(Figure 4.1). Some cases will present with ulcerated lesions either instead of or in addition to the classic swelling (Figure 4.2). Self-trauma from pruritis is often significant and may result in further damage to the skin, conjunctiva, and corneas that may confound both diagnosis and therapy. Chronic inflammation of the lids can result in eyelid distortion with cicatrix formation leading to either entropion or ectropion and secondary corneal and conjunctival irritations (Peña and Leiva 2008; Bistner 1994). Damage to the meibomian glands or their ducts can impair the production and secretion of lipids from the eyelid glands resulting in a tear quality deficiency, rapid tear fluid evaporation, and clinical signs of exposure keratitis and dry eye (Samuleson 2013).

There are innumerable causes of blepharitis, from infectious etiologies (parasites, bacteria, fungi, Leishmania) to allergies to immune-mediated disease, trauma, and neoplasia (Peña and Leiva 2008, Bistner 1994; Peiffer 1980; Lindley, Boosinger, and Cox 1990; Yamaki and Ohono 2008). Diagnostics to rule out the more easily treated conditions would include skin scrapings and cytology to look for infectious agents and biopsy for histopathology and microbiologic culture and susceptibility. The cases that most commonly take on a protracted or chronic course are usually allergic or immune-mediated in nature. Animals with allergic blepharitis are

Chronic Disease Management for Small Animals, First Edition. Edited by W. Dunbar Gram, Rowan J. Milner and Remo Lobetti.
© 2018 John Wiley & Sons, Inc. Published 2018 by John Wiley & Sons, Inc.

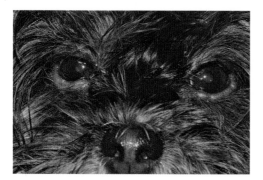

Figure 4.1 Chronic immune-mediated blepharitis in a mixed-breed dog. This case was steroid responsive.

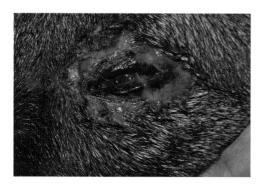

Figure 4.2 Immune-mediated blepharitis in a German Shepherd Dog. This case presented with ulcerated lesions rather than the nodular swellings seen in Figure 4.1 and had lesions at sites distant to the eyes.

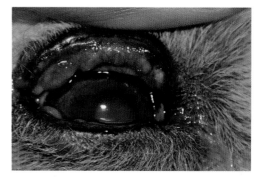

Figure 4.3 Meibomianitis in a Shih Tzu. Note the accumulations of glandular secretions in the subconjunctival space.

usually pruritic and also exhibit signs distant to the eyes, especially the ears and feet (Peña and Leiva 2008). Treatment of any secondary infections should be initiated along with allergy testing and elimination therapy or desensitization therapy to address the underlying cause. Supportive care with topical anti-inflammatories for the eyelids and the associated conjunctivitis is usually helpful and may be required intermittently for flare-ups. Immune-mediated blepharitis can take several forms and may be accompanied by ocular or multi-organ disease (Peña and Leiva 2008; Bistner 1994; Peiffer 1980; Lindley, Boosinger, and Cox 1990; Yamaki and Ohono 2008). The pemphigus complex diseases, discoid and systemic lupus erythematosus, and uveodermatologic syndrome

are examples of autoimmune conditions that often affect the eyelids as well as distant sites, often with depigmentation, ulceration, and crusting (Peña and Leiva 2008; Lindley, Boosinger, and Cox 1990; Yamaki and Ohono 2008). Biopsy is required to confirm diagnosis of these conditions and chronic (often life-long) systemic therapy is necessary. Uveodermatologic syndrome, sometimes referred to as Vogt-Koyanagi-Harada syndrome, is a condition in which tissues heavily-laden with pigment (melanin) are the target of disease and the uveitis that develops is usually severe and can lead to secondary glaucoma and vision loss (Lindley, Boosinger, and Cox 1990; Yamaki and Ohono 2008). These immune-mediated diseases require systemic therapy with immunosuppressive or immune-modulating therapy.

Meibomianitis is an inflammation of the meibomian glands located within the eyelids at the margins (Samuleson 2013). Inflammation of these glands causes eyelid swelling and often an observable enlargement of the meibomian glands and chalazions seen when the eyelids are everted to reveal the palpebral conjunctiva (Figure 4.3). This condition is often secondary to a bacterial infection or hypersensitivity. However, it can become chronic and will lead to reduction of tear film lipid and ocular surface inflammation and damage. Topical and systemic antibiotics, selected based upon culture of the exudate from the glands, are indicated as well as systemic corticosteroids if an allergic or immune-mediated etiology is suspected. Warm compresses may provide some relief to the patient.

Eyelid Neoplasia

Neoplasia of the eyelids is very common in dogs, less so in cats. Dog eyelids exhibit a variety of neoplasms of the eyelids that are usually benign and typically responsive to conservative surgical procedures. Many small eyelid tumors are slow growing and do not initiate any clinical signs. Others, however, may cause a considerable amount of ocular surface irritation that will become chronic if not addressed. Meibomian adenomas, epitheliomas, and papillomas are the most common types of neoplasia, however, melanomas, mast cells tumors, basal cell tumors, and fibroma/fibrosarcomas are noted occasionally (Aquino 2007; Roberts, Severin, and Lavach 1986).

Eyelid neoplasia in cats, however, tends to be aggressive and often malignant, requiring intervention before a chronic condition can be established. Squamous cell carcinoma is by far the most common type of eyelid neoplasia in the cats, most often seen in older felines with light-colored hair coats and minimally pigmented skin (Aquino 2007; Roberts, Severin, and Lavach 1986). The lesions tend to be erosive or ulcerated wounds rather than proliferative masses. Early intervention is recommended to minimize local extension. Other tumors that have been reported in the eyelids of cats include mast cell tumors, papillomas, adenoma/adenocarcinomas, basal cell tumors, fibrosarcomas, and peripheral nerve sheath tumors (Aquino 2007; Roberts, Severin, and Lavach 1986).

Ocular Surface Disorders

The Preocular Tear Film

The preocular tear film consists of lipid, aqueous, and mucin components (Samuleson 2013). The most superficial layer is a lipid secreted by the meibomian glands that acts to slow or prevent evaporation of the aqueous portion of the tear film. The lipid portion promotes a stable, optical smooth layer of tears over the cornea. The aqueous component of tears is secreted by lacrimal glands of the orbit and nictitating membrane and accounts for most of the total tear volume. It consists of water, electrolytes, glucose, urea, surface-active polymers, glycoproteins, and tear proteins, including immunoglobulins and other factors involved in immune surveillance and antimicrobial efforts. The final layer of tears is mucin, which is produced by the goblet cells of the conjunctiva. This mucin keep the aqueous tear fluid attached to the corneal epithelium and fills in any irregularities of the corneal surface. A deficiency of any of these three components will result in clinical signs of dry eye.

Keratoconjunctivitis sicca

Keratoconjunctivitis sicca (KCS) is unfortunately an all too common ocular disease in the dog and it is generally a lifelong condition requiring chronic and diligent therapy and monitoring (Figure 4.4). The incidence of KCS in dogs is great with roughly 1% of the general population affected (Giuliano 2013). Quantitative or "classic" KCS is characterized by a deficiency of the aqueous tear fluid which results in desiccation and inflammation of the conjunctiva and cornea. Ocular pain and progressive corneal disease, with subsequent reduction in vision, occur.

The reduction or absence of lacrimal secretions may result from a single disease process or a combination of conditions affecting the lacrimal glands. The most common etiology is an immune-mediated inflammation of the lacrimal glands which results in dysfunction and impaired production of the aqueous fraction of tears (Giuliano 2013; Kaswan, Martin, and Dawe 1985; Hendrix *et al.* 2011; Barachetti *et al.* 2015). A variety of other etiologies have been identified, however, including neurogenic causes, toxic changes within the glands due to drug or chemical exposure, and metabolic

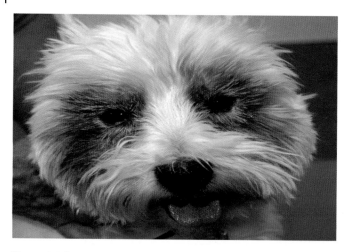

Figure 4.4 Keratoconjunctivitis sicca in a West Highland White Terrier. Note the discoloration of the facial fur. This is common in many types of tear and ocular surface disorders. Also note the mucoid discharge present.

alterations (Giuliano 2013). Several breeds are disproportionately affected by acquired KCS, thus suggesting a genetic predisposition (Table 4.1). The diagnosis of KCS is made on the basis of typical clinical signs and decreased Schirmer tear test (STT) results. In the clinical setting, STT I readings in dogs are generally interpreted as follows: ≥ 15 mm/min = normal production; 11–14 mm/min = early or subclinical KCS; 6–10 mm/min = moderate or mild KCS; and ≤ 5 mm/min = severe KCS (Table 4.2). Acute onset KCS is occasionally seen, wherein an eye becomes acutely and severely painful and usually exhibits axial corneal ulceration (Figure 4.5). If not addressed promptly, these cases may develop suppurative inflammation which exacerbates the progressive nature of the corneal disease with stromal malacia, descemetocele formation, and iris prolapse. Fortunately, in most cases, the onset of KCS is more gradual, with increasing severity over a period of several weeks (Giuliano 2013). These eyes initially present for redness and appear inflamed, with intermittent mucoid or mucopurulent discharge (Figure 4.6). As the severity and chronicity of the KCS increases, the ocular surface becomes lackluster, the conjunctiva becomes progressively more hyperemic, and persistent

tenacious mucopurulent ocular discharge develops. The keratitis, which progresses if left untreated, is usually characterized by extensive corneal vascularization and pigmentation (Figure 4.7 and Figure 4.8). This corneal opacification can lead to vision deficits or loss.

Treatment of quantitative dry eye has two primary goals: 1) stimulate the patient to produce organic tears and 2) supplement the patient with topical lubricants (artificial tear preparations). Additionally, depending upon the presence and severity of other clinical signs, topical anti-inflammatory medications, usually corticosteroids, may be necessary to control initial or intermittent surface inflammation. Topical antibiotics maybe necessary to control secondary bacterial conjunctivitis. Dry eye is the foremost reason for bacterial conjunctivitis to develop. It is rare for primary bacterial conjunctivitis to occur in small animals without an antecedent condition. The use of a mucolytic agent may facilitate administration of other topical medications and may make cleaning and removal of the mucoid discharge easier.

Since most cases of KCS are immune-mediated in origin, the most commonly employed tear stimulating drugs are the immunomodulating agents, cyclosporine (0.2–2.0%) and tacrolimus (0.02–1.0%), both of which work by targeting T-helper cells and decreasing the inflammatory response

Table 4.1 Breed predisposition to chronic ocular disease.

KCS	Zonular Instability	Primary Glaucoma
Cavalier King Charles Spaniel	Jack/Parsons Russell Terrier	American and English Cocker Spaniels
English Bulldog	Fox Terriers	Bassett Hound
Lhasa Apso	Sealyham Terrier	Chow Chow
Shih Tzu	Miniature Bull Terrier	Shar-Pei
Pug	Tibetan Terrier	Boston Terrier
West Highland White Terrier	Shar-Pei	Norwegian Elkhound
Bloodhound	Border Collie	Siberian Husky
American Cocker Spaniel	German Shepherd	Beagle
Pekingese	Lancashire Heelers	Miniature and Toy Poodles
Boston Terrier	Italian Greyhound	Samoyed
Miniature Schnauzer	Chinese Crested Dog	Cairn Terrier
Samoyed		Shih Tzu
		Australian Cattle Dog
		Akita
		Jack Russell Terrier
		Bichon Frise
		Fox Terriers
		Border Collie
		Lhasa Apso
		Pekingese
		Bouvier des Flandres
		Brittany Spaniel
		Dalmatian
		English and Welsh Springer Spaniels
		Italian Greyhound
		Dachshund
		Chihuahua

within the lacrimal glands (Giuliano 2013; Kaswan, Martin, and Dawe 1985; Hendrix *et al.* 2011; Barachetti *et al.* 2015). They also have a separate lacrimogenic effect separate from their anti-inflammatory effects that is not as yet well understood. The choice of drug to initiate therapy with is generally a matter of clinician preference. If, however, therapy with cyclosporine fails to resolve clinical signs and return STT values to the normal range, it is worth trying tacrolimus, as there is a subset of animals that does not respond to cyclosporine but will respond to this alternative. With the exception of the 0.2% commercially available ointment preparation of cyclosporine, both drugs must be compounded for topical use. Recently, biodegradable slow release cyclosporine episcleral implants have become available (Barachetti *et al.* 2015). These are helpful both in refractory cases and those that have an underwhelming response to therapy due to poor compliance. A small percentage of patients develop neurogenic

Table 4.2 Interpretation of STT I values and treatment recommendations.

STT I value	Diagnosis	Treatment options
≥15 mm/minute	Normal	
11–14 mm/minute	Early or subclinical KCS	Cyclosporine 0.2–1.0% q12–24 h or Tacrolimus 0.02% q12–24 h and Artificial Tears q8–12 h
6–10 mm/minute	Mild to moderate KCS	Cyclosporine 1.0–2.0% q12h or Tacrolimus 0.02–.03% q12h and Artificial Tears q4–6 h +/– Dexamethasone 0.01% q8–24 h +/– Acetycysteine 5.0% q8–12 h
≤5 mm/minute	Severe KCS	Cyclosporine 1.0–2.0% q8–12 h and/or Tacrolimus 0.03%–1.0% q8–12 h and Artificial Tears q2–6 h +/– Dexamethasone 0.01% q8–24 h +/– Acetycysteine 5.0% q6–12 h +/– Pilocarpine (if neurologic origin is suspected) +/– Episcleral CsA implants +/– Parotid duct transposition +/– Buccal mucosal graft

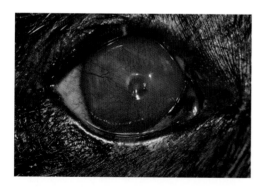

Figure 4.5 A deep stromal corneal ulcer that has resulted from dry eye. The axial location is typical for ulcers that develop from exposure and KCS.

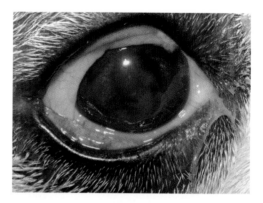

Figure 4.6 Mild to moderate KCS with early corneal changes and mucoid discharge.

KCS, wherein the innervation to the lacrimal glands is disrupted (Giuliano 2013). If the KCS has developed due to a neurogenic insult, the addition of pilocarpine may be helpful to supplement the absent neurotransmitter and stimulate aqueous tear production from the glands. It may be given orally (1–2 drops of the 2% topical preparation per 10 kg body weight PO in the food q12h, increasing in one drop intervals if no improvement is noted until clinical signs of hypersalivation, vomiting, or diarrhea occur; or a dilute preparation (0.1%) given topically q12h).

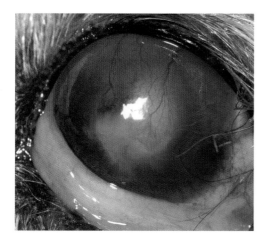

Figure 4.7 Keratitis in a Shih Tzu secondary to moderate dry eye. Note the corneal vascularization and superficial pigmentation.

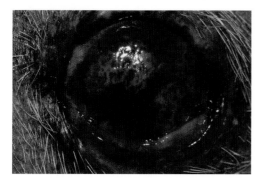

Figure 4.8 Severe KCS with extensive corneal pigmentation and fibrosis in a Chinese Crested Dog.

If the KCS fails to respond to medical therapy, surgical options exist. Parotid duct transposition wherein the salivary duct is repositioned into the ventral conjunctival fornix will supply the ocular surface with lubrication, however, it may be associated with undesirable consequences such as excessive "epiphora," facial dermatitis and mineral accumulation on the cornea or eyelids (Giuliano 2013). It can dramatically improve patient comfort, however. Recently, the use of buccal mucosal grafts has been advocated to improve patient comfort. In this procedure, a free graft of mucosa from the oral cavity is sutured into the conjunctival fornix. It is believed that the transplantation of glandular tissue from the mouth to the eye provides something in the way of additional lubrication, although the STT values remain unchanged. Some report a dramatic improvement in patient comfort.

Qualitative Tear Deficiencies (Qualitative Dry Eye)

If either the lipid produced by eyelid meibomian glands or the mucin produced by conjunctival goblet cells components of the tear film are absent or decreased in quantity, clinical signs of KCS will develop even if STT measurements are within the normal range (Giuliano 2013). This is known as qualitative dry eye. This condition most often occurs secondary to disruption or inflammation of the target tissues that produce either the mucin or lipid fractions of the tears. Chronic conjunctivitis or chronic blepharitis or meibomianitis will result in a reduction of mucin and lipid, respectively. When the tear quality is impaired, aqueous tears will evaporate too quickly and will not be able to stay distributed evenly and adequately across the ocular surface, essentially creating a functional dry eye. The diagnosis is confirmed with either of the vital dyes, rose Bengal or Lissamine green, which localize to areas of the cornea where the mucin fraction is insufficient. Additionally, the tear film break-up time will help determine if the tear film is unstable and evaporating too quickly (Giuliano 2013). When fluorescein stain is applied to the ocular surface in high concentrations, it will saturate the tear film. After blinking to evenly distribute the dye, the patient's eyelids are held open manually (to prevent blinking) and the time is counted in seconds until the homogenous green color on the ocular surface begins to develop dark splotches, indicating areas where the tear film has "broken up," or become unstable and started to evaporate or dissipate. If this break up occurs before 10 seconds of elapsed time, the tear film is described as unstable and of poor quality.

Treatment is aimed at improving the quality and amount of mucin and/or lipid and supplementing with artificial tears, essentially the same approach used in quantitative dry eye. Medical treatment with cyclosporine or tacrolimus will in most cases normalize or improve tear lipids and mucin and result in an improvement of clinical signs. Artificial tears will bridge the gap while tear quality is on the mend. Compounding the immunomodulators in an oily base will help with clinical signs. The addition of essential fatty acids to the diet is thought by some to be helpful in improving tear quality.

Conjunctivitis

Conjunctivitis can be a particularly frustrating condition when it becomes chronic. Conjunctival hyperemia, chemosis and discharge ranging in character from clear and serous to mucoid or mucopurulent are the most common clinical signs seen (Figures 4.9 and 4.10). With chronicity, the patient may develop conjunctival follicles which are semi-transparent, bubble-like aggregates of lymphoid tissue, the result of chronic antigenic stimulation (Figure 4.11). The most common etiologies for chronic conjunctivitis in dogs are tear film abnormalities (see earlier discussion) and allergies. A thorough ocular examination with evaluation of the quantity and quality of the tear film is necessary to determine the etiology. Allergic conjunctivitis is a rule-out diagnosis that is made if the tear film is sufficient and there are no other signs or indications of ocular or systemic disease (Peña and Leiva 2008; Bistner 1994; Peiffer 1980; Lourenço-Martins *et al.* 2011). Treatment of allergic conjunctivitis is best achieved with identification and removal of the offending antigen. If this is not possible, symptomatic treatment with the least amount of drug necessary to control clinical signs will be necessary. Topical corticosteroids, cyclosporine, or antihistamines may be considered (Lourenço-Martins *et al.* 2011). It may be challenging to find the right "cocktail" of empiric medications for some individual patients. Topical lubricants (artificial tears) may be helpful for short-term comfort.

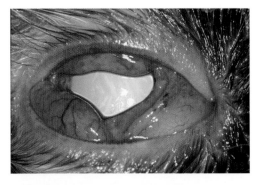

Figure 4.10 Herpetic keratitis is a cat with profound conjunctival chemosis and hyperemia.

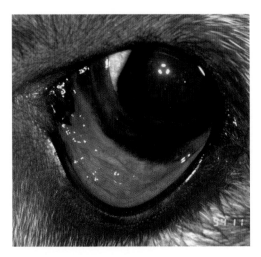

Figure 4.11 Chronic conjunctivitis in this Labrador Retriever has resulted in follicle formation.

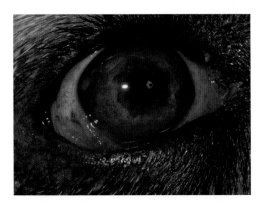

Figure 4.9 Allergic conjunctivitis in a mixed breed dog. Note the conjunctival hyperemia and chemosis.

Conjunctivitis in cats is most often initiated by an infectious agent. Feline herpesvirus-1 (FHV-1) is the most common infectious agent responsible for conjunctivitis in cats (Peiffer 1980; Malik *et al.* 2009). *Chlamydophila felis* and mycoplasmal organisms are also implicated, but less often. When cats develop chronic conjunctivitis, it may be difficult to implicate FHV-1 because the classic respiratory signs associated with primary infections are usually absent. However, since the virus establishes itself and develops latency, it may contribute to active conjunctivitis and keratitis at any time, particularly during periods of stress. In some cats, the immune system will mount a response to the presence of viral antigen and cause ocular surface inflammation without the cytolytic contributions of viral replication. Additionally, FHV-1 may initiate the development of KCS in cats, so clinical chronic conjunctivitis in cats may be due to a multitude of related problems (Giuliano 2013). The establishment of causation is difficult to prove considering most cats have been exposed to FHV-1 and many become carriers and can shed virus without clinical signs. The presence of the virus detected via indirect fluorescent antibody staining or PCR will not necessarily be diagnostic (Sjödahl-Essén *et al.* 2008). Neither will conjunctival cytology be helpful in diagnosing FHV-1, however, it may be helpful for diagnosing chlamydophilal (cytoplasmic inclusions), mycoplasmal (organisms seen), or eosinophilic conjunctivitis (eosinophils, mast cells), all of which may occur as concurrent conditions or co-infections with FHV-1. Treatment can be very frustrating to both cats and their owners. Generally, if an infectious agent is suspected, a course of antimicrobial agents is recommended. If chlamydophilal or mycoplasmal organisms are present or suspected, a course of topical (oxytetracycline, chloramphenicol or erythromycin q6h for 2–3 weeks) and/or systemic tetracyclines or macrolides (doxycycline 5 mg/kg PO q12h or azithromycin 5 mg/kg PO q24h) may be helpful, but may not be effective at eliminating a carrier state. Herpetic keratoconjunctivitis is somewhat more difficult to control. The minimal amount of medical intervention should be employed. Often, particularly in mild cases, topical lubricants may be sufficient to help minimize discomfort until the flare-up subsides on its own. A short course of systemic non-steroidal therapy (meloxicam 0.1 mg/kg PO q24h or robenacoxib 1 mg/kg PO for 3 days) may be helpful initially as well. In severe or refractory cases, or those in which there is also corneal involvement, anti-viral therapy may be indicated. Antiviral therapy with topical agents will limit the extent of systemic side effects, but may be challenging due to the fact that effective drugs are not commercially available and must be produced by a compounding pharmacy (cidofovir 0.5% q12h or idoxuridine 0.1% q4h) (Figure 4.12). If topical agents aren't successful in decreasing the severity of clinical signs or if there are systemic signs or dermatologic involvement, systemic antiviral may be used (famciclovir 10–90 mg/kg q24h) (Sjödahl-Essén *et al.* 2008). Antivirals are usually given until clinical signs resolve and then are discontinued, rather than tapered in frequency. A few cats require chronic administration, rather than interval therapy during an active bout, and these cats should be monitored regularly with complete blood counts and serum chemistries to determine if any bone marrow or renal toxicity is developing.

Cats will also develop non-infectious conjunctivitis. Eosinophilic conjunctivitis, with or without keratitis, typically presents with the classic signs of conjunctivitis (hyperemia, chemoisis, and discharge) but may also exhibit raised, irregular, or roughened lesions resembling granulation tissue in the bulbar, palpebral or nictitans conjunctiva or on the cornea (Allgower, Schaffer, and Stockhaus 2001) (Figure 4.13). Cytology of these lesions reveals the presence of eosinophils and mast cells. Tear production may be decreased in these cats secondary to obstruction of lacrimal ductules by the

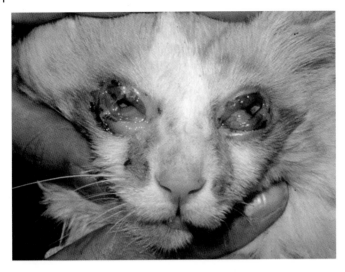

Figure 4.12 Severe herpetic blepharokeratoconjunctivitis in an eldery feline.

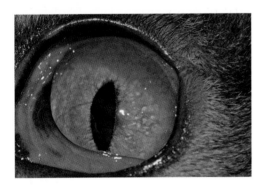

Figure 4.13 Eosinophilic keratoconjunctivitis conjunctivitis in a cat.

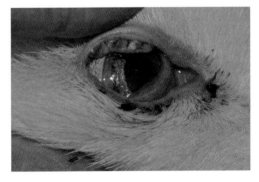

Figure 4.14 Lipogranulomatous conjunctivitis in a cat.

conjunctival swelling. Treatment is aimed at decreasing the inflammatory response and usually requires an extended course of treatment with a very slow taper of frequency. Lipogranulomatous conjunctivitis is an unusual form of conjunctivitis occurring in older cats as non-ulcerated white nodules in the palpebral conjunctiva (Kerlin and Dubielzig 1997) (Figure 4.14). Histopathology of the lesions describes macrophages and multinucleated giant cells filled with lipid. Surgical excision of the nodules may be curative, otherwise chronic therapy with corticosteroids is necessary to minimize the inflammation and improve patient comfort.

Corneal Disease

Corneal Ulcers

Most chronic cases of corneal ulceration are in actuality cases of refractory or recurrent ulceration due to some other form of chronic ophthalmic disease, such as KCS, corneal degeneration, or chronic intraocular disease that disrupts the integrity of the cornea. Please see other sections of this chapter for a discussion of the diagnosis and treatment of these other conditions. Treatment for these secondary corneal ulcers should always occur concurrently to treatment for the underlying condition, if possible, or at least in recognition of the impact the underlying etiology has on

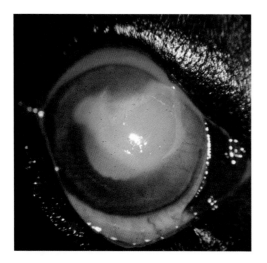

Figure 4.15 Refractory, or indolent ulcer, in a dog. Not the loose lip of epithelium and the fluorescein that has seeped underneath this non-adherent tissue.

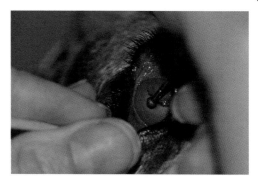

Figure 4.16 Diamond burr debridement of a refractory superficial corneal ulcer in a dog.

the wound healing potential of the cornea. Therapy for a corneal ulcer should aim to 1) sterilize the wound bed (i.e., treat an infection if present, prevent an infection if not), 2) address the concurrent anterior uveitis present, 3) stop or prevent further breakdown of corneal collagen, 4) provide analgesia, and 5) provide structural stabilization if the ulcer is deep or perforating.

Many cases of refractory or indolent ulcers develop due to a defect or degeneration in corneal epithelial cell adhesion and/or the anterior stroma and are quite common in older dogs (Bentley and Murphy 2004; Gosling, Labelle, and Breaux 2013; Nevile *et al.* 2015; Sansom and Blunden 2010; da Silva *et al.* 2011; Michau *et al.* 2003) (Figure 4.15). In addition to the goals of therapy outlined above, these cases require mechanical debridement to remove any abnormal tissue from the ocular surface and to encourage reattachment of the overlying epithelium. Several forms of debridement are possible. Simple debridement of any non-adherent or "lipped" epithelial tissue can and should be performed with a dry, sterile, cotton-tipped applicator. After application of a topical anesthetic agent, such as proparacaine or tetracaine, the cotton-tipped

applicator should be used in a circular motion to peel away the loose epithelium from the margins of the wound. If this is insufficient to encourage re-epithelialization, more aggressive debridement with either a diamond burr or a small gauge needle (grid keratotomy or multiple punctate keratotomy) may be necessary. A diamond burr will polish the exposed stroma and create an improved area for epithelial attachment (da Silva *et al.* 2011) (Figure 4.16). Keratotomies disrupt the exposed stroma or any membranes that have formed atop it to allow epithelial adhesion. None of these procedures should be performed on corneal ulcers that are not superficial due the risk of progression of the wound and perforation. Diamond burr debridement is also useful to remove superficial mineral deposits from the exposed stroma in cases of corneal degeneration or band keratopathy (Nevile *et al.* 2015; Sansom and Blunden 2010).

The addition of a bandage contact lens may improve the comfort of a patient with a superficial ulcer, especially if some adnexal irritation, such as trichiasis, entropion, or an adjacent eyelid mass, is exacerbating the problem, and facilitate reepithelialization (Gosling, Labelle, and Breaux 2013).

Keratitis

Corneal inflammation regardless of etiology has a very similar set of clinical signs, typically corneal vascularization, pigmentation, and occasional cellular infiltrate. Most of the immune-mediated forms of keratitis, including chronic superficial keratitis, also known as pannus, eosinophilic keratitis, pigmentary keratitis, and KCS are chronic conditions that require longstanding therapy to slow or prevent progression of the corneal lesions and maintenance of corneal clarity (Andrew 2008) (Figure 4.17). The mainstay therapy for immune-mediated keratitis is topical anti-inflammatory medication, either an immunomodulator such as cyclosporine or tacrolimus, or a steroidal or non-steroidal anti-inflammatory. Often steroids and either

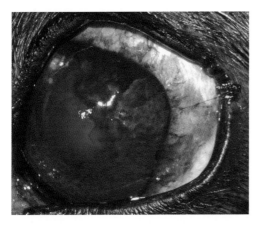

Figure 4.17 Chronic superficial keratitis, or pannus, in a Greyhound.

cyclosporine or tacrolimus are used in concert to control the inflammation through different mechanisms. This often achieves better control than sequential therapy. Steroids are generally more potent and will work faster to control clinical signs, while the immunomodulators have a slower onset of action but are safer for long-term control and generally have fewer untoward side effects. Limiting exposure to UV radiation may decrease the severity or slow the progression of some forms of keratitis, particularly chronic superficial keratitis in German Shepherd Dogs and Greyhounds (Figure 4.18).

A deeper form of keratitis affecting the corneal endothelium presents with corneal edema and sometimes keratitic precipitates on the endothelial surface (Andrew 2008). This condition often becomes chronic since damage to the corneal endothelium is usually irreversible due to the limited regenerative potential of the endothelium. Immunomodulators do not penetrate the cornea well, so topical steroids are generally the preferred treatment. Topical hyperosmotic agents, such as 5% sodium chloride solution or ointment, may facilitate removal of excess fluid in the corneal stroma and are particularly helpful if fluid has coalesced into

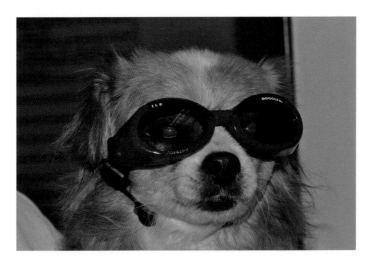

Figure 4.18 Goggles may limit exposure to UV radiation. They may also be helpful for protecting the eyes of visually impaired animals that may be injured or at risk.

bullae within the anterior stroma or the epithelium. Bullae rupture will result in corneal ulceration, which is painful and necessitates the discontinuation of topical steroid therapy. Corneal ulcers that accompany endotheliitis or endothelial degeneration are often refractory or slow to healing.

Corneal Degenerations

Corneal degenerations are secondary pathologic changes. They may occur in the epithelium and anterior stroma or in the endothelium. The specific cell type affected determines the form and clinical signs that develop (Samuleson 2013). Once the process of corneal degeneration begins, it is generally not curable, but may be manageable. Degenerations may be unilateral or bilateral, but are often asymmetric when bilateral. Epithelial disruption with subsequent ulceration and vascularization is common.

In the superficial form, lipids, cholesterol, calcium, or a combination thereof are deposited in the anterior stroma secondary to inflammation, vascularization, and tissue weakness. The age-related form of this condition is common in aged dogs and can lead to chronic pain and recurrent and refractory corneal ulcerations (Figure 4.19). The form that occurs secondary to chronic ocular inflammation resembles band keratopathy

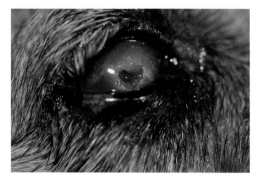

Figure 4.19 Corneal degeneration in an aged dog. Some of the corneal stroma and deposits have slough leaving a deep stromal corneal ulcer. Note the white, crystalline opacities surrounding the defect and the corneal vascularization.

wherein mineral deposits accumulate in the subepithelial space or in the anterior stroma and prevent proper adhesion of the corneal epithelium. The gritty and irregular deposits may cause the epithelium to erode. The rough feeling of the underlying deposits is terribly uncomfortable to the patient as the eyelids rub over the surface with every blink. Routine medical therapy for an ulcer should be begun along with the addition of a chelating agent, usually some form of EDTA, to try to remove some of the deposits or at least decrease their accumulation. The ulcers that develop are often refractory to healing and repeated manual debridement is often necessary to facilitate epithelial adhesion. Cotton tipped applicator debridement followed by diamond burr keratectomy can be most beneficial to the healing process (Gosling, Labelle, and Breaux 2013; Nevile *et al.* 2015; Sansom and Blunden 2010; da Silva *et al.* 2011). However, if epithelialization and adhesion is not achieved after several attempts, lamellar keratectomy may be necessary to facilitate healing and improve comfort. However, it should not be performed repeatedly because the stroma may not regenerate to full thickness in aged and diseased corneas.

The corneal degenerations secondary to endothelial disease present with corneal edema, usually starting from the temporal aspect of the cornea. They occur most frequently in the Boston Terrier, Dachshund, and Chihuahua breeds (Figure 4.20, Figure 4.21, and Figure 4.22). The disease progresses until complete edema, occasionally complicated with recurrent corneal bullae formation, and visual impairment to blindness occurs. Medical therapy with topical osmotic agents (5% NaCl) is helpful but does not clear the cornea completely and will become less effective at managing corneal bullae as the disease progresses. Surgical treatment is more definitive, but not curative. It may include thermokeratoplasty wherein the superficial corneal stroma is cauterized with thermal energy to coagulate the corneal collagen and decrease potential space between the lamellae for fluid accumulation,

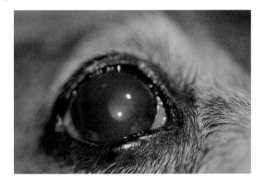

Figure 4.20 Corneal endothelial degeneration in a Chihuahua. In this breed, the condition is inherited. Note the mid-range pupil. Pupil size and responsiveness may help differentiate endothelial disease from glaucoma, which is one of the differentials for corneal edema.

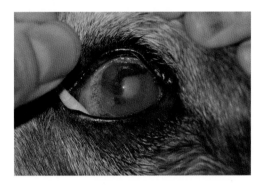

Figure 4.21 Corneal endothelial degeneration in a Bassett Hound. Note the corneal vascularization present that was the response to a long-standing superficial corneal ulcer. Microbullae form within the stroma and epithelium when significant corneal edema is present which may rupture resulting in ulceration that may be slow or refractory to healing.

superficial keratectomy with Gunderson conjunctival pedicle grafts or full-thickness keratoplasty (Michau *et al.* 2003) (Figure 4.23). Keratoplasties are essentially corneal transplants which replace the disease endothelium with viable endothelial cells from a healthy donor eye. Endothelial degeneration predisposes the patient to refractory and recurrent ulcerations as bullae form from the accumulation of edema fluid in the corneal stroma then rupture through the epithelium.

Intraocular Disease

Glaucoma

Glaucoma is perhaps the most frustrating ocular disease for the practicing small animal veterinarian, client, and patient. It is an insidious disease that occurs in many breeds of dog (including mixed-breeds) and is associated with an increase in intraocular pressure (IOP) that is incompatible with the health of the eye. Loss of vision results in time and the acute and sustained pressure spikes that occur are quite frequently very painful for the veterinary patient. Glaucoma is a leading cause of blindness in dogs, affecting approximately 2% of the canine population, and uncontrolled IOP can threaten life quality as a result of the discomfort that results (Gelatt and MacKay 2004a, 2004b).

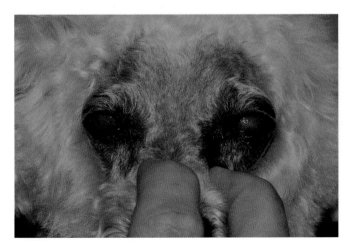

Figure 4.22 Bilateral corneal edema in a Bichon Frise from endothelial degeneration.

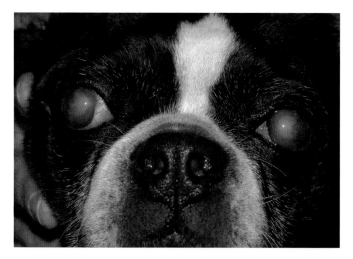

Figure 4.23 This Boston Terrier has had bilateral keratectomies and Gunderson conjunctival flaps placed laterally in an attempt to minimize the progression and complications from endothelial decompensation.

Aqueous humor is essential to the health of the eye in that it functions to provide oxygen and nutrition to the avascular structures of the eye and acts as a waste sink for the products of metabolic breakdown. Aqueous humor is produced in the ciliary body by active secretion and ultrafiltration of plasma (Samuleson 2013). The enzyme carbonic anhydrase participates in the energy-dependent secretory phase of aqueous production. Most of the aqueous humor flows from the posterior chamber, through the pupil, to the anterior chamber, and exits at the iridocorneal angle into the intrascleral venous plexus. A small percentage of the outflow in dogs and cats, known as the uveoscleral or nonconventional pathway, exits through the iris, ciliary body, choroid, and sclera. The balance between formation and drainage of aqueous humor maintains IOP within a normal range of approximately 15 to 25 mmHg. Due to conformational differences, brachycephalic animals tend to have slightly higher IOPs than mesocephalic and dolichocephalic individuals, hence the wide range. With most modern instruments for estimating IOP, the normal IOP is in the low to middle teems.

Glaucoma is a set of diseases that all have the common risk factor of IOP elevation. Essentially increased IOP with associated visual deficits due to damage to and death of the retinal ganglion cells and their axons are the hallmarks of the disease. IOP-independent alterations such as excitotoxic amino acids, defects in the optic nerve head microcirculation, and extracellular matrix abnormalities of the iridocorneal angle and optic nerve may also contribute to damage in glaucoma. In most cases in dogs and cats, glaucoma is caused by obstruction or stenosis of the aqueous humor outflow pathways. It remains a challenge to the veterinarian to detect the early subtle disturbances of glaucoma and to effectively treat this condition. Delayed or inadequate therapy can lead to irreversible blindness and a painful, cosmetically unacceptable eye.

When a patient presents with a painful, red eye, glaucoma should be ruled out among the possible diagnoses of conjunctivitis, uveitis, or keratitis. Pain may manifest as depression, anorexia, rubbing at the eye, or squinting. However, in chronic cases wherein the patient has had time to acclimatize to the IOP elevation, overt signs of pain or discomfort may be absent. All ocular tissues are affected by an elevated IOP. Clinical signs include a "red eye," the result of congestion of episcleral vessels, corneal edema, mydriasis, blepharospasm, blindness, and buphthalmos

(Figure 4.24). With the exception of buphthalmos, which is a finding in the chronic condition, the remainder of these clinical signs may occur at any stage of glaucoma (Figure 4.25). Pupillary light reflexes may be normal, slow, or absent in early glaucoma, depending on the functional status of the iris sphincter muscle, retina, and optic nerve and the IOP. Acute elevations of IOP above 45 mm Hg cause paralysis of the iris sphincter muscles and subsequent mydriasis. Buphthalmos, or enlargement of the globe, may occur more rapidly in young dogs and cats, due to the elastic nature of young globes. Rupture of the cornea's Descemet's membrane may accompany elevated corneal tension and buphthalmos to produce multiple, linear corneal striae. Persistent corneal

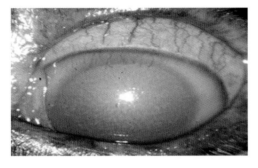

Figure 4.24 Acute glaucoma in a dog. Note the episcleral injection, corneal edema and mydriasis.

endothelial damage can result in permanent corneal edema. Buphthalmos causes increased tension on the lens zonules, which in turn can result in zonular disinsertion and lens subluxation or luxation. Prolonged or recurrent elevations of IOP lead to degeneration of the retina and optic nerve, with cupping or atrophy of the optic nerve head. The onset of clinical signs of glaucoma in cats is often insidious, as this species is less likely to demonstrate the acute intense corneal edema and episcleral congestion exhibited by dogs. Clinical signs of the glaucomas depend on the stage of disease and, to some extent, on the type of glaucoma. The signs of glaucoma may be asymmetric in the same patient, with different stages occurring in different eyes. The signs of the secondary glaucomas are like those of the primary glaucomas, but clinical signs of the antecedent etiology, such as an anterior uveitis, an intraocular mass, or a lens luxation, will be present as well. The congenital glaucomas affect young animals, usually within the first 3 to 6 months of life. Often, the first clinical sign in these animals is rapid onset of buphthalmia and lagophthalmos, or the inability to completely close the palpebral fissure.

A diagnosis of glaucoma is made based upon clinical signs and an index of suspicion for the disease. It can be confirmed or supported with

(a)   (b)

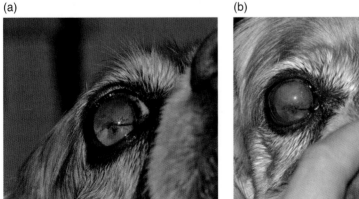

Figure 4.25 a and b Chronic glaucoma in a Cocker Spaniel. Note the buphthalmos, corneal edema, fibrosis and pigmentation. The tapetal reflection is bright, indicating likely retinal degeneration secondary to chronic elevations of IOP or segmental vascular infarcts.

tonometry, or an estimate of IOP that is above the reference range of normal. Tonometry in the outpatient clinic provides only a "snapshot," and diurnal variations in IOP occur, but it is the easiest way to monitor the progression and response of the disease. In the dog, the higher levels occur in the early morning and the lowest readings in the early evening. The most common tools for tonometry in the veterinary clinic are the TonoPen, an applanation tonometer that measures the amount of force necessary to indent a fixed surface area of the cornea, and the TonoVet, a rebound tonometer that measures the rebound force and velocity that a pin returning from contacting the cornea has (von Spiessen *et al.* 2015; Görig *et al.* 2006). Both instruments have similar accuracies and the choice of which to use is mostly based upon clinician preference. IOP must be accurately measured to diagnose and monitor glaucoma.

Types of Glaucoma

Glaucoma is classified on the basis of the probable cause, the appearance of the drainage angle and the stage or duration of the condition (Gelatt and MacKay 2004a, 2004b) (Table 4.3). In the primary glaucomas, there is an inherited anatomic or functional defect in drainage of the aqueous humor in the absence of concurrent ocular disease (Komáromy and Petersen-Jones 2015). It is common in some breeds of dog and is always bilateral, although development of clinical disease is usually asymmetric (Table 4.1). Siamese cats also have an inherited form of primary glaucoma (Dietrich 2005). In the secondary glaucomas, the increase in IOP is associated with some known antecedent or concurrent ocular disease that results in physical obstruction of an outflow pathway (Gelatt and MacKay 2004b; Johnsen, Maggs, and Kass 2006). These cases are not inherited and may be unilateral or bilateral, depending upon the presence of the underlying condition in each eye. Many of the conditions that initiate these forms of glaucoma may be genetically determined in certain breeds, such as cataract or zonular dysplasia (lens luxation). The secondary glaucomas are nearly as prominent in the canine population as are primary forms, so making the distinction between the two forms is critical. Clinical management of the secondary glaucomas, however, is often more clear-cut, because the cause of the increased IOP can usually be ascertained and the prognosis for development of glaucoma in the non-affected eye is clear. Secondary glaucoma may be initiated by uveitis, cataract development and its resultant uveitis, lens luxations, or intraocular neoplasia (Figure 4.26 and Figure 4.27). Medical or surgical treatment of the secondary glaucomas is directed toward removing, if possible, the cause of the elevated IOP. Secondary glaucoma is by far more common in cats than is primary glaucoma. Congenital glaucomas are rare in dogs and cats and usually occur due to

Table 4.3 Types of Glaucoma.

Primary	Secondary	Congenital
Open/normal angle	Uveitis	Anterior segment dysgenesis
Narrow/closed angle	Lens luxation	
	Lens-induced (chronic cataract, intumescent cataract, phacolytic uveitis, phacoclastic uveitis)	
	Hyphema	
	Intraocular neoplasia	
	Pigmentary/melanocytic proliferation	

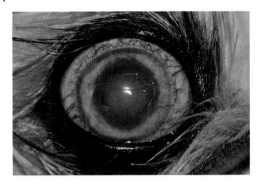

Figure 4.26 Secondary glaucoma in a dog. Note the episcleral injection, peripheral corneal vascularization, and edema. The pupil is mid-range, which is commonly noted when uveitis is present concurrently.

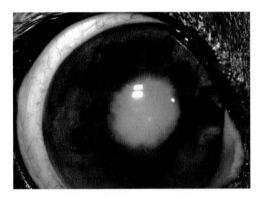

Figure 4.27 Chronic lens-induced uveitis has resulted in considerable intraocular damage, including 360 degree posterior synechia.

developmental abnormalities of the aqueous humor outflow pathways. The extent of the angle anomaly may affect the time of onset for the elevation of IOP. The more severe the defect, the sooner the elevation in IOP occurs.

Therapy for Glaucoma

There is no cure for glaucoma unless the condition is secondary and the initiating condition or insult can be removed or corrected promptly. The goals of therapy are retention of vision as long as possible and elimination of pain, since glaucoma can cause remarkable discomfort when IOP elevation is uncontrolled. Glaucoma is a progressive condition and requires regular and frequent monitoring to determine if current medical therapies are sufficiently controlling IOP.

IOP is the primary risk factor in glaucoma and the easiest aspect of the disease to monitor, therefore it has become the main target of therapy (von Spiessen *et al.* 2015; Görig *et al.* 2006). In general, it is desirable to achieve the "target" or "safe" IOP for each canine eye that is at or lower than the bottom of the reference range of normal IOP. An IOP reduction to levels that decrease retinal ganglion cell (RGC) loss from glaucoma to normal, age-related levels is usually lower than what would be considered a normal IOP in a normal animal. To achieve this reduction of IOP, a means of either decreasing the production of aqueous humor or increasing the outflow or drainage of fluid from the eye must be found. It is critically important that "prophylactic" therapy be initiated in the normotensive fellow eye when primary glaucoma has been diagnosed in one eye, since studies have demonstrated that early therapy in the normotensive eye may delay the onset of IOP elevation for a considerable amount of time (up to a mean of 30 months) (Miller *et al.* 2000). In secondary glaucoma, the inciting cause is identified and either removed or suppressed and anti-hypertensive medical therapy is usually indicated concurrently.

Both medical and surgical options for glaucoma therapy are available, however, as with any condition that has a multitude of treatment options, there exists no single gold standard treatment (Table 4.4). Therapy should be individualized and will change as the stage of the disease advances and whether or not vision is still present. Medical therapy for the narrow- and closed-angle glaucomas is usually short term when employed alone, because eventually, the outflow becomes so impaired that effects of drugs become inadequate. Some clinical studies suggest that there are higher long-term success rates for controlling IOP and maintenance of vision if surgery is performed earlier in the glaucoma process (Gelatt and MacKay 2004a;

Table 4.4 Treatment of Glaucoma.

Control stage	Treatment
Initial control	IV mannitol (1–2 g/kg IV) or Glycerine (1–2 g/kg PO)
	Prostaglandin analogues (SID-BID) (in the absence of uveitis or lens luxations)
	Aqueocentesis (when medical therapies fail to lower IOP)
	Address concurrent or causative ocular condition (when glaucoma is secondary)
	Initiate topical maintenance medications in affected and fellow eye
Short-term control	Beta-blockers or other adrenergics (BID-TID)
	CAIs (topical dorsolamide or brinzolamide BID-TID)
	Prostaglandin analogues (SID-BID)
	Neuroprotective drugs – memantine, amlodipine
	Laser cyclophotocoagulation
	Gonioshunt
Long-term control	Laser cyclophotocoagulation
	Gonioshunt
	Supplement with medical control
Salvage control	Enucleation
	Evisceration with intraocular prosthesis
	Chemical ciliary body ablation

Miller *et al.* 2000; Sapienza and van der Woerdt 2005; Hardman and Stanley 2001).

In most cases, multiple drug therapy to decrease IOP by reducing production of aqueous humor and diminishing the resistance to aqueous humor outflow will be necessary, even if surgical options are pursued. Beta-adrenergic antagonists, such as timolol and betaxalol, act by decreasing production of aqueous humor (Plummer, MacKay, and Gelatt 2006). Although the exact mechanism by which it is decreased is unknown, and will lower IOP only a few millimeters, therefore they are not good single agent drugs for the control of IOP in eyes that have documented elevations (Plummer, MacKay, and Gelatt 2006). They do, however, work synergistically to lower IOP even greater than the additive effect would be when used in combination with carbonic anhydrase inhibitors (Plummer, MacKay, and Gelatt 2006). They are also inexpensive options for prophylactic therapy of the fellow eye that has not yet developed ocular hypertension. Carbonic anhydrase inhibi-

tors (methazolamide, acetazolamide) reduce ciliary body production of aqueous humor (Gelatt and MacKay 2001a). These drugs when given systemically can cause metabolic acidosis, and the dosage should be carefully adjusted to minimize side effects, which include panting, nausea, and vomiting. Topical formulations (dorsolamide, brinzolamide) have been developed that do not typically cause these untoward side effects and are more efficacious at lowering IOP (Plummer, MacKay, and Gelatt 2006; Gelatt and MacKay 2001a). These drugs make up the mainstay of chronic medical therapy for glaucoma and may be formulated in combination with a beta-blocker drug. Prostaglandin analogues (latanaprost, bimatoprost) decrease IOP by increasing the percentage of aqueous humor outflow through the uveoscleral or unconventional drainage pathway (Gelatt and MacKay 2001b). These drugs have become a go-to for emergency treatment of severe hypertensive episodes. In many instances, they will lower IOP abruptly within 15–30 minutes. However, they may exacerbate any uveitis present and will result in profound miosis that may make examination of the posterior segment difficult or impossible. They should not be used when anterior lens luxations are present since the miosis that results behind the lens can cause a condition called malignant glaucoma wherein the IOP rises due to further occlusion of aqueous drainage. Topical parasympathomimetic drugs (pilocarpine, demecarium bromide) act primarily to cause ciliary muscle contraction, increasing the outflow of aqueous humor (Gelatt *et al.* 1983). This action is independent of their effect on the iris sphincter muscle. Parasympathomimetics are contraindicated in glaucoma associated with anterior uveitis and they should be used with caution in glaucoma associated with anterior lens luxations. These drugs are not single agent treatments since they do not lower IOP dramatically and are most often used to augment therapy already instated. Sympathomimetic drugs (dipivefrin, brimonidine) reduce IOP by increasing production of aqueous humor and increasing outflow (Gelatt *et al.* 1983; Gelatt and MacKay 2002). These drugs, too, are not employed as single agents and are most effective in reducing IOP when combined with parasympathomimetics. Brimonidine may have some neuroprotective effects (Gelatt and MacKay 2002).

Oral and intravenous hyperosmotic agents (mannitol, glycerin) lower IOP rapidly by osmotically reducing the volume of the vitreous (Dugan, Roberts, and Severin 1989). They are used in the emergency treatment of acute glaucoma but are ineffective or impractical for long-term or maintenance therapy.

Intravitreal glutamate levels are elevated in canine glaucoma. Glutamate is extremely toxic to the retinal ganglion cells, resulting in their overstimulation. Glutamate excitotoxicity is mediated by intraneuronal calcium influx. Intraneuronal homeostatic imbalance induces apoptosis and cell death (Almasieh *et al.* 2012). The use of glutamate receptor antagonists (memantine) and calcium channel blocking drugs (amlodipine) for

neuroprotection is being studied and may become standard care in the future.

Since glaucoma once established (any primary cases and many secondary cases if the damage is considerable or the primary cause has not been eliminated) is a progressive condition, frequent and diligent monitoring is necessary. It is generally recommended that "stable" patients have their IOP measured every 2–3 months in perpetuity.

Surgical Treatment for the Glaucomas

With the narrow-angle and angle-closure glaucomas in dogs, surgical treatment is recommended early (Gelatt and MacKay 2004a; Sapienza and van der Woerdt 2005; Hardman and Stanley 2001; Almasieh *et al.* 2012). Medical treatment usually provides a few months of effective IOP control. Surgical intervention is recommended to augment the effects of medical therapy, however, these will neither cure nor prevent the possibility of progression. Anterior chamber shunts (i.e., gonioimplants) and laser cyclophotocoagulation appear to offer the longest periods of successful IOP control (Sapienza and van der Woerdt 2005; Hardman and Stanley 2001; Almasieh *et al.* 2012; Westermeyer, Hendrix, and Ward 2011; Bras, Robbin, and Wyman 2005). Targeted laser ablation with the aid of endoscopic visualization may improve our ability to decrease aqueous humor production and lower IOP for longer periods of time (Bras, Robbin, and Wyman 2005). If the glaucoma is secondary in origin, surgical therapy will be aimed at removing the offending cause (i.e., lens extraction with luxated or subluxated lenses).

Treatment for Blind, End-Stage Glaucoma

Salvage procedures to prevent ocular pain, to reduce the enlarged and blind globe to near-normal size, and to provide a cosmetically acceptable eye include pharmacologic destruction of the ciliary body with intravitreal injection of gentamicin, intraocular prosthesis, in which a silicone ball is placed in an eviscerated globe, and enucleation (i.e., surgical removal of the globe).

Conditions of the Uvea

Uveitis

The most common acquired condition of the uvea is inflammation, referred to as uveitis. Anterior uveitis involves the iris and ciliary body; posterior uveitis affects the choroid and by natural extension the retina since the choroid and the retina are so intimately associated. When both the anterior and posterior segments of the eye are involved, it is termed panuveitis. Intraocular inflammation is a non-specific response to a wide variety of insults and etiologies, ranging from trauma, to infectious or neoplastic disease (local or systemic), to immune-mediated conditions (Massa *et al.* 2002; van der Woerdt, Nasisse, and Davidson 1992). Typically when uveitis becomes chronic, it is because the primary insult has not been removed or eliminated or the condition is primary or perpetuated by an auto-immune assault.

Acute uveitis typically presents with a degree of pain, manifested as blepharospasm, episceral injection, corneal edema, miosis, aqueous flare and sometimes with anterior chamber hyphema, fibrin or hypyon (Figure 4.28). Chronic uveitis will often result in iris color change, usually hyperpigmentation,

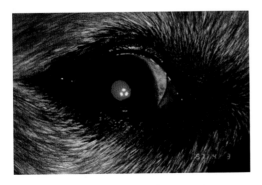

Figure 4.28 Acute uveitis in a dog. Note the episcleral injection and miosis.

and may cause permanent scarring in the ocular interior.

When uveitis is diagnosed, symptomatic therapy should be initiated as soon as possible and a workup looking for causative or concurrent conditions should be performed. A thorough ophthalmic examination may reveal local disease such as the presence of cataract, which invariable results in lens-induced uveitis or an intraocular neoplasm, although the severity may vary considerably (Massa *et al.* 2002; van der Woerdt, Nasisse, and Davidson 1992). If no causative lesion is noted within the eyes, a thorough physical examination may reveal other sites of disease. Survey labwork (complete blood count, serum biochemical profile, and urinalysis), along with serology for infectious agents common to the species or geographic locale and imaging of the thorax and abdomen may be necessary to elucidate an etiology. Cats should be tested for feline leukemia and feline immunodeficiency virus, even if they previously tested negative for the viruses when healthy, and possibly for exposure to feline coronavirus (if clinical signs and chemistry results support this) and toxoplasmosis. Auto-immune uveitis is a diagnosis of exclusion and every effort should be made to identify a cause in order to implement directed therapy.

However, regardless of the cause, anti-inflammatory therapy is critical to eliminate or minimize the damage that unchecked inflammation within the eye will cause (Zarfoss *et al.* 2010). Severe or chronic uveitis may result in corneal edema, vascularization and fibrosis, anterior and posterior synechia, cataract formation, the development of secondary glaucoma and, if the uveitis involves the posterior segment, retinal edema, detachment and degeneration (Figure 4.29). All of these lesions will affect ocular clarity and will negatively impact the potential for sight. Uveitis is also a profoundly painful condition. Anterior uveitis is best treated with topical medications. Steroids are generally more effective at addressing and controlling uveitis than are

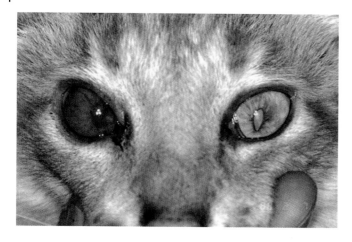

Figure 4.29 Chronic uveitis in a cat. Note the iris color change, iridal neovascularization and cataract.

non-steroidal anti-inflammatory agents, however, care must be taken to choose a topical steroid preparation that will be capable of penetrating the cornea and acting within the eye. Prednisolone acetate is the preferred steroid for intraocular inflammation, because the acetate formulation allows for effective penetration. Dexamethasone is, of course, more potent than prednisolone, but its penetration is less. Avoid hydrocortisone and sodium phosphate formulations of prednisolone. The frequency of delivery will depend upon the severity of the condition. Therapy should continue for at least one month following resolution of all clinical signs, but in most cases of chronic uveitis must be continued indefinitely with the goal of decreasing medication to the least amount necessary to keep the condition under control. Chronic topical steroids may result in impaired corneal healing and local immunosuppression and may result in crystalline deposits within the corneal stromal. For these reasons, controlled cases of chronic uveitis secondary to cataract (or following cataract removal surgery) may be switched to topical NSAIDs for maintenance therapy, which may be slightly safer for long-term use. Additionally, cases of anterior uveitis usually benefit from the application of a cycloplegic medication such as atropine which will help to stabilize the blood-aqueous barrier, dilate the pupil, which will minimize the development of synechia, and decrease ciliary spasm, which causes significant pain. Atropine, however, is contraindicated if the IOP is elevated as it may exacerbate IOP elevations.

Posterior uveitis must be addressed with systemically administered anti-inflammatory or immunosuppressive medications since topicals alone will be insufficient to control posterior segment disease. Systemically administered steroids may suppress the inflammation, but are associated with untoward systemic side effects, so long-term therapy may be switched to immunomodulating agents such as cyclosporine, azathioprine, or leflunomide. Uveodermatologic syndrome, also known as VKH syndrome, is an example of an autoimmune panuveitis that requires systemically administered medications, as well as topical medications (Lindley, Boosinger, and Cox 1990; Yamaki and Ohono 2008) (Figure 4.30). This condition is most frequently encountered in the arctic breeds of dog and has a very high incidence of secondary glaucoma. Cases of chronic uveitis should be monitored frequently (q2–6 months), even once seemingly well-controlled, for continued responsiveness and IOP trends.

Pigmentary Uveitis in the Golden Retriever

Recently, a chronic form of primary uveitis has been described in the Golden Retriever breed (Sapienza, Simó, and Prades-Sapienza 2000). It is referred to as either pigmentary uveitis (PU) or Golden Retriever uveitis

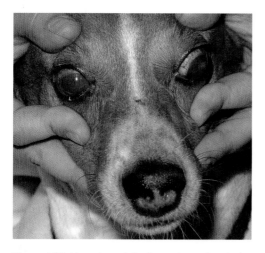

Figure 4.30 Uveodermatologic syndrome in a Jack Russell terrier. This dog has severe uveitis and secondary glaucoma as well as lesions on the nasal planum.

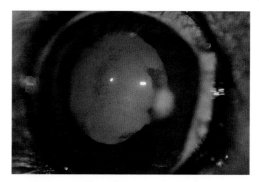

Figure 4.31 Pigmentary uveitis in the Golden Retriever. Not the pigment deposition on the anterior lens capsule and the hyperpigmented iris.

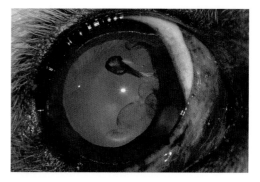

Figure 4.32 Uveal cysts in a Golden Retriever. This dog has no other active signs of pigmentary uveitis, but should be monitored closely.

(GRU) and is characterized by low-grade inflammation and pigment changes within the eye (Sapienza, Simó, and Prades-Sapienza 2000; Holly *et al.* 2015; Esson *et al.* 2009). The iris will often become hyperpigmented and there will be radially oriented deposits of pigment on the anterior lens capsule (Figure 4.31). Fibrin may accumulate in the anterior chamber and posterior synechia is common. Uveal cysts are often present, but their role in the disease has yet to be firmly established (Figure 4.32). Secondary glaucoma is common and may result in blindness in many, if not most patients over time. Signs of inflammation are generally confined to the anterior segment, but damage to the optic nerve and retina will occur once the IOP begins to rise. The condition typically progresses despite extensive topical and systemic therapy. Early diagnosis and intervention in the form of topical steroids and NSAIDs may slow changes but will not prevent them. Regular monitoring for IOP elevation is warranted.

Uveal Neoplasia

Uveal neoplasia may form as either a primary (local condition) or the result of a metastatic lesion. In most cases, the course of disease is rather short once it is recognized with uveitis and secondary glaucoma, usually necessitating removal of the globe. Most cases of intraocular melanoma develop as raised, nodular lesions arising from the iris or ciliary body. Feline diffuse melanosis and melanoma are the exceptions. Melanoma is the most common primary intraocular neoplasm in most species, but its appearance and behavior can vary. Cats may have a form that manifests as a progressive pigmentation of the iris which occurs over several months to several years (Kalishman *et al.* 1998; Acland *et al.* 1980) (Figure 4.33 and Figure 4.34). The pigmentation often develops simultaneously in several areas of the iris and over time will cause an increase in thickness of the iris and changes to the pupil shape and mobility. Eventually the tumor will invade the drainage apparatus and result in secondary glaucoma, but these changes often occur very slowly. The point at

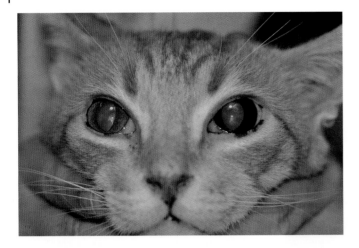

Figure 4.33 Diffuse iris melanoma in a cat.

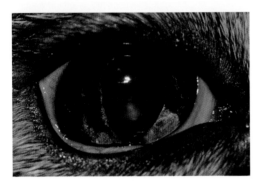

Figure 4.34 Diffuse iris melanoma in a cat.

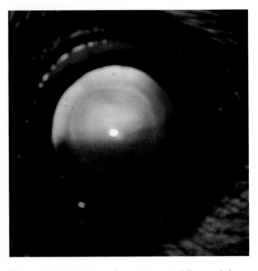

Figure 4.35 Nuclear sclerosis in a middle aged dog. Note the homogenous spherical structure in the central lens and the unobstructed tapetal reflex.

which benign pigment cell proliferation on the surface of the iris transforms into invasive melanoma cells is difficult to define, which is problematic for prognostication and treatment recommendations. Once the tumor cells are in the iridocorneal angle and the scleral venous plexus, metastasis is likely, however (Kalishman *et al.* 1998). Frequent monitoring with photography of pigment progression and measurement of IOP is warranted until involvement of the angle, elevations of IOP or pupillary changes are noted or the client comes to terms with the prospect of enucleation (Acland *et al.* 1980).

Lenticular Changes

Nuclear Sclerosis

Nuclear sclerosis is a consistent finding in dogs older than 7 years that occurs from progressive lens fiber formation and internal compression of older lens fibers, especially those in the lens nucleus (Samuleson 2013). The change is associated with senescence and alters the optical properties of the compressed central lens fibers causing light-scattering. The result is a clinically apparent, whitish-blue or gray appearance to the nucleus on diffuse illumination of the lens. Distant diffuse illumination, however, will reveal an intact and normal tapetal or fundic reflex (Figure 4.35). The nucleus will appear as a clear, homogenous circular ring in the axial lens. Visual examination of the fundus via direct or indirect ophthalmoscopy is possible through the central lens, except in the most severe of examples in which there may be a subtle decrease in fine detail. In contrast, early or immature cataracts appear as dark structures with distant retroillumination or as irregular opacities that typically obscure visualization of the fundus. The patient's functional sight is not typically significantly affected when nuclear sclerosis develops, although depth perception may be affected in older animals or in those who participate in speed and agility competition (Murphy, Zadnik, and Mannis 1992).

Cataract

Cataracts classified as "senile" or "age-related" are commonly seen in the aged dog. They are typically classified as senile if no other antecedent etiology is known or apparent. The age of onset at which a cataract should be considered to be age related is arbitrary (usually greater than 6–7 years of age) and related to the breed. It was reported in one study, however, that all dogs over 13 years of age had some degree of cataract formation (Williams, Heath, and Wallis 2004). The clinical appearance and progression rate of age-related cataracts can vary, but they often appear as punctate or linear opacities in the axial lens concurrent with or after the development of nuclear sclerosis. Cortical cataractous changes, often in a wedge or spoke pattern in the peripheral lens, may also occur to varying extents.

Other etiologies of cataract in the dog include heredity (by far the most common cause of cataract development in canines), diabetes mellitus, and intraocular disease, such as uveitis or glaucoma (Williams, Heath, and Wallis 2004; Gelatt and Mackay 2005; Basher and Roberts 1995; Oberbauer *et al.* 2008). In cats, the majority of cataracts are secondary to uveitis or some other intraocular condition (Stiles 2013). Inherited cataracts and metabolic cataracts do occur sporadically in cats, but not nearly with the frequency of uveitis cataracts (Stiles 2013). Thorough physical and ophthalmic examinations and minimum data base collection should be performed to look for potential underlying systemic or metabolic disease when a diagnosis of cataract has been made.

If an owner is interested in cataract removal surgery for their pet, an early referral to a veterinary ophthalmologist should be made in order to determine eligibility for surgery and to counsel the owners about the pre- and post-operative requirements of cataract surgery. Patients that have had cataract removal surgery will require regular examinations of the eyes and intraocular pressure monitoring and often topical medical therapy for the rest of their lives. Patients that are not candidates for cataract removal, will also require regular eye examinations. Cataracts invariably initiate the development of uveitis, often referred to as lens-induced uveitis (LIU), which can result in either subclinical or overt and severe clinical signs (van der Woerdt, Nasisse, and Davidson 1992; Wilcock and Peiffer 1987). If left untreated, many cataractous eyes will develop synechia (adhesions of the iris to the lens or the peripheral cornea) and preiridal fibrovascular membranes which interfere with normal drainage of aqueous humor with subsequent elevation of intraocular pressure and eventual overt secondary glaucoma (Zarfoss *et al.* 2010; Wilcock and Peiffer 1987). Topical therapy with steroidal or nonsteroidal anti-inflammatories is necessary to prevent or delay the consequences of LIU. Diligent monitoring of IOP, as well as for the signs of anterior uveitis, is strongly recommended at least 2–3 times annually.

Lens Luxations and Subluxations

Lens luxations develop due to an inherited dysplasia of the zonules that suspend the lens in its normal location or secondary to chronic inflammation or another insult that is damaging to these zonules (Gould *et al.* 2011; Morris and Dubielzig 2005). Lens luxations in the terrier breeds and some others are common due to zonular dysplasia, and these dogs may present with either unilateral or bilateral and acute or chronic secondary glaucoma (Table 4.1). The glaucoma is either associated with the iridocyclitis that results from microtrauma between the unstable lens and iris, with resultant increases of aqueous humor fibrin, proteins, and inflammatory cells, which can clog the drainage apparatus

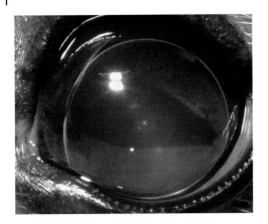

Figure 4.36 Anterior lens luxation of a clear, non-cataractous lens in a Chinese Crested dog.

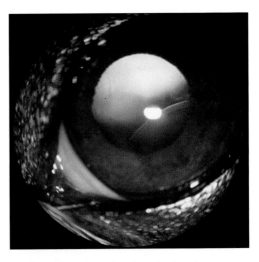

Figure 4.38 Posterior lens luxation in a dog.

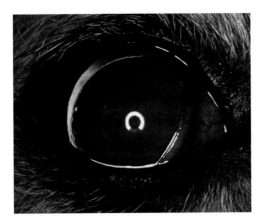

Figure 4.37 Lens subluxation in a mixed-breed dog. Note the dorsolateral aphackic crescent.

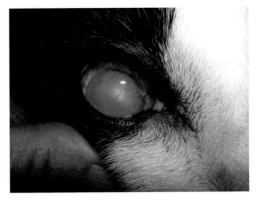

Figure 4.39 Anterior lens luxation of a mature cataract in a cat. Note the iridal neovascularization that had adhered to the nasal aspect of the lens. This luxation was secondary to chronic uveitis.

and contribute to the formation of preiridal fibropupillary membranes and synechiae or due to mechanical impairment of aqueous humor passage through the pupil by and anteriorly luxated lens (Wilcock and Peiffer 1987).

A completely luxated lens can remain in the patella fossa, luxate into the anterior chamber, or move posteriorly through the torn anterior vitreal face and into the vitreous (Figure 4.36, Figure 4.37, Figure 4.38, and Figure 4.39). A large number of animals with partial or complete lens luxations, both anterior and posterior, will develop glaucoma (Gelatt and MacKay 2004b; Dietrich 2005; Johnsen, Maggs, and Kass 2006; Glover *et al.*

1995). Regardless of the direction of lens displacement, anterior uveitis is invariably present and is one of the targets of medical therapy. When a patient presents with anterior lens luxation, the displaced lens will in many cases be in contact with the corneal endothelium resulting in focal edema. If there is significant elevation of IOP or moderate to severe uveitis, there may be diffuse corneal edema. It may be difficult to accurately assess IOP with the lens in such close proximity to the cornea. Care should be taken not to indent the cornea so that it presses into the lens; the IOP in that case may be falsely elevated.

Early removal of displaced lenses, particularly in Terriers, has the highest possibly of success for retention of vision and prevention of secondary glaucoma (Gelatt and MacKay 2004b; Dietrich 2005; Johnsen, Maggs, and Kass 2006; Glover *et al.* 1995). The primary objective of lens extraction is to prevent or treat secondary glaucoma and to diminish inflammation. Early referral to a veterinary ophthalmologist for counselling and surgical therapy is recommended. Medical therapy should consist of topical anti-inflammatory medications (prednisolone acetate 1%, dexamethasone 0.1% q6-12 h; or an NSAID if the cornea is compromised) and topical anti-hypertensive medications, depending upon the measured IOP. In some cases of posterior lens luxation or subluxation when surgery is not possible or is declined, it may be helpful to use a miotic agent such as demecarium bromide to prevent anterior movement of the lens (Binder, Herring, and Gerhard 2007). Due to the high risk of secondary glaucoma, these patients should be monitored regularly for elevations in IOP (q2–6 months).

Posterior Segment Disease

Retinal Degeneration

Most cases of chronic posterior segment disease (trauma, inflammation, hypertension) will result in some degree of retinal degeneration, which can be recognized by tapetal hyperreflectivity, retinal vessel attenuation, depigmentation and pigment clumping, the appearance of choroidal vasculature or the contours of such (particularly when they previously were not able to be visualized) and optic nerve atrophy. There exist a great many forms of inherited retinal degeneration and dystrophy that occur at various ages in companion animals. These, too, will result in progressive decline in retinal structure and function. Presently, there are no available treatments that will reverse or slow these types of changes once they occur in veterinary

patients. Some clinicians advocate the use or oral antioxidant supplements to support eye health (Kador *et al.* 2014).

Hypertensive Retinopathy

Animals with systemic hypertension often develop ocular signs that include retinal detachments and ocular hemorrhage. Any animal with acute vision loss, mydriasis, impaired pupillary light reflexes, retinal detachments, and/or ocular hemorrhage should be evaluated for systemic hypertension and, if indicated, its underlying etiology (Maggio *et al.* 2000; Sansom, Rogers, and Wood 2004) (Figure 4.40). Treatment for hypertensive retinopathy requires normalization of the systemic blood pressure. Retinal detachments occur because hydrostatic pressure within the choroidal vasculature causes fluid leakage with accumulation in the subretinal space. If the pressure is lowered, the fluid will be reabsorbed and the retina will reattach as long as it has not become torn. Vision may be restored if the detachment resolved rapidly. The longer the retina is away from the choroid, the source of its oxygen and nutrition, the greater the likelihood of permanent damage and degeneration. Hemorrhage

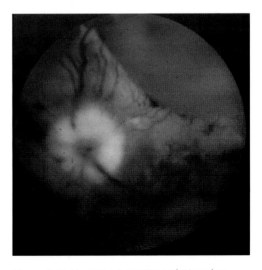

Figure 4.40 Hypertensive retinopathy in a dog secondary to renal disease. Note the multifocal retinal detachments and retinal hemorrhages.

within the eye causes uveitis, so in addition to systemic therapy for the hypertension, therapy for concurrent uveitis may ne indicated.

Blindness

The great majority of companion animals that have visual deficits or have lost sight completely can still have wonderful, happy and healthy lives as long as their human caregivers recognize their pet's limitations and take steps to ensure the animal's safety and comfort. It is important to recognize that many of the conditions that result in loss of vision are painful. When vision is lost, there may still remain the need to continue treatment and monitoring to control or restore the patient's comfort.

With a period of adjustment, visually impaired animals will acclimate to their environments and compensate with their other senses. Consideration of the patient's environment and senses of smell, hearing, and place are important when learning to live with a visually impaired pet. First and foremost, the animal's environment must remain or be made safe for an unsighted pet. Dogs and cats that cannot see will "map" their environments if given time and support. In many cases, they will develop such a sense of place and the confidence necessary to negotiate in such a way that visitors unfamiliar with the pet's deficits may not even recognize the lack of sight. If the pet is reticent or if the environment is novel, leading the pet on a short leash around and from room to room and providing treats and positive reinforcement will facilitate adjustment. Picking up cats or small dogs and carrying them around the house should be avoided as it prevents the pet from mapping the home and can be confusing to the pet if they are set down in another part of the home. It is critically important that the environment be examined for dangers that are at pet-level and that sharp edges and other hazards be removed. Baby gates may be employed to block access to swimming pools, stairs or hazards that cannot be removed.

For dogs, the leash should become an important safety tool. Keeping the pet on a short leash whenever outside of his/her home range will impart some degree of confidence and keep the pet within reach if an unexpected danger presents itself. Training the pet with new commands such as "watch," "step up," "step down," "left," "right," and "stop," may improve the pet's engagement and safety. Clicker training may be helpful for some pets as well. Continue to walk the dog to keep them physically and mentally fit. It is advisable to exchange a collar for a harness that provides somewhat more control and permits greater guidance. Remember that when presented with another animal, the visually impaired pet will not be able to read the body signals and visual cues that animals usually give to one another. Supervision is necessary when introducing new animals until a hierarchy and understanding has been established. Once accustomed to one another, sighted and blind companions often interact very well. Some sighted dogs become a great help to the impaired pet and will act as a form of "seeing eye" guide.

Keeping the pet's bowls and bedding in the same place can be helpful for orientation. If the pet becomes confused but can return to his/her personal effects and home-base, re-orientation will be easier. Refraining from moving the furniture, or recognizing that that will require the pet to re-orient him/herself, and keeping the house picked up and things in their normal places is helpful as well. Carpet runners or non-slip pads, especially on slick surfaces or in doorways can provide landmarks, as can different textures (mulch, pebbles, varied surfaces).

Many blind pets will have heightened senses for hearing and smell. It is possible take advantage of this to help the pet's security. Talk to your pet often and let him/her know when you are approaching or about to touch him/her. Keeping a radio on and in the same place will provide the pet with a landmark and provides some level of comfort and security when a human caretaker is absent. Placing windcharms on the porch, by the outside door or in a particular area of the yard may help a dog keep its bearings outside. Other pets in the house may wear jingling tags or bells to alert the impaired pet to their presence and location. Water fountains for drinking work very well for blind pets since the burbling sound of the water helps the pet locate the water source. Switching to or adding toys that have bells or squeakers may encourage or permit a pet to continue active play which is important to both the physical and mental health of the pet. Pets can and do learn the names of certain toys. This may be a way to engage the pet in play.

Employing scents or pheromones in different parts of the home may be helpful for placing, particularly if used and corners or junctions in the home. Toys that are scented or have holes for treats can engage and keep a pet's interest.

It is helpful if the human companion maintains an upbeat and positive attitude with their visually impaired pet, especially if the vision loss is recent or acute. A human that feels sorry for themselves or their pet will transmit that sense of sadness or despair and may cause or increase a pet's anxiety. Speaking to the pet in a normal, cheerful voice and providing positive reinforcement will ease the pet's transition.

References

Acland GM, McLean IW, Aguirre GD, Trucksa R. Diffuse iris melanoma in cats. Journal of the American Veterinary Medical Association. 1980; 176(1): 52–56.

Allgower I, Schaffer EH, Stockhaus C. Feline eosinophilic conjunctivitis. Veterinary Ophthalmology. 2001; 4: 69–74.

Almasieh M, Wilson AM, Morquette B, Cueva Vargas JL, Di Polo A. The molecular basis of retinal ganglion cell death in glaucoma. Progress in Retinal Eye Research. 2012; 31(2): 152–181.

Andrew SE. Immune-mediated canine and feline keratitis. The Veterinary Clinics of North America: Small Animal Practice. 2008; 38(2): 269–290.

Aquino SM. Management of eyelid neoplasms in the dog and cat. Clinical Techniques in Small Animal Practice. 2007; 22(2): 46–54.

Barachetti L, Rampazzo A, Mortellaro CM, Scevola S, Gilger BC. Use of episcleral cyclosporine implants in dogs with keratoconjunctivitis sicca: pilot study. Veterinary Ophthalmology. 2015; 18(3): 234–241.

Basher AW, Roberts SM. Ocular manifestations of diabetes mellitus: diabetic cataracts in dogs. The Veterinary Clinics of North America: Small Animal Practice. 1995; 25(3): 661–676.

Bentley E, Murphy CJ. Thermal cautery of the cornea for treatment of spontaneous chronic corneal epithelial defects in dogs and horses. Journal of the American Veterinary Medical Association. 2004; 224(2): 250–253, 224.

Binder DR, Herring IP, Gerhard T. Outcomes of nonsurgical management and efficacy of demecarium bromide treatment for primary lens instability in dogs: 34 cases (1990–2004). Journal of the American Veterinary Medical Association. 2007; 231(1): 89–93.

Bistner S. Allergic- and immunologic-mediated diseases of the eye and adnexae. The Veterinary Clinics of North America: Small Animal Practice. 1994; 24(4): 711–734.

Bras ID, Robbin T, Wyman M. Diode endoscopic cyclophotocoagulation in canine and feline glaucoma. Veterinary Ophthalmology 2005: 8: 449.

da Silva EG, Powell CC, Gionfriddo JR, Ehrhart EJ, Hill AE. Histologic evaluation of the immediate effects of diamond burr debridement in experimental superficial corneal wounds in dogs. Veterinary Ophthalmology. 2011; 14(5): 285–291.

Dietrich U. Feline glaucomas. Clinical Techniques in Small Animal Practice. 2005; 20(2): 108–116.

Dugan SJ, Roberts SM, Severin GA. Systemic osmotherapy for ophthalmic disease in dogs and cats. Journal of the American Veterinary Medical Association. 1989; 194(1): 115–118.

Esson D, Armour M, Mundy P, Schobert CS, Dubielzig RR. The histopathological and immunohistochemical characteristics of pigmentary and cystic glaucoma in the Golden Retriever. Veterinary Ophthalmology. 2009; 12(6): 361–368.

Gelatt KN, MacKay EO. Changes in intraocular pressure associated with topical dorzolamide and oral methazolamide in glaucomatous dogs. Veterinary Ophthalmology. 2001a; 4(1): 61–67.

Gelatt KN, MacKay EO. Effect of different dose schedules of latanoprost on intraocular pressure and pupil size in the glaucomatous Beagle. Veterinary Ophthalmology. 2001b; 4(4): 283–288.

Gelatt KN, MacKay EO. Effect of single and multiple doses of 0.2% brimonidine tartrate in the glaucomatous Beagle. Veterinary Ophthalmology. 2002; 5(4): 253–262.

Gelatt KN, MacKay EO. Prevalence of the breed-related glaucomas in pure-bred dogs in North America. Veterinary Ophthalmology. 2004a; 7(2): 97–111.

Gelatt KN, MacKay EO. Secondary glaucomas in the dog in North America. Veterinary Ophthalmology. 2004b; 7(4): 245–259.

Gelatt KN, Mackay EO. Prevalence of primary breed-related cataracts in the dog in North America. Veterinary Ophthalmology. 2005; 8(2): 101–111.

Gelatt KN, Gum GG, Brooks DE, Wolf ED, Bromberg NM. Dose response of topical pilocarpine-epinephrine combinations in normotensive and glaucomatous Beagles. American Journal of Veterinary Research. 1983; 44(11): 2018–2027.

Giuliano E. Diseases and surgery of the canine lacrimal secretory system. In: KN Gellat, Ed. Veterinary ophthalmology. John Wiley and Sons. 2013: 912–944.

Glover TL, Davidson MG, Nasisse MP, Olivero DK. The intracapsular extraction of displaced lenses in dogs: a retrospective study of 57 cases (1984-1990). Journal of the American Animal Hospital Association. 1995; 31(1): 77–81.

Görig C, Coenen RT, Stades FC, Djajadiningrat-Laanen SC, Boevé MH. Comparison of the use of new handheld tonometers and established applanation tonometers in dogs. American Journal of Veterinary Research. 2006; 67(1): 134–144.

Gosling AA, Labelle AL, Breaux CB. Management of spontaneous chronic corneal epithelial defects (SCCEDs) in dogs with diamond burr debridement and placement of a bandage contact lens. Veterinary Ophthalmology. 2013; 16(2): 83–88.

Gould D, Pettitt L, McLaughlin B, et al. ADAMTS17 mutation associated with primary lens luxation is widespread among breeds. Veterinary Ophthalmology. 2011; 14(6): 378–384.

Hardman C, Stanley RG. Diode laser transscleral cyclophotocoagulation for the treatment of primary glaucoma in 18 dogs: a retrospective study. Veterinary Ophthalmology. 2001; 4(3): 209–215.

Hendrix DV, Adkins EA, Ward DA, Stuffle J, Skorobohach B. An investigation comparing the efficacy of topical ocular application of tacrolimus and cyclosporine in dogs. Veterinary Medicine International. 2011. DOI: 10.4061/2011/487592

Holly VL, Sandmeyer LS, Bauer BS, Verges L, Grahn BH. Golden retriever cystic uveal disease: a longitudinal study of iridociliary cysts, pigmentary uveitis, and pigmentary/cystic glaucoma over a decade in western Canada. Veterinary Ophthalmology. 2015. DOI: 10.1111/vop.12293

Johnsen DA, Maggs DJ, Kass PH. Evaluation of risk factors for development of secondary glaucoma in dogs: 156 cases (1999–2004). Journal of the American Veterinary Medical Association. 2006; 229(8): 1270–1274.

Kador PF, Guo C, Kawada H, Randazzo J, Blessing K. Topical nutraceutical Optixcare EH ameliorates experimental ocular oxidative stress in rats. Journal of Ocular Pharmacology and Therapeutics. 2014; 30(7): 593–602.

Kalishman JB, Chappell R, Flood LA, Dubielzig RR. A matched observational study of survival in cats with enucleation due to diffuse iris melanoma. Veterinary Ophthalmology. 1998; 1(1): 25–29.

Kaswan RL, Martin CL, Dawe DL. Keratoconjunctivitis sicca: immunological evaluation of 62 canine cases. American Journal of Veterinary Research. 1985; 46(2): 376–383.

Kerlin RL, Dubielzig D. Lipogranulomatous conjunctivitis in cats. Veterinary and Comparative Ophthalmology. 1997; 7: 177–179.

Komáromy AM, Petersen-Jones SM. Genetics of canine primary glaucomas. The Veterinary Clinics of North America: Small Animal Practice. 2015; 45(6): 1159–1182.

Lindley DM, Boosinger TR, Cox NR. Ocular histopathology of Vogt-Koyanagi-Harada-like syndrome in an Akita dog. Veterinary Pathology. 1990; 27(4): 294–296.

Lourenço-Martins AM, Delgado E, Neto I, Peleteiro MC, Morais-Almeida M, Correia JH. Allergic conjunctivitis and conjunctival provocation tests in atopic dogs. Veterinary Ophthalmology. 2011; 14(4): 248–256.

Maggio F, DeFrancesco TC, Atkins CE, Pizzirani S, Gilger BC, Davidson MG. Ocular lesions associated with systemic hypertension in cats: 69 cases (1985–1998). Journal of the American Veterinary Medical Association. 2000; 217(5): 695–702.

Malik R, Lessels NS, Webb S, et al. Treatment of feline herpesvirus-1 associated disease in cats with famciclovir and related drugs. Journal of Feline Medicine and Surgery. 2009; 11(1): 40–48.

Massa KL, Gilger BC, Miller TL, Davidson MG. Causes of uveitis in dogs: 102 cases (1989–2000). Veterinary Ophthalmology. 2002; 5(2): 93–98.

Michau TM, Gilger BC, Maggio F, Davidson MG. Use of thermokeratoplasty for treatment of ulcerative keratitis and bullous keratopathy secondary to corneal endothelial disease in dogs: 13 cases (1994–2001). Journal of the American Veterinary Medical Association. 2003; 222(5): 607–612.

Miller PE, Schmidt GM, Vainisi SJ, Swanson JF, Herrmann MK. The efficacy of topical prophylactic antiglaucoma therapy in primary closed angle glaucoma in dogs: a multicenter clinical trial. Journal of the American Animal Hospital Association. 2000; 36(5): 431–438

Morris RA, Dubielzig RR. Light-microscopy evaluation of zonular fiber morphology in dogs with glaucoma: secondary to lens displacement. Veterinary Ophthalmology. 2005; 8(2): 81–84.

Murphy CJ, Zadnik K, Mannis MJ. Myopia and refractive error in dogs. Investigative Ophthalmology and Visual Science. 1992; 33(8): 2459–2463.

Nevile JC, Hurn SD, Turner AG, Morton J. Diamond burr debridement of 34 canine corneas with presumed corneal calcareous degeneration. Veterinary Ophthalmology. 2015. DOI: 10.1111/vop.12304

Oberbauer AM, Hollingsworth SR, Belanger JM, Regan KR, Famula TR. Inheritance of cataracts and primary lens luxation in Jack Russell Terriers. American Journal of Veterinary Research. 2008; 69(2): 222–227.

Peiffer RL. Ocular immunology and mechanisms of ocular inflammation. The Veterinary Clinics of North America: Small Animal Practice. 1980; 10(2): 281–302.

Peña MA, Leiva M. Canine conjunctivitis and blepharitis. The Veterinary Clinics of North America: Small Animal Practice. 2008; 38(2): 233–249.

Plummer CE, MacKay EO, Gelatt KN. Comparison of the effects of topical administration of a fixed combination of dorzolamide-timolol to monotherapy with timolol or dorzolamide on IOP, pupil size, and heart rate in glaucomatous dogs. Veterinary Ophthalmology. 2006; 9(4): 245–249

Roberts SM, Severin GA, Lavach JD. Prevalence and treatment of palpebral neoplasms in the dog: 200 cases (1975-1983). Journal of the American Veterinary Medical Association. 1986; 189(10): 1355–1359.

Samuleson DA. Ophthalmic anatomy. In: KN Gelatt, Ed. Veterinary Ophthalmology. John Wiley and Sons. 2013: 39–170.

Sansom J, Blunden T. Calcareous degeneration of the canine cornea. Veterinary Ophthalmology. 2010; 13(4): 238–243.

Sansom J, Rogers K, Wood JL. Blood pressure assessment in healthy cats and cats with hypertensive retinopathy. American Journal of Veterinary Research. 2004; 65(2): 245–252.

Sapienza JS, Simó FJ, Prades-Sapienza A. Golden Retriever uveitis: 75 cases (1994–1999). Veterinary Ophthalmology. 2000; 3(4): 241–246.

Sapienza JS, van der Woerdt A. Combined transscleral diode laser cyclophotocoagulation and Ahmed gonioimplantation in dogs with primary glaucoma: 51 cases (1996–2004). Veterinary Ophthalmology. 2005; 8(2): 121–127.

Sjödahl-Essén T, Tidholm A, Thorén P, et al. Evaluation of different sampling methods and results of real-time PCR for detection of feline herpes virus-1, Chlamydophila felis and Mycoplasma felis in cats. Veterinary Ophthalmology. 2008; 11(6): 375–380.

Stiles J. Feline ophthalmology. In: KN Gelatt, Ed. Veterinary Ophthalmology. John Wiley and Sons. 2013: 1477–1559.

van der Woerdt A, Nasisse MP, Davidson MG. Lens-induced uveitis in dogs: 151 cases (1985-1990). Journal of the American Veterinary Medical Association. 1992; 201(6): 921–926.

von Spiessen L, Karck J, Rohn K, Meyer-Lindenberg A. Clinical comparison of the TonoVet(®) rebound tonometer and the Tono-Pen Vet(®) applanation tonometer in dogs and cats with ocular disease: glaucoma or corneal pathology. Veterinary Ophthalmology. 2015; 18(1): 20–27.

Westermeyer HD, Hendrix DV, Ward DA. Long-term evaluation of the use of Ahmed gonioimplants in dogs with primary glaucoma: nine cases (2000–2008). Journal of the American Veterinary Medical Association. 2011; 238(5): 610–617.

Wilcock BP, Peiffer RL. The pathology of lens-induced uveitis in dogs. Veterinary Pathology. 1987; 24(6): 549–553.

Williams DL, Heath MF, Wallis C. Prevalence of canine cataract: preliminary results of a cross-sectional study. Veterinary Ophthalmology. 2004; 7(1): 29–35.

Yamaki K, Ohono S. Animal models of Vogt-Koyanagi-Harada disease (sympathetic ophthalmia). Ophthalmic Research. 2008; 40(3–4): 129–135.

Zarfoss MK, Breaux CB, Whiteley HE, et al. Canine pre-iridal fibrovascular membranes: morphologic and immunohistochemical investigations. Veterinary Ophthalmology. 2010; 13(1): 4–13.

5

Heart Disease

Simon Swift

Introduction

Heart disease in dogs and cats can vary from mild disease that will not affect the lifespan of the patient to disease that can cause premature death, through heart failure or sometimes acutely with sudden cardiac death. Apart from dilated cardiomyopathy and degenerative valve disease, there is little evidence that therapy in the asymptomatic stages of heart disease delays the onset of heart failure or prolongs life. Heart failure can be described as a syndrome whereby the heart is unable to maintain blood pressure or can only do so with elevated filling pressures. Once dogs and cats develop heart failure, their clinical signs can often be managed medically in the long term. Unfortunately, many diseases are progressive and so eventually the signs return and may not be amenable to control. In considering heart disease in small animals, it helps to recall the classification scheme:

Class A: Animals with no evidence of heart disease but a predilection to develop it, for example, a 6-year-old cavalier King Charles spaniel with no murmur, or a Maine coon cat with the myosin binding protein abnormality and no structural changes.

Class B: This class can be subdivided:
- **Class B1:** Evidence of heart disease but no structural changes or clinical signs, for example, a cavalier King Charles spaniel with a heart murmur suggestive of degenerative mitral valve disease but no chamber enlargement.
- **Class B2:** Evidence of heart disease and structural change but no clinical signs, for example, a cavalier King Charles spaniel with a heart murmur and left atrial enlargement or a Doberman with dilated cardiomyopathy with evidence of left ventricular dilation and systolic dysfunction on echocardiography.

Class C: Evidence of congestive heart failure or on treatment for congestive heart failure (compensated).

Class D: Severe congestive heart failure requiring hospitalization and intensive care that is refractory to conventional medications.

Patients progress from one class to the next but cannot move in the reverse direction, in other words, once a patient develops heart failure, they stay in class C even when compensated. Not every patient will develop heart failure but for those that do, treatment has two phases and goals. Initial treatment of acute congestive heart failure is aimed at ensuring that the patient does not die. In the case of acute pulmonary edema, this effectively involves stopping the patient from drowning and treatments are aimed to achieve this even if their effects may be detrimental in the long run. However, once this is achieved, the goal moves to controlling

Chronic Disease Management for Small Animals, First Edition. Edited by W. Dunbar Gram, Rowan J. Milner and Remo Lobetti.
© 2018 John Wiley & Sons, Inc. Published 2018 by John Wiley & Sons, Inc.

clinical signs and extending longevity. In doing this, it should be remembered that heart failure is a neurohormonal disease that involves the activation of a number of hormones that may be beneficial in the setting of acute blood loss but are detrimental in patients with heart failure and stimulation of the adrenergic system. Activation of the renin-angiotensin-aldosterone system results in increases in levels of angiotensin II and aldosterone both of which have harmful effects chronically. Angiotensin II causes vasoconstriction, increased aldosterone levels, sodium retention, increased thirst and myocardial remodeling. Increased aldosterone levels result in increased sodium and water retention with potassium loss, as well as sympathetic potentiation. Aldosterone is also responsible for myocardial fibrosis and cell death. Furthermore, the sympathetic system itself is stimulated and again, chronic stimulation is harmful causing increased heart rate and contractility, vasoconstriction. Baroreceptor reflexes become blunted and there is down-regulation of beta receptors.

While the benefits of angiotensin converting enzyme (ACE) inhibitors and aldosterone antagonists have been demonstrated in dogs and to a lesser extent in cats, the benefits of beta blockage have yet to be convincingly demonstrated. In humans, they are commonly used to treat congestive heart failure and disease due to ischemic myopathy. However in veterinary patients who suffer from different diseases, it may be that survival times are too short to show advantage.

Treatment of Acute Heart Failure

Regardless of the cause of left heart failure with pulmonary edema, the treatment is similar. The emergency presentation of a patient in acute congestive heart failure requires prompt and appropriate investigation and treatment. Detailed investigation may have to be delayed due to the unstable nature of the patient and treatment instituted urgently.

Patients can vary in their presentation depending on the severity from mildly tachypneic to severely dyspneic, coughing up the pink froth of pulmonary edema. Initial treatment involves stabilization of the patient (Figure 5.1 and Figure 5.2). The following protocol is a guide:

1) *Cage rest*: This reduces oxygen consumption by the tissues.
2) *Oxygen supplementation:* This can be delivered using an oxygen cage. If the temperature is not regulated, large dogs tend to become hyperthermic. A nasal oxygen tube, nasal prongs or flow by may also be used (Figure 5.3). In cats, a brief thoracic ultrasound is appropriate, as if a large pleural effusion is detected, it must be drained by thoracocentesis. This can be life-saving in severely dyspneic cats.
3) *Diuretic:* Typically a loop diuretic such as furosemide is given intravenously. This route is used as it is faster acting and the furosemide has a venodilating action. In fractious patients when catheter placement would be too stressful, an intramuscular route can be used pending control of heart failure. Doses of 2–4 mg/kg furosemide are used initially. The patient's respiratory rate should be reviewed at 30 minutes and then one hour. If the rate has not decreased, repeat the dose or consider using a continuous rate infusion of furosemide at 1 mg/kg/hr. As soon as the respiratory rate starts to fall this dose rate should be decreased or serious side effects could occur.
4) *Positive inotrope:* Pimobendan should be given at 0.3 mg/kg p.o. as patients benefit from inotropic support. In Europe, an intravenous preparation is available. However, given orally, it is rapidly active.
5) *Monitor:* Recording the respiratory rate and effort is a good guide to response. As the pulmonary edema resolves, the respiratory rate and effort should decrease. The production of a large volume of dilute urine is also a sign that the diuretics are effective. Radiographs can also be helpful, showing resolution of pulmonary edema.

(a)

(b)

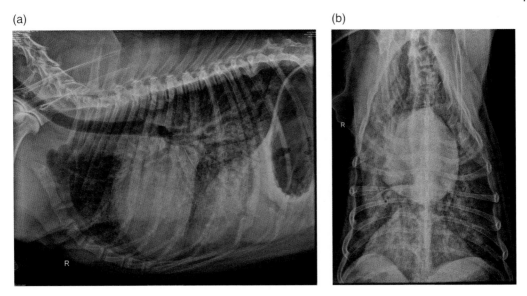

Figure 5.1 X-ray of acute pulmonary edema pre treatment. Lateral and DV radiographs of a 7 year old Doberman pinscher with dilated cardiomyopathy dog with pulmonary edema and after treatment. In Figure 5.1a, the extensive interstitial/alveolar pattern can be seen especially in the perihilar region on the lateral and in the right caudal lung field on the DV.

(a)

(b)

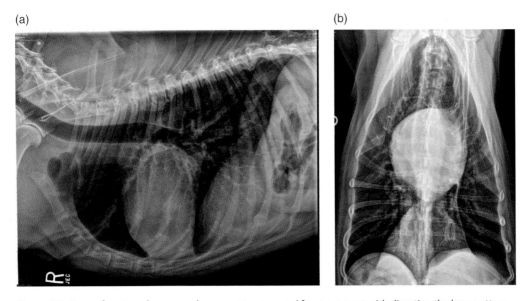

Figure 5.2 X-ray of acute pulmonary edema post treatment. After treatment with diuretics, the lung pattern has normalized and the outline of the left atrium is clearer as it is now surrounded by air. Notice the heart size is smaller.

6) *Blood pressure:* Assessing blood pressure may help in decision making regarding ongoing treatment options. Generally the optimum blood pressure in acute congestive heart failure is 90–100 mmHg and vasodilators can help decrease the afterload, encouraging forward flow and offloading the ventricle. Sodium nitrosside, hydralazine, and an ACE inhibitor can help. Sodium nitroprusside is the most

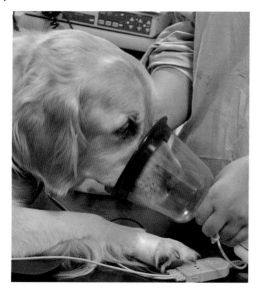

Figure 5.3 A dog with acute heart failure being administered oxygen. It is important that this does not stress the dog or cat.

effective and is given as a constant rate infusion with the dose titrated to blood pressure. Unfortunately, cost makes it prohibitive in most settings and the patient needs careful monitoring. If the blood pressure is low as in some DCM dogs, a pressor may be needed to increase pressure as well as provide inotropic support. In these cases, a constant rate infusion of dobutamine is often helpful. Venodilators such as nitroglycerine used to be recommended to decrease the preload although recent evidence suggests that they are not effective. The effect of ACE inhibitors on blood pressure is minimal with a decrease of 5–10 mmHg expected.

7) *Sedation:* Some patients are stressed by their disease or hospitalization. Opiates can help alleviate this anxiety and reduce oxygen consumption although low doses are preferred due to their depression of the respiratory centers. Buprenorphine or butorphanol are frequently chosen.

As the patient improves, the oxygen concentration can be gradually decreased to that of room air with monitoring of the respiratory rate and the medication switched to oral drugs for discharge. Radiographs are helpful to document to resolution of the pulmonary edema.

Management of Chronic Congestive Heart Failure

After discharge, frequency of revisits is determined by the stability of the patient and response to treatment. With standard cases, it is common to extend the reexamination period. Typically cases are seen at one week, one month, and then every 3 months indefinitely. At the reevaluations, blood samples are taken to assess electrolyte levels and renal function. Blood pressure should also be checked. Other tests such as chest radiographs, echocardiography, and ECG are only requested if there is a change in the patient's condition as tests are only indicated if they change the prognosis or the treatment recommendations.

Patients with congestive left heart failure are usually discharged with:

- *Diuretics*: Furosemide is the usual diuretic at 0.5–2 mg/kg PO TID-BID. The dose range is adjusted to control the resting breathing rate to less than 40 per minute at rest. Higher doses of diuretics are required to get heart failure under control than to maintain control. As a result the initial dose can be decreased with time and the owner's cooperation in monitoring and dose adjustment is vital for long-term management. The main side effects are increased thirst and urination but dehydration and electrolyte depletion can be seen at higher doses especially if the patient becomes anorexic. Ultimately, renal failure can develop and this can be a dose limiting consequence.

- *Calcium inodilator:* Pimobendan causes vasodilation via phosphodiesterase 3 action and the positive inotropic action is due to increasing the affinity of troponin C for calcium. In both DCM and degenerative valve disease, pimobendan has been shown to extend survival times. Dose are 0.1–0.3 mg/kg BID but the top end of the dosage range is preferred. The drug should not be administered with food as this will limit absorption.

- *ACE inhibitor:* ACEi have been shown to prolong life in dogs with DCM and degenerative valve disease. Furosemide and heart failure are potent stimuli of the renin-angiotensin-aldosterone system. Increased angiotensin II has a number of deleterious effects including water and sodium conservation, vasoconstriction and myocardial remodeling. Enalapril at 0.5 mg/kg SID to BID and benazepril at 0.25–0.5 mg/kg SID are the common agents used although ramapril and quinapril are also available in some countries.

- *Spironolactone:* This potassium sparing diuretic is used mainly for its anti-aldosterone action. Aldosterone levels increase in heart failure due partly to elevated angiotensin II levels. Although the evidence for the use of aldosterone antagonists is not complete, it is compelling enough to warrant its inclusion. These drugs prolong life but are unlikely to cause a significant change in clinical signs. As a result, they do not have to be added at the initial stages but rather at the one week or one month recheck, especially with client who may become confused with multiple medications and administration times. This drug is fat soluble so administration with food increases absorption.

Other drugs are added as required – see specific diseases.

Specific Heart Diseases

Degenerative Valve Diseases

Brief Review of Diagnostics
Degenerative valve disease affects mainly the mitral and tricuspid valves. It is also called myxomatous mitral valve disease due to the pathology and endocardiosis although this term has fallen out of favor as it does not help describe the disease. It is the leading cause of heart disease being responsible for 75% of all cases of heart disease seen in general practice and may affect up to 8 million dogs in the United States. It is most prevalent in small breed dogs and the cavalier King Charles spaniel is particularly prone, developing the disease at a young age with 50% of all cavaliers developing a murmur by 6 years. In this breed, a genetic predisposition has been documented.

As the mitral valve is most commonly affected, the disease has a reliable biomarker, the presence of a left apical systolic murmur. Typically initially, this is quiet, grade 1 or 2, with little evidence of cardiac remodeling, but as the disease progresses, the murmur becomes louder often radiating to the right. In a third of cases, the tricuspid valve is also affected and a right apical systolic murmur can be appreciated.

Blood samples: In asymptomatic dogs, these are usually normal but with the onset of heart failure mild elevation of renal parameters is often seen due to the pre-renal renal failure caused by the poor cardiac output. Biomarkers such as atrial natriuretic peptide (ANP) and brain natriuretic peptide (BNP) rise in the few months prior to heart failure and in the dyspneic dog, a high level of BNP is strongly suggestive of heart failure.

ECG findings: These are usually non-specific. A tall or wide R wave can represent left ventricular enlargement and a wide P wave can suggest left atrial enlargement. Arrhythmias are not uncommon. Atrial or supraventricular premature complexes (SVPC) are seen and atrial fibrillation (AF) is occasionally found especially in larger dogs secondary to the left atrial dilation. Ventricular arrhythmias can be found but isolated ventricular premature complexes (VPC) are more common than runs of ventricular tachycardia (VT).

Radiographs are very helpful to document progression of the disease and confirm the presence of congestive heart failure.

In asymptomatic dogs, the heart and lungs can be normal in class B1. The pulmonary vasculature should also be normal. Once cardiac remodeling develops, dogs enter class B2 and left atrial and ventricular enlargement can be seen on the radiographs due to the volume overload of the regurgitation. This is typically observed with tracheal elevation which suggests left ventricular enlargement and a triangular soft tissue density on the caudodorsal margin of the cardiac silhouette on the lateral radiographs. On the DV radiograph, a bulge at the 2–3 o'clock position suggests enlargement of the left auricle. As left atrial pressures start to rise, the pulmonary vein dilates and this can be used as a sign that heart failure is imminent. Once heart failure develops, an interstitial/alveolar pattern develops in the caudodorsal lung fields on the lateral and the right caudodorsal lung field first, obscuring the outline of the left atrium. This is particularly evident in the left lateral view where the right lung is uppermost and should be filled with air.

Echocardiography can be used to confirm the etiology of the murmur. The thickened mitral valve leaflets can be seen and volume overload of the left ventricle and left atrium can be assessed. The left atrium to aorta ratio is a reliable way to document left atrial enlargement as the disease progresses. The disease affects the chordae tendineae and if these rupture, valve prolapse or a flail leaflet may be seen. Color flow with variance mapping will show the turbulent jet of mitral regurgitation and mitral regurgitation can been seen on echocardiography before a murmur is audible. The size of this jet can be used to roughly assess severity (Figure 5.4). As the blood is pumped back into the low pressure left atrium, most echocardiographic parameters for systolic function are elevated as they are affected by the low afterload. For example the fractional shortening is usually 25–30%, but in advanced mitral valve disease when 50–75% of the output of the left ventricle returns to the left atrium, the fractional shortening

may be as high as 40–50%. However, this does not mean that systolic function is normal and dogs with advanced disease benefit from inotropic support.

There are few differential diagnoses for a left apical systolic murmur and in an older small breed dog, degenerative valve disease is the likely cause. In younger animals, mitral valve dysplasia is seen particularly in the bull terrier breed. Co-morbidities are mainly those of an aging dog. Renal failure presents a significant problem as it may reduce the dosage of diuretic that can be used.

Therapeutics Acute, Chronic, and Expected Outcome

See section on treatment of acute and chronic left sided congestive heart failure

Trials involving angiotensin converting enzyme inhibitors (ACEi) and beta blocker have not demonstrated a delay in the onset of congestive heart failure in asymptomatic dogs. A recent trial showed that the calcium inodilator, pimobendan, delayed the onset of congestive heart failure by 15 months when used in dogs with stage B2 degenerative mitral valve disease. The entry criteria were strict including a large heart on x-ray and echocardiography as well as a loud murmur. Current recommendations for asymptomatic dogs include avoiding a high sodium diet and the use of omega 3 fatty acids. The recommended dose of DHE and EPA are 25 mg/kg and 40 mg/kg respectively.

Once heart failure is controlled and the patient returns home, heart failure can recur after a period for a number of reasons:

1) *Rupture of a chordae tendinae* – this is probably the most common cause and can result in acute death. It can be visualized with echocardiography. The patient is treated as for acute congestive heart failure although the dose of diuretics especially will need to be increased. The sudden increase in left atrial pressure causes the return of heart failure and it may take several days for the left atrium to dilate and adapt to the increased pressure.

(a)

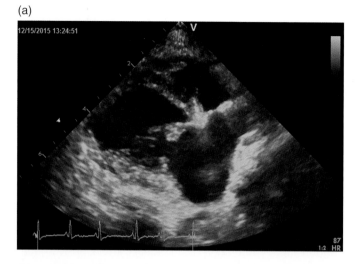

(b)

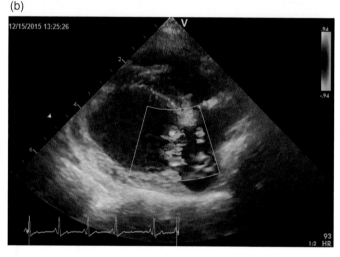

Figure 5.4 Echocardiogram of a dog with advanced degenerative mitral valve disease. This right parasternal long axis 2D view (Figure 5.4a) shows the thickened mitral valve especially the anterior leaflet. The left atrium and left ventricle show eccentric hypertrophy due to the volume load. On color flow (Figure 5.4b), the green turbulent jet of mitral regurgitation can be seen filling the left atrium during systole.

2) *Development of an arrhythmia usually AF.* When AF develops, the dogs lose the atrial component of left ventricular filling and the heart rate increases, decreasing diastolic filling. Rate control is usually sufficient to bring the failure under control.

3) *Left atrial tear* – the mitral regurgitant jet produces fibrous scars on the left atrial wall, so called "jet lesions" and can eventually puncture the left atrial wall causing a hemopericardium. These are difficult to treat as the pericardium should not be drained unless the cardiac tamponade is life threatening. Then a small volume is withdrawn. The pressure in the pericardium helps reduce the leak which, in some cases, can heal. Cage rest and drugs to reduce blood pressure to 90–100 mmHg are used to reduce the afterload and hence regurgitant fraction and left atrial pressures. Recurrence is not uncommon.

4) *Increasing systolic dysfunction* – the volume-loaded left ventricle becomes unable to eject blood into the circulation without elevated filling pressures and pulmonary edema. This may be seen with a gradual increase in breathing rate necessitating changes in medications. For patients that have recurrence of heart failure with none of the previous three causes, treatment is continued as:

a) *Optimize medications*: Ensure the drugs are given correctly, for example, every 12 hours for twice daily medication, ensure spironolactone is given with food which enhances its absorption and pimobendan is given on an empty stomach. The dose of pimobendan should be increased to closer to 0.3 mg/kg to ensure its effect. Some cardiologists increase the dose of pimobendan to three times daily although there is no evidence this is beneficial.

b) *Change medications*: If furosemide is being given twice daily, increase frequency to 3 or 4 times as it has a relatively short duration of action. Alternatively, a parenteral route can be considered if the owner is able to inject the furosemide subcutaneously twice daily. This can be more effective for patients who have concomitant right heart failure and so may not be absorbing medications well. If this is ineffective consider adding a thiazide diuretic to encourage sequential nephron blockade. Beware when adding in thiazide diuretics as dehydration and electrolyte depletion can easily occur. Start at the lower end of the dose range and titrate up to effect. Alternatively, consider switching to a more potent loop diuretic such a torsemide. The starting dose of torsemide is typically 1/10 of the total daily dose of furosemide. That dose is halved and given twice daily. For example if a dog is receiving 10 mg furosemide three times daily, the starting dose of torsemide would be 1.5 mg twice daily. Again electrolyte depletion and dehydration are common side effects and may necessitate dose reduction.

Another complication of advanced degenerative mitral valve disease is the development of pulmonary hypertension. Dogs with pulmonary systolic pressures over 55 mmHg have a worse prognosis than those with lower pressures. While syncope can be a sign, lethargy and other non-specific signs are common. Treatment with a phosphodiesterase 5 inhibitor, for example, sildenafil 2–3 mg/kg BID – TID, often reduces clinical signs although a reduction in pulmonary artery pressure may be hard to document with increased flow.

Low sodium diets rich in omega 3 fatty acids have been advocated but there is little evidence in veterinary literature regarding their benefit. Moderate sodium restriction would be prudent and a calorie dense diet will help mitigate cardiac cachexia. Often, if the dog is eating a good quality diet, it should continue on this rather than try to change diet to one that may be less palatable.

Prognosis is variable with degenerative mitral valve disease, making prediction of survival time difficult. Some dogs with mild disease never develop congestive failure, while others have a more rapid progression of their disease. Patients with class B1 disease can be monitored with an annual echocardiogram or radiograph to assess cardiac size. Patients in class B2 warrant closer monitoring with a review every 6 months. It is helpful to actively enroll the owner in monitoring their pet. Counting their resting respiratory rate has been shown to be one of the most effective ways of detecting the onset of heart failure. Rates less than 30 breath/minute are normal while rates over 40 require further investigation. When patients are in the compensated stage of congestive heart failure (class C) continuing to monitor breathing rate is a useful way of monitoring the effectiveness of diuretics and guide dose adjustments.

Once heart failure develops, the mean survival time is 9–12 months. However as chordal rupture, for example, may cause acute decompensation at any time, predicting the lifespan of an individual dog is impossible. There are certain parameters that are associated with poorer prognosis such as larger LA:Ao ratio, high E wave velocities of mitral inflow or larger LV but ultimately they suggest that the more advanced the disease, the poorer the prognosis.

Quality of Life with Euthanasia Decision

Initially once heart failure is controlled, quality of life is usually normal with few clinical signs and reasonable exercise tolerance. However with more advanced disease, quality of life deteriorates and increasing doses of diuretics are required to control the congestive heart failure. The high doses of diuretics produce electrolyte depletions which can predispose the patient to weakness and arrhythmias. In addition elevation of urea and creatinine suggest increasing renal compromise. This can cause the patients to have poor appetites which contributes to their cardiac cachexia and electrolyte depletion. Ultimately, for some patients, the heart failure cannot be controlled without producing unacceptable renal failure. Sudden death is uncommon but can occur. It may be due to a malignant ventricular arrhythmia or rupture of a major chordae and fulminant pulmonary edema.

Cardiomyopathies

Cardiomyopathies refer to the primary heart muscle diseases suffered by dogs and cats. As a result, all secondary causes must be ruled out to make the diagnosis. Secondary causes include:

- Hyperthyroidism especially cats
- Tachycardiomyopathy where a sustained fast heart rate can lead to a dilated poorly contractile ventricle, for example, supraventricular tachycardia.
- Drug toxicity such as doxorubicin
- Infections, for example, trypanosomiasis
- Hypertension or increased growth hormone as a cause of LV hypertrophy

- Nutritional deficiencies. Both taurine and carnitine deficiencies have been report in dogs as a cause of heart disease with a DCM phenotype and taurine deficiency in cats. American cocker spaniels and Newfoundlands may be predisposed but taurine levels should be assayed in any unusual breeds with a DCM phenotype as supplementation can be curative. Blood carnitine levels reflect poorly myocardial levels so supplementation can be attempted with an improvement in systolic function expected in 2–3 months.

In dogs, the most common disease seen is dilated cardiomyopathy (DCM). The ventricle (mainly left) becomes dilated and poorly contractile and on histology the myofibers have a wavy appearance. Certain breeds such as the Doberman and Irish wolfhound are predisposed. Boxers have a variant with mainly right ventricular origin VPCs called arrhythmogenic right ventricular cardiomyopathy (ARVC) or perhaps better, arrhythmogenic cardiomyopathy. On histology both the left and right ventricles have a fibrofatty infiltration similar to the human disease.

Cats are more likely to develop hypertrophic cardiomyopathy (HCM) with a spontaneous increase in the thickness of the ventricular walls, usually the left ventricle so that the thickness exceeds 5.5 mm in diastole. This may start with papillary muscles abnormalities which in some cats develop into symmetrical hypertrophy of the left ventricle. In other cats, the hypertrophy is more asymmetrical with discrete bulges. If these occur in the left ventricular outflow tract, a dynamic murmur can be appreciated. A murmur may also be caused by mitral regurgitation which can also develop due to systolic anterior motion (SAM) of the anterior mitral leaflet.

Cats can also suffer from DCM although this is rare since feline diets are now supplemented with taurine. Restrictive cardiomyopathy (RCM) is also seen. In this disease, the ventricle becomes fibrotic unable to relax and fill with blood. The muscle walls may have a normal thickness but the atria are usually very dilated. ARVC in cats is similar to the boxer form of the disease and if the heart muscle disease does not fit into any of these categories, it is called unclassified cardiomyopathy. Most of the discussion will be restricted to HCM as it is the most common feline cardiomyopathy.

Dilated Cardiomyopathy

Brief Review of Diagnostics

Dogs have a long asymptomatic period where echocardiographic changes are evident although in some breeds such as the boxer and Doberman, a Holter analysis of the heart rhythm over 24 hours can be more helpful. Over 500 VPCs in 24 hours or the presence of ventricular couplets is suggestive of the disease although other causes such as abdominal disease may have to be ruled out.

Blood Samples: As for degenerative valve disease, serum biochemistry is usually in the reference range in asymptomatic patients although renal parameters rise with heart failure. The pattern with ANP and BNP is also similar to degenerative valve disease with values rising at or just prior to heart failure. Troponin may be elevated especially in patients with frequent ventricular arrhythmias and may have prognostic utility as patients with higher troponin have a poorer prognosis.

ECG findings: These can be variable with some dogs having a normal rhythm but may show the wide P wave and tall R wave suggestive of left atrial and ventricular enlargement respectively. In others atrial and ventricular premature complexes can be seen and the later can vary from isolated complexes to bigeminy to runs of ventricular tachycardia. Atrial fibrillation (Figure 5.5) is not uncommon and often precipitates the onset of heart failure with the reduced diastolic filling and loss of the atrial component of LV filling. Irish wolfhounds may develop slow atrial fibrillation without concurrent myocardial disease, so

called lone atrial fibrillation although many go on to develop DCM later in life. Holter monitoring may be the most sensitive and specific way to diagnose this disease is some breeds.

Radiographs: In the asymptomatic stage, the cardiac silhouette maybe enlarged although this can be difficult to document especially in breeds such as the Doberman. Once heart failure develops, an interstitial/alveolar pattern is seen in the caudodorsal lung lobes, especially the right due to the presence of pulmonary edema (see Figure 5.1). The pulmonary veins are usually distended. In some dogs, a pleural effusion is also seen. If right-sided heart failure is also present, a ground glass appearance to the abdomen suggests ascites and this will obscure the hepatomegaly. A distended caudal vena cava would support this.

Echocardiography: The presence of a dilated thin walled poorly contractile left ventricle and dilated left atrium are seen in advanced cases and in those with heart failure. In dogs with asymptomatic disease, the changes are more subtle and reference to breed standards or an allometric scaling system such as Cornell may be needed. The right ventricle and right atrium may also be affected especially in ARVC in boxers. In clinical cases the various measures of systolic function would be expected to be depressed. These include fractional shortening, ejection fraction, systolic time intervals, and E point septal separation as well as tissue Doppler parameters. On color flow Doppler, a small jet of mitral regurgitation is often seen which explains the soft left apical systolic murmur. This is caused by dilation of the mitral annulus which drags the leaflet tips apart, leading to incompetence (Figure 5.6).

Therapeutics Acute, Chronic, and Expected Outcome

Both pimobendan and ACE inhibitors have been shown to be beneficial in the asymptomatic case delaying the onset of heart failure. Asymptomatic dogs with frequent arrhythmias may be given anti-arrhythmic medication

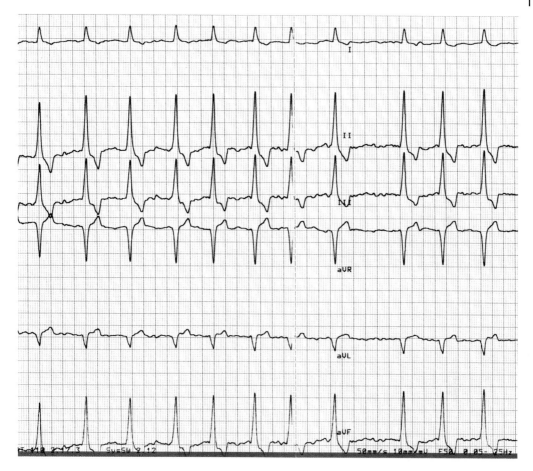

Figure 5.5 ECG from an 8-year-old Labrador with atrial fibrillation. This ECG shows the hallmarks of this rhythm abnormality: tachycardia, irregularly irregular, no P waves and a narrow supraventricular QRS. Note the irregular baseline which represents the atrial fibrillation. This movement, called F waves, can be fine or coarse. 50 mm/s and 1 cm/mV.

especially if the coupling interval is very short (R on T phenomenon) which may suggest ventricular fibrillation is likely. Although, there is no evidence that drug therapy makes sudden death less likely, it may reduce syncopal episodes. Once a dog is started on anti-arrhythmic medication, the Holter monitor should be repeated after one month to assess response, as all anti-arrhythmic drugs have the potential to be pro-arrhythmic. Once stable, the Holter monitor is usually repeated every 6 months and again one month after any drug change.

Treatment for acute heart failure is as previously described. Some patients with poor myocardial function may have low blood pressure and require positive inotropic support with dobutamine. Patients with atrial fibrillation require careful reduction of their heart rate as they may be relying on this elevated heart rate to maintain output. Often resolving their heart failure will reduce heart rate as it reduces the sympathetic drive. At discharge, dogs receive the same 3 or 4 medications as described previously as well as medication to control heart rate if necessary.

Atrial fibrillation requires drugs to slow the heart rate as the underlying mechanism for its development is atrial enlargement which cannot be addressed. As a result, the beneficial effects of cardioversion to sinus

(a)

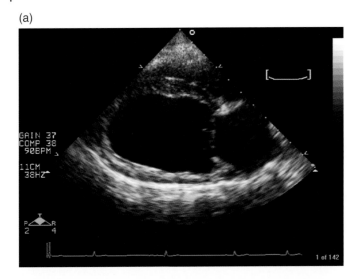

(b)

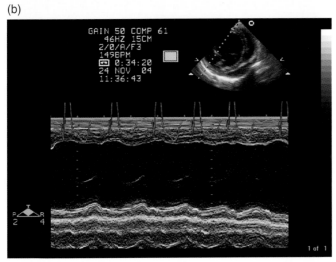

Figure 5.6 Echocardiogram of dog with dilated cardiomyopathy. The left atrium and left ventricle are dilated and the ventricle appears thin walled (Figure 5.6a). On M mode (Figure 5.6b), the reduced fractional shortening can be appreciated and this is consistent with reduced contractility.

rhythm are likely to be short lived. Digoxin, calcium channel blockers (diltiazem) and beta blockers (usually atenolol) can all be used to slow heart rate. Beta blockers tend to have more negative inotropic effects which are usually dose related so are less frequently used. Diltiazem also has some negative inotropic effects but this is less severe. Digoxin acts centrally via vagal centers to slow heart rates. A combination of digoxin and diltiazem has been shown to provide better rate control than either drug alone and presumably this will

translate into longer survival. The optimum heart rate for patients with atrial fibrillation has yet to be determined but rates of 140–160 bpm in the clinic and 120–140 bpm on Holter monitor have been reported.

Quality of Life with Euthanasia Decision

As for degenerative valve disease, dose escalation of diuretics and ACE inhibitors is seen with progressing disease. The owner should be advised that many dogs with DCM are at risk of sudden death especially if they have frequent VPCS or runs of ventricular tachycardia. Options for patients who are diuretic resistant include:

- More frequent administration of furosemide
- Parenteral administration of furosemide
- Addition of a thiazide diuretic
- Switching to the more potent loop diuretic, torsemide, as described previously

Right heart failure can contribute to the development of cardiac cachexia. Severe weight loss is not uncommon in dogs with chronic disease. This can be caused by increased catabolism (heart failure is an inflammatory disease), poor nutritional intake with poor appetite, poor absorption and poor metabolism from the under-perfused liver. Poor appetite can be due to:

- Advancing renal failure
- Altered taste sensations with medications
- Digoxin toxicity

Use of a calorie dense food can help to mitigate weight loss. Supplementation with omega 3 fatty acids has been shown to be beneficial in human patients with cardiac cachexia and the same is likely to be true in dogs. The dose of omega 3 fatty acids is as described previously.

Balancing diuretic requirements between controlling heart failure and not exacerbating renal failure is an act that will ultimately be lost with advancing renal failure in the face of increased diuretic requirements. Sudden cardiac death is always a possibility.

Hypertrophic Cardiomyopathy

Brief Review of Diagnostics

Cats can have a long asymptomatic period and although 30% of cats may have a murmur with 50% of those having structural heart disease, many cats never go on to develop heart failure. For cats with mild left ventricular hypertrophy and no left atrial enlargement, annual evaluations are sufficient as the disease is slowly progressive. The only way to assess disease stage is with echocardiography. However, once left atrial enlargement is documented, heart failure is likely to occur and more frequent re-evaluation is prudent.

There is no firm evidence that treatment prior to the onset of heart failure is beneficial. However, if the hypertrophy is severe or there is significant left atrial dilation, treatment is often started.

Blood samples: In the asymptomatic patients, routine blood work will be normal. Biomarkers may be helpful especially in cats with other signs of heart disease such as murmur or gallop. Elevated BNP would increase the suspicion of cardiac disease and prompt further evaluation with an echocardiogram. Once heart failure develops, pre-renal renal failure causes elevations of urea and creatinine.

ECG: This may be normal or consistent with left ventricular hypertrophy – tall or wide R wave. Atrial or ventricular premature complexes may be present but malignant arrhythmias are uncommon. A particular branch block is recognized in cats and its detection again increases the suspicion of cardiomyopathy. A left anterior fasicular block is seen in cats where the R wave is negative in leads 2 and 3 but positive in lead 1. When cats develop heart failure, their rate does not increase as dramatically as dogs.

Radiographs: The hypertrophy is concentric so the cardiac silhouette can be normal even in significantly affected cats. However if atrial dilation is present a discrete enlargement can be caudodorsally. If biatrial enlargement is present, the cardiac silhouette can have a Valentines's shape on the DV. When cats develop heart failure the interstitial alveolar pattern can occur anywhere in the lung fields (Figure 5.7). Cats in heart failure can also develop significant pleural effusions that may warrant treatment. Thick pulmonary veins support the diagnosis of heart failure. Ascites is rare in cats with heart failure

Echocardiography: This is the definitive test that allows the diagnosis and disease

(b)

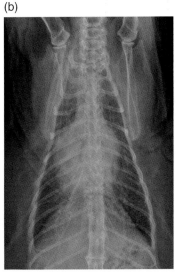

(a)

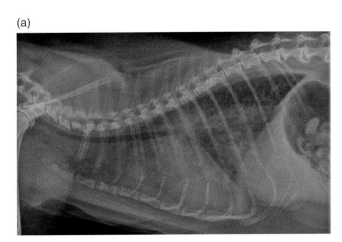

Figure 5.7 Lateral (Figure 5.7a) and DV (Figure 5.37b) chest radiograph from a 13-year-old DSH cat with congestive heart failure. A moderate pleural effusion is present and patches of pulmonary edema. In cats, these can occur anywhere in the lungs unlike the perihilar distribution seen in dogs.

severity to be identified. The hypertrophy of the left ventricle can be visualized and the size of the left atrium assessed. The left ventricular walls should be less than 5.5 mm in diastole and the left atrial diameter under 16 mm in long axis. In addition, the LA:Ao ratio should be under 1.6. In some cats, mitral regurgitation due to SAM or dynamic left ventricular outflow tract obstruction (DLVOTO) is present. The left auricle can be examined for the presence of a thrombus (Figure 5.8). Also, the presence of spontaneous echo contrast in the left atrium which looks like swirling smoke suggests an increased likelihood of thrombosis and would warrant the introduction of antithrombotic medication.

Therapeutics Acute, Chronic, and Expected Outcome

There is no good evidence currently that medication of asymptomatic cats is beneficial. Previously it was believed that cats with DLVOTO benefited from beta blockage. However, recent evidence suggests this is not the case. If the left ventricle thickness exceeds 9 mm in places, the addition of an ACE inhibitor can be tried due to the effects on myocardial remodeling. If the left atrium is very large, over 19 mm, the cat is at increased risk of a thromboembolic event. The sluggish blood flow in the left atrium predisposes cats to this. The recent FAT CAT (feline aortic thromboembolism clopidogrel v. aspirin trial) study indicated that clopidogrel is superior to aspirin in prevention of re-thrombosis. Clopidogrel is administered as 75 mg ¼ tablet once daily. It is bitter and can be administered in a gel capsule to improve palatability. The dose of aspirin is more variable with doses as high as 10–25 mg/kg every 48 hours but for platelet inhibition, 0.5 mg/kg is probably sufficient.

Cats with cardiomyopathy can develop heart failure with pulmonary edema and/or pleural effusion. However they can also have a thromboembolic event. Pulmonary edema is treated as for canine left heart failure with oxygen, cage rest, and furosemide. Pimobendan can be given if inotropic support is needed. Cats are particularly sensitive to the stress of further investigations so these may be delayed until the disease is under control. It is also easy to create electrolyte

(a)

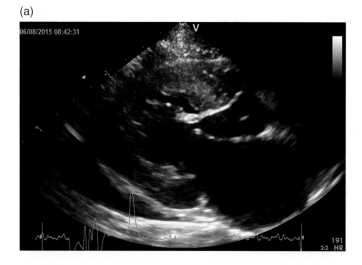

(b)

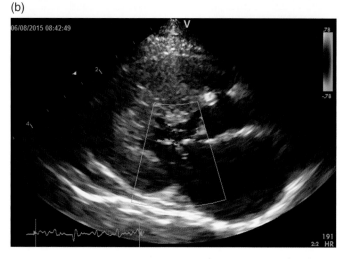

Figure 5.8 Echocardiogram from a cat with hypertrophic cardiomyopathy. The right parasternal long axis view (Figure 5.8a) shows the thickened left ventricular walls and dilated left atrium. During systole (Figure 5.8b) color flow shows the green turbulence shows high velocity flow in the left ventricular outflow tract caused by dynamic obstruction with end systolic cavity obliteration. There is also a jet of mitral regurgitation secondary to systolic anterior motion (SAM) of the anterior mitral valve leaflet.

and renal abnormalities with high diuretic dose and this should be carefully monitored. Once the respiratory rate and effort start to decrease, the cat can be switched to oral medications.

If a cat has a pleural effusion, thoracocentesis is indicated to obtain a sample and to therapeutically remove the fluid. No amount of diuresis will reduce the pleural effusion in the short term but treatment including diuretics is aimed at slowing the recurrence of the fluid. Thoracic ultrasound can be used to confirm the clinical suspicion of a pleural effusion and to guide location for drainage. A butterfly or over the needle catheter is advanced into the pleural cavity and suction applied with a three way tap. As much fluid as possible should be drained from each side. In cats with severe life threatening dyspnea, this can be life-saving although it may have to be performed in two stages. The first procedure removes a small amount of fluid with minimum restraint and stress. The cat can then recover in oxygen for 30 minutes before a second procedure to remove the rest of the fluid. Even the removal of a little as 20 ml in the first procedure can make a significant difference to the respiratory effort of the cat.

Thromboembolic events are life threatening for cats as recovery is often poor with up to 50% of cats not surviving to discharge despite appropriate intensive care. The terminal aortic trifurcation is the most common site with the classic signs of paresis, pallor, lack of pulse, and pain. The stress can also precipitate the onset of heart failure which can complicate treatment. Other arteries can be affected including the renal, cerebral, and forelimb, usually the right. For these arteries, the prognosis is better with cats with forelimb thromboses recovering within a week. Aortic thromboembolism requires prompt treatment. The heart failure should be managed as previously. Pain is often the most severe problem and can be difficult to control even with appropriate opiate analgesia. Use of thrombolytic medication such as tissue plasminogen activator is associated with high fatality rate probably because the cat is not presented early in the course of its disease. Beyond 6 hours, high levels of potassium and toxic metabolites such as myocardial depressant factors build up in the ischemic tissues and sudden release of these into the circulation can cause sudden death. Instead, heparin or low molecular weight fragments such as dalteparin may be used to help clot dissolution. The dose of heparin is 250–300 IU/kg TID while the dose of dalteparin is less well established with 100 IU/kg every 8 to 12 hours often used. Symptomatic treatment is provided which may include management of the heart failure and pain and encouraging feeding. Hospitalization for at least 7 days is required in severe cases and at the end of that period, cats that are likely to survive, will show some improvement in hind limb function although this is often unilateral initially. Weak pulses may be felt, the limb is slightly warmer and some return of function is seen although knuckling is common. Some cats develop a dry gangrene of the limb and the lower portion becomes hard and dry resembling mummification. For these cats, amputation is required.

Quality of Life with Euthanasia Decision

If a cat is presented with a severe aortic thromboembolism, the owner needs to be involved in the decision making process as treatment is not inexpensive and the outcome is often poor. If pain cannot be adequately managed, euthanasia should be considered. A brief echocardiogram is helpful as if further thrombi are identified in the left auricle, recurrence in a short period is likely. Large thrombi can result in sudden death. Anorexic cats in heart failure rapidly develop electrolyte abnormalities and increasing renal parameters further depress appetite creating a downwards spiral which is difficult to treat. Cats that survive to discharge are at risk of recurrence although clopidogrel will help to reduce that risk. Most owners are unwilling to allow their cat to be treated for a recurrence.

Cats with compensated congestive heart failure have an average survival of 9–12 months depending on the severity of their heart disease. Recurrence of heart failure with escalating doses of diuretics is common as the disease progresses and as with dogs, the balance between renal and heart failure often determines ultimate outcome. Cats seem to be more sensitive to the addition of a thiazide diuretic or switching to torsemide.

Congenenital Cardiac Diseases

Dogs and cats with congenital heart disease can vary in the severity of their signs from those that are minimally affected with normal life expectancies although they should not be used for breeding to those with severe disease who will die prematurely from heart failure or sudden cardiac death. While the most common congenital heart disease seen in cats is probably a ventricular septal defect, this section will discuss the three most common congenital cardiac diseases seen in dogs:

- Subaortic stenosis
- Pulmonic stenosis
- Patent ductus arteriosus (PDA)

Brief Review of Diagnostics

The presence of a heart murmur in a young puppy is the clinical sign that should raise suspicion of congenital heart disease. Subaortic and pulmonic stenoses both have a left basilar murmur. However while subaortic stenosis is associated with a murmur that radiates up the carotid arteries and weak femoral pulses, the murmur of pulmonic stenosis tends to radiate dorsally on the chest wall. The murmur of a PDA is also left basilar but characteristic as it is continuous, waxing and waning during the entire cardiac cycle but reaching a peak in systole. Pulses tend to be bounding due to the increased difference between systolic and diastolic pressures. As PDA and pulmonic stenosis are potentially treatable diseases, it is important to have a definitive diagnosis so that treatment can be recommended as appropriate.

Blood samples: Routine hematology and biochemistry would be expected to be normal in dogs with congenital heart disease that is not cyanotic unless heart failure develops. However, in right to left shunting PDAs, polycythemia can develop due to the caudal cyanosis. Biomarkers are usually unremarkable until heart failure develops.

ECG: In PDAs, the ECG is usually normal. In subaortic stenosis, the pattern can suggest left ventricular hypertrophy with a tall, wide R wave. The ECG appearance of pulmonic stenosis is more helpful. In severe cases right axis deviation is seen with a negative lead 1 and positive leads 2 and 3. This, together with deep negative S waves in leads 1, 2, and 3, is the characteristic of right ventricular hypertrophy. This finding in a puppy with a left basilar systolic murmur increases the suspicion of pulmonic stenosis and should prompt referral.

Radiographs: Radiographic changes can vary depending on the severity of the lesion. Dogs with mild disease may have normal thoracic radiographs. In dogs with moderate to severe stenosis, the radiographic changes are often disappointing as there is concentric hypertrophy so the evidence of left or right ventricular hypertrophy may be hard to identify. However, the DV view is helpful as the post stenotic dilation of the main arteries can be identified. The post stenotic bulge of the aorta can be visualized at the 12–1 o'clock position in cases of aortic stenosis whereas that of the pulmonary artery is seen at 1–2 o'clock in pulmonic stenosis. The typical left to right shunting PDA causes volume overload of the left atrium and ventricle. As a result, a left-sided enlargement pattern would be expected. However, while cardiomegaly is usually documented the typical appearance of left atrial enlargement with a triangular soft tissue density extending from the caudodorsal border of the heart is not seen. Instead on the DV a classic appearance of three bulges may be seen, the aorta and pulmonary artery at the 12–1 and 1–2 o'clock positions respectively. The third bulge is the left auricle which is at 2–3 o'clock. However the three knuckles are seen in about 25% of cases. Perhaps more useful is documenting the overcirculation of the lungs. Both the pulmonary artery and vein should be dilated and this is perhaps best seen by the ability to follow these vessels far into the periphery beyond where they would normally fade.

Echocardiography

- *Aortic stenosis*: In mild to moderate cases, the changes can be minimal with little to no left ventricular hypertrophy. However, in these cases, a small ridge under the aortic valve is usually visible. With increasing severity a fibrous ring may be seen causing various degrees of stenosis and there may be a change in the aortoseptal angle which may have a role in the etiology (Figure 5.9). The left ventricle becomes increasingly hypertrophied

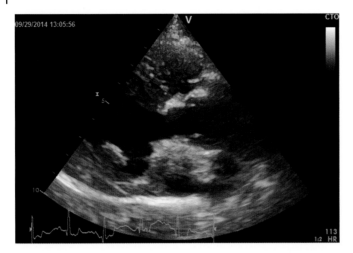

Figure 5.9 Echocardiogram from a 1 year old Chow Chow with subaortic stenosis. In this right parasternal 5 chamber view optimized for the left ventricular outflow tract, the discrete sub valvular ridge can be seen. The left ventricle shows concentric hypertrophy due to the pressure load.

and hyperechoic areas may been seen especially in the papillary muscles suggesting fibrosis which is probably the result of hypoxia. On Doppler examination, a high speed turbulent jet can be seen in the left ventricular outflow tract. Aortic regurgitation may also be seen but is not usually significant. The assessment of aortic regurgitation can be difficult and can vary from assessment of the size of the jet to measuring the pressure half-life. The severity of subaortic stenosis is determined by the pressure gradient (Table 5.1), which is related to the velocity by the modified Bernoulli equation:

$$\text{Pressure gradient}\,(\text{mmHg}) = 4 \times \text{velocity}^2\,(\text{m/s})$$

To assess the velocity accurately, it is critically important that the ultrasound beam is correctly aligned with flow. Hence although the left apical long axis view can be used, higher velocities are often obtained from the subcostal angle so this should always be interrogated to accurately assess severity.

- *Pulmonic stenosis:* Again, in mild to moderate cases, the changes can be min-

Table 5.1 Severity of aortic regurgitation.

Severity	Velocity in m/s	Pressure gradient (mmHg)
Normal	Less than 2.2	Less than 20
Mild	2.2–3.5	20–50
Moderate	3.5–4.5	50–80
Severe	Over 4.5	Over 80

imal. With increasing severity, the right ventricle becomes hypertrophied. As pressures in the right ventricle exceed those in the left ventricle the septum becomes flattened and the right ventricle may become dominant with the septum moving towards the right side in systole – paradoxical septal motion. Pulmonic stenosis is usually valvular and is more common in small breed dogs especially the bulldog (Figure 5.10; Figure 5.11). Two types are recognized although there is significant overlap. In type A, the valve leaflets are normal but appear fused together along the commisures. In type B, the valve leaflets are more thickened and dysplastic. The pulmonary artery may also be

(a)

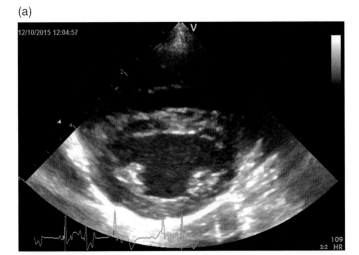

(b)

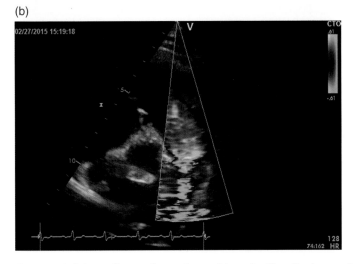

Figure 5.10 Echocardiogram from a 2 year old cavalier King Charles spaniel with severe pulmonic stenosis. In the right parasternal short axis view (Figure 5.10a), the right ventricular free wall is hypertrophied due to the increased pressure with flattening of the interventricular septum as the pressures in the the right ventricle near or exceed those in the left ventricle. On color flow (Figure 5.10b), the green jet of turbulent flow can be seen starting at the valve and the pulmonary artery is dilated post stenotically.

hyperplastic. In bulldogs, an abnormal arrangement of the coronary arteries may complicate the stenosis. In these dogs, the left coronary artery arises as a branch of the single right coronary artery. This left coronary artery then circles round the pulmonary artery to reach the left ventricle. This R2A anomaly may contribute to the stenosis. Again, alignment with flow is critical for accurate assessment of severity. Maximal velocities

should be obtained from both the right and left short axis views and the higher value used. In severe cases hypertrophy in the outflow tract can cause a dynamic stenosis where the thickened muscle crushes the outflow tract. This can complicate the Bernoulli equation causing underestimation of pressure gradients. Pulmonic regurgitation is not uncommon but is rarely significant. The tricuspid valve may become incompetent and

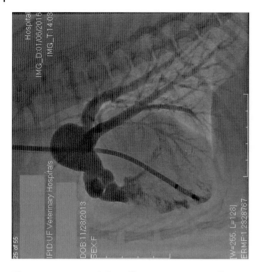

Figure 5.11 Lateral chest fluoroscopic image from a small breed dog with pulmonic stenosis showing contrast being injected into the right ventricle. The right ventricle is hypertrophied with prominent papillary muscles and the outflow tract can be visualized. The discrete valvular stenosis and the post stenotic dilation can be seen.

assessing the speed of the regurgitant jet can help confirm severity. Fortunately in most dogs the degree of tricuspid regurgitation remains small as this valve protects the right atrium and systemic veins from the high pressures present in the right ventricle.

- *PDA:* The volume overload of the left side of the heart can be documented in moderate and severe disease. The dilated left atrium and left ventricle can be seen and the left ventricle can appear to have depressed systolic function with a reduced fractional shortening although this is not significant in the long term. The dilated left side can lead to secondary mitral regurgitation due to dilation of the annulus. On the short axis, the pulmonary artery is dilated and color flow confirms the turbulent flow arising from the ductus heading towards the transducer as it enters the pulmonary artery. In most cases, the ductus can be visualized and measured and

importantly the size of the narrow ending as the ductus enters the pulmonary artery, assessed (Figure 5.12).

Therapeutics Acute, Chronic, and Expected Outcome

Aortic and pulmonic stenosis: Dogs with mild to moderate aortic and pulmonic stenosis do not usually require treatment and may not require further evaluation. As disease severity moves into the moderate/severe category, there is a potential for the disease to progress and those dogs may benefit from annual re-evaluations with an echocardiogram.

Aortic stenosis: In dogs with severe disease, beta blockers are initially used to reduce the risk of arrhythmias and sudden death. For subaortic stenosis, this is continued long term although more recent evidence has questioned the benefit of beta blocking agents. Valve replacement and infundibular myectomy has not been shown to prolong survival and is no longer performed. Cutting and high pressure balloon dilation of the subvalvular region has been described and although the pressure gradient may decrease in the immediate post-operative period, there are no long-term data to indicate this is translated into increased survival and many dogs experience an increase in their gradients over time. Clinical experience suggests that beta blockers reduce the risks of sudden death and syncopal episodes which usually occur at exercise.

Pulmonic stenosis: For dogs with severe pulmonic stenosis, balloon dilation of the obstruction has been shown to reduce gradients and prolong survival. Beta blockers are usually administered for 2 weeks prior to the procedure to reduce dynamic obstruction and reduce the risk of serious arrhythmias during the procedure. This is performed under general anesthesia with fluoroscopic guidance. The diameter of the pulmonary artery can be measured on fluoroscopy and the obstruction visualized. Balloons measuring 1.2 to 1.5 times the

(a)

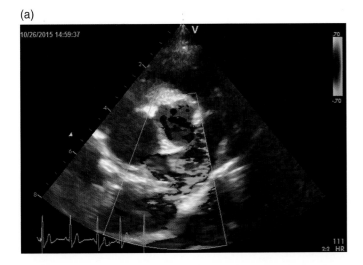

(b)

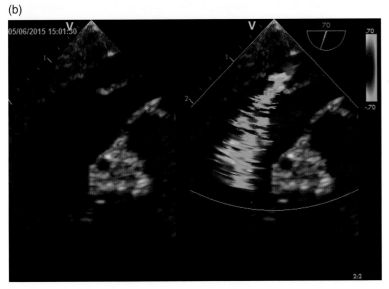

Figure 5.12 Echocardiogram from a dog with a patent ductus arteriosus. This left parasternal cranial view (Figure 5.12a) shows the pulmonary artery with blood flowing away from the transducer coded blue. The ductus enters the pulmonary artery distally and the red flow of blood in the ductus flowing toward the transducer changes to a green turbulent jet when it enters the pulmonary artery. The pulmonary artery is dilated. The transesophageal view (Figure 5.12b) shows the blood from the ductus on top entering the main pulmonary artery. In this color compare view the shape of the ductus can be appreciated as it narrows at the pulmonary artery entrance.

diameter of the pulmonary artery are selected and a reduction of the pressure gradient of 50% would be a successful result. Higher pressure balloons and the use of a double balloon technique in larger dogs may improve outcomes. In dogs with type A pulmonic stenosis, 95% would be expected to respond well. In dogs with type B, the results are poorer due to the thickened leaflets and hypoplastic pulmonary artery with about 2/3 expected to improve. Dogs are followed with a repeat echocardiogram to assess gradients in 2–3 months and then as necessary depending on the pressure gradient. Dogs that return to mild disease, can be weaned off their beta blockers once right ventricular hypertrophy has resolved but if dogs remain in the moderate to severe category, beta blockage may be needed for life. Some dogs especially type B initially respond well but restenosis can recur presumably because the stenotic lesion is stretched rather than torn. For dogs that have a restenosis or respond poorly, beta blockage should be maintained. Further treatment involves the patch graft technique where a patch is sewn over the stenosis and the entire area opened up during brief inflow occlusion. Severe incompetence of the pulmonic valve is created but dogs seem to cope well with this despite the risk of chronic right-sided volume overload. At the University of Florida, we have been placing a bare metal stent across the stenosis with a similar effect.

PDA: Dogs with small PDAs may not require treatment if the volume of blood is so small it is hemodynamically insignificant. However, these dogs may be at increased risk of developing infective endocarditis and prophylactic antibiotics should be given as needed. Dogs with larger ductuses will die prematurely if their ductus is not closed with 75% not surviving to one year of age. Closure can be achieved two ways. Either a thoractomy and surgical ligation can be performed or a minimally invasive technique used to close the ductus. Both have similar success rates with 95% of dogs expected to survive. Recovery is faster from the minimally invasive technique but it is usually more expensive due to the implants used. These include coils, vascular plugs and more recently the Amplatz canine duct occluder (Figure 5.13; Figure 5.14). Such techniques require the use of fluoroscopy although more recently, transesophageal echocardiography has reduced this requirement and allows visualization of ductus in detail. After closure, an echocardiogram is repeated in 1 month to assess closure and remodeling. A small

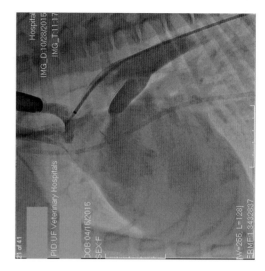

Figure 5.13 This lateral chest fluoroscopic image shows a catheter in the aorta injecting contrast. The PDA can be visualized as a finger like projection extending ventrally towards the pulmonary artery. It narrows at the pulmonary artery entrance and the pulmonary artery is dilated. This is the most common type of PDA and is amenable to closure with an Amplatz canine duct occluder (ACDO).

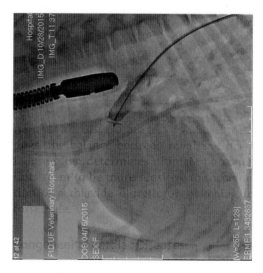

Figure 5.14 Lateral chest fluoroscopic image showing an ACDO deployed in the ductus. The first disc is in the pulmonary artery and the second in the ductus itself. Contrast is injected to check placement and lack of flow through the ductus.

percentage suffer from residual flow especially if the ductus is large. If this is small-volume, low-velocity flow, it may close eventually but if it remains open, there should be no long-term consequence, although there may be an increased risk of infective endocarditis. If there is significant residual flow, the procedure may have to be repeated.

For dogs with a large PDA in which the ductus is not closed there are two possible outcomes:

- If the ductus remains left to right shunting, left heart failure can develop with pulmonary edema and breathlessness. Treatment is as for other causes of congestive heart failure with diuretics, usually furosemide, an ACE inhibitor, pimobendan possibly with spironolactone. The ductus can still be closed at this stage but the long-term outlook is poorer compared to dogs that have their ductus closed prior to the onset of heart failure.
- In some dogs, a reactive change occurs in the pulmonary arteries and pulmonary hypertension develops. As the pressure in the pulmonary artery rises, the velocity of blood flow across the PDA decreases until eventually the murmur disappears. Ultimately, they can become right to left shunting with de-oxygenated blood entering the descending aorta causing caudal mucous membrane (differential) cyanosis. These dogs present with signs of exercise intolerance or due to signs associated with their polycythemia. The kidney responds to the de-oxygenated blood by producing more erythropoietin. The development of polycythemia is very variable and unpredictable. Unfortunately, once the PDA becomes right to left shunting, it cannot be closed as this will lead to the death of the patient – the PDA is acting as a pressure release valve for the pulmonary circulation. Drugs like the phosphodiesterase V inhibitor, sildenafil can be used to try to reduce pulmonary artery pressure but generally have limited effect because the changes to the pulmonary arteries are structural. As the clinical signs are mainly due to polycythemia, repeated phlebotomies may be needed to control clinical signs. The amount of blood removed depends on the PCV and size of the dog. For dogs where the intervals between phlebotomies is short or who are resistant to the treatment, hydroxyurea can be used to reduce red cell production. The rate at which the PCV can change is variable so it is difficult to give precise guidelines for each dog. Generally the PCV is checked one month then 3 monthly after phlebotomy. This interval can be lengthened depending on the rate of rise of the PVC

Quality of Life with Euthanasia Decision

For dogs with small PDAs and mild aortic and pulmonic stenosis, these dogs should have a normal life expectancy. For dogs with large PDAs that are occluded at a young age and certainly before heart failure develops, again life expectancy should be normal. For dogs with significant cardiomegaly and poor systolic function, the prognosis is more guarded but these patient will have significant prolongation of life expectancy if the PDA is closed, surviving to middle to old age. Untreated dogs with a large PDA have a poor life expectancy and should be treated for heart failure as described when it occurs.

Dogs with severe pulmonic stenosis that is not treated or do not respond to balloon dilation and severe aortic stenosis should remain on beta blockers to try to prevent sudden death and decrease the dynamic obstruction. Dogs with severe disease have hypertrophied ventricles which may be poorly oxygenated especially during exercise. This can cause ventricular arrhythmias and result in collapse or, if ventricular fibrillation develops, sudden death. If dogs do not experience sudden cardiac death, they can survive to middle to old age even with severe disease. Ultimately the dogs develop systolic dysfunction due to the severe chronic pressure overload and this can be seen with a dilating left ventricular chamber on echocardiogram. When left heart failure develops, treatment is similar to other causes of congestive heart failure. There is a concern that positive inotropes such as pimobendan should be avoided as they may exacerbate the dynamic obstruction but in practice these seems to be more than balanced by the positive effects on contractility. Sub-aortic stenosis tends to be poorly responsive to the usual treatments for congestive heart failure because of the underlying etiology. Hence progression is more rapid and the time before the heart failure becomes unresponsive to therapy short. For canine subaortic stenosis there seems to be a supersevere category with dogs that have gradients of 80–130 mmHg surviving to 8.3 years but those with gradients over 130 mmHg having a median survival of 2.8 years.

Arrhythmias

Both bradycardias and tachycardias can result in clinical signs. Signs often include exercise intolerance or lethargy and collapse. While the syncopal episodes can have the classic anamnesis of occurring at exercise with flaccid paralyisis and short duration with rapid recovery, this is not always the case. Cerebral hypoxia due to the cardiac event can cause seizure like activity. The normal heart rate for dogs is extremely variable with average rates of 65–95 bpm over 24 hours. However, within that, the heart rate can vary from 40–50 bpm at rest to 250 bpm when exercising. In addition, pauses of up to 4 seconds at rest are not uncommon.

The important bradycardias include:

- Advanced (high grade) second degree AV block
- Third degree AV block
- Sick sinus syndrome (SSS)
- Persistent atrial standstill (PAS)

Significant tachycardias include:

- Atrial and supraventricular tachycardia (SVT)
- Atrial flutter
- Atrial fibrillation (AF)
- Ventricular tachycardia (VT)

Dogs with VT tend to be more symptomatic than dogs with SVT as the ventricular complex does not use the normal conduction pathways to the ventricle so the contraction is less efficient at ejecting blood.

Brief Review of Diagnostics

If an arrhythmia is detected, an ECG is essential to determine the exact rhythm abnormality. An echocardiogram can be helpful to confirm any structural changes and routine hematology and biochemistry can also be useful especially in collapsing dogs to rule out medical causes of collapse.

Second degree AV block has two forms. In type 1 (Wenckbach) the P-R length varies with subsequent complexes until there is an unconducted P wave. This usually represents high vagal tone and is atropine responsive. In type 2, the P–R interval is constant with occasional unconducted P waves. This suggests disease of the conduction system – fibrosis or degeneration – and is more likely to progress to third degree heart block in which there is no communication between the atria and the ventricles (Figure 5.15). The atria have their rate which is faster than the slow ventricular escape rhythm that keeps the dog alive.

Sick sinus syndrome (SSS) is a disease where impulse formation fails in the SA node as well as in other cardiac tissue so long pauses are seen (Figure 5.16). The disease is rarely fatal but dogs can be very symptomatic with it. Breeds typically affected include the West Highland white terrier and Miniature Schnauzer. The Miniature Schnauzer can get a particular form of SSS with periods of bradycardia and tachycardia. Often the bradycardia needs to addressed before medication given to control the tachycardia.

Atrial standstill can be caused by primary atrial myocardial disease but more commonly by hyperkalemia. As a result patients with atrial standstill should be screened for hyperkalemia. Common causes include urethral obstruction usually in cats and Addison's disease. PAS is caused by atrial myocardial disease. The ECG is characterized by a lack of P waves (Figure 5.17).

Supraventricular arrhythmias usually have a normal narrow complex appearance to the QRS as they use the conduction pathways of

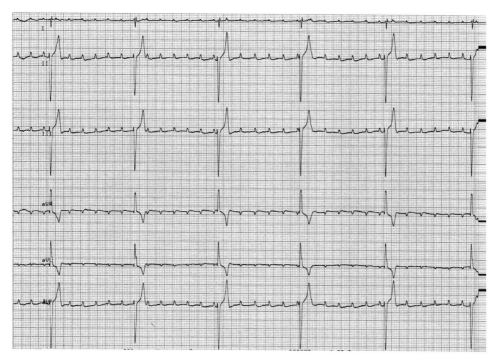

Figure 5.15 ECG from a dog with 3 degree AV block. The P waves continue through the ECG with no relation to the QRS – every P-R interval is different. The QRS are wide and bizarre as they are ventricular escape complexes. The atrial rate is 180 bpm and the ventricular rate is 30 bpm. The atrial rate is fast as the intrinsic mechanisms are trying to increase the heart (ventricular) rate. 25 mm/s and 1 cm/mV.

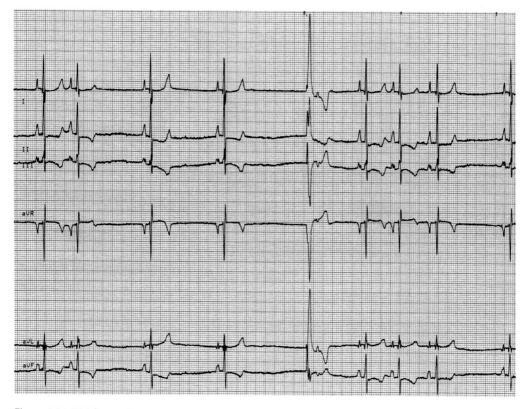

Figure 5.16 ECG from a dog with sick sinus syndrome. There are long pauses and ventricular escape complexes. 50 mm/s and 1 cm/mV.

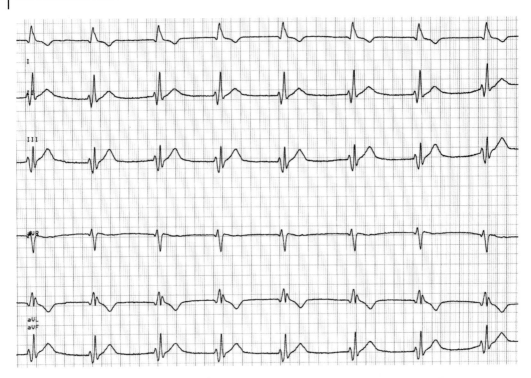

Figure 5.17 ECG from a dog with persistent atrial standstill due to atrial myocardial disease. There are no P waves on any leads. The QRS is narrow suggesting a supraventricular origin and this is because the SA node is still active with the impulse transmitted to the AV node via intermodal tracts. 50 mm/s and 5 mm/mV″ as the rate is not slow.

the ventricles while ventricular arrhythmias tend to be wide and bizarrely shaped. The latter can be positive if the origin is in the right ventricle and negative if they originate in the left ventricle. SVT is caused by either a focal atrial tachycardia, an area of the atrial myocardium that spontaneously depolarizes or an accessory pathway which is an embryological remnant of muscle that bridges the valvular fibrous ring allowing connection between the atria and ventricles outside the AV node. The P wave can be abnormal or hidden in the preceding QRS complex. However the complexes appear narrow like the sinus complexes (Figure 5.18).

Atrial flutter (Figure 5.19) and AF are particular atrial tachycardias. In atrial flutter, a macro re-entry circuit revolves round the tricuspid valve. Hence the ECG has a saw-tooth like appearance to the baseline. Atrial fibrillation is a micro re-entry circuit with at least fine or six small wavelets causing circuit rhythms in the atria (Figure 5.5). For these to

be sustained, the atria must be a certain size, hence it is more common in larger breed dogs and with atrial enlargement.

While ventricular arrhythmias (Figure 5.20; Figure 5.21) can suggest primary heart muscle disease, the underlying cause is more likely to be extracardiac. Extra cardiac causes include:

- Abdominal neoplasia especially splenic
- Gastric dilation/volvulus
- Septicemia
- Pyometra

Basically, anything that irritates the heart muscle may cause VPCs.

Therapeutics Acute, Chronic, and Expected Outcome

If possible identify the underlying cause and correct if possible. If a bradycardia is caused by high vagal tone, ocular, CNS, gastrointestinal, or respiratory disease should be suspected. In patients with hyperkalemia, the likely

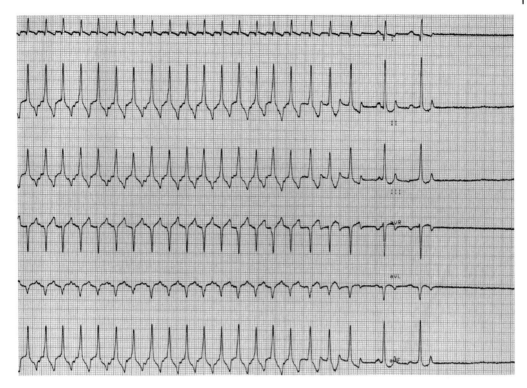

Figure 5.18 ECG from a young Labrador with supraventricular tachycardia. The complexes are narrow suggesting their supraventricular origin and the rhythm is regular. Vagal maneuvers help confirm the mechanism when the rhythm breaks to sinus. 50 mm/s and 1 cm/mV.

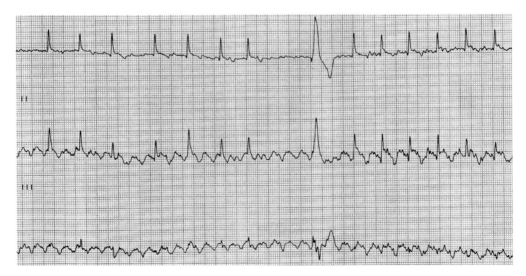

Figure 5.19 ECG from a miniature schnauzer with atrial flutter and one ventricular complex. The QRS complexes are narrow suggesting a supraventricular origin and the rhythm is irregular. A regular saw tooth like pattern can be seen on the baseline which represents the flutter wave going round the, usually tricuspid, annulus. 50 mm/s and 1 cm/mV.

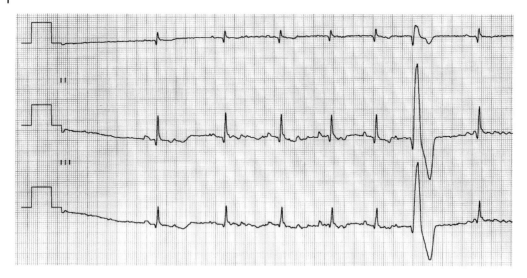

Figure 5.20 ECG from a boxer with arrhythmogenic right ventricular cardiomyopathy showing sinus rhythm and an isolated VPC. The VPC is upright in lead 2 suggesting a right ventricular origin. 50 cm/s and 1 cm/mV.

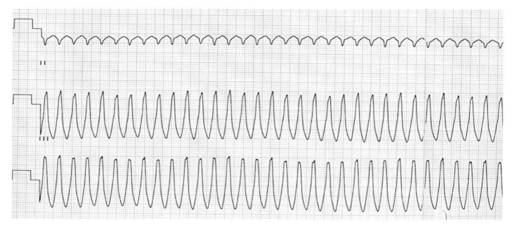

Figure 5.21 ECG from a dog with dilated cardiomyopathy showing ventricular tachycardia. The rhythm is fast and regular and the complexes are wide and bizarre suggesting a ventricular origin. This responded to lidocaine. 50 mm/s and 1 cm/mV.

causes usually include Addison's disease and urinary tract obstruction. If no underlying cause can be identified, therapies to increase heart rate may be indicated. These include:

- Drugs to decrease vagal tone: atropine or oral propantheline
- Drugs to increase sympathetic tone: iso-proterenol or terbutaline
- Drugs that increase heart rate through other mechanisms: theophylline
- Pacemaker implantation

Patients with sick sinus syndrome occasionally respond to atropine and that can translate into response to oral anticholinergic agents. Unfortunately, the response can be variable and some patients continue to be symptomatic either because of poor rate response or an increase in heart block. Patients with SSS can remain symptomatic for months to years so it seems to be relatively benign, rarely resulting in sudden death. However, it is progressive and those patients that respond initially may relapse in the future.

Dogs with high grade second degree AV and third degree AV block generally do not respond to anticholinergic drugs as there is no vagal innervation of the ventricles. They may improve temporarily with sympathomimetic agents but this increase in heart rate declines with changes in the beta receptor population. These patients ultimately require pacemaker implantation as otherwise they are at risk of sudden death. In dogs, the pacemaker is implanted dorsally over the right neck with the endocardial lead introduced into the right ventricle via the jugular vein. In cats and small dogs, an epicardial lead is used with the pacemaker implanted in the abdomen. Endocardial leads tend to cause chylous thoracic effusions in cats perhaps because of the small jugular diameter relative to the lead diameter. Potential problems include lead infection, dislodgement, and seroma formation. In dogs, if the heart block is cause by fibrosis of the conduction pathway, the life expectancy should be normal with good quality of life. However, if neoplasia or myocardial disease is documented, the prognosis is poorer. In cats, pacemaker implantation seems to have little effect on longevity. However, the cats become less symptomatic.

Tachycardias are treated with one of the four classes of anti-arrhythmia agents:

1) Class 1 – sodium channel blockers
   a) Quinidine and procainamide
   b) Lidocaine and mexiletine
   c) Flecainide and propafenone
2) Class 2 – beta blockers, for example, atenolol, propranolol, and esmolol
3) Class 3 – potassium channels blockers, for example, sotalol and amiodarone
4) Class 4 – calcium channel blockers, for example, diltiazem

Generally, class 1 and 3 are effective against ventricular arrhythmias and class 2 and 4 act on the SA and the AV node. Drugs can be combined as they have different actions so it is common to use both a class 1 and class 3 agent together to control ventricular arrhythmias. However, calcium channel blockers should not be combined with beta blockers as both agents have negative inotropic effects and the results on myocardial contractility can be significant.

SVT can be controlled with sotalol alone or in combination with a class 1 agent such as mexiletine although digoxin may be used. In patients where it is difficult to obtain control, continued lethargy may be seen but syncope is uncommon. For these patients, a tachycardiomyomathy can develop where the sustained tachycardia ultimately causes the heart muscle to become dilated and poorly contractile and they usually present in right heart failure. If the tachycardia can be controlled, these changes can reverse. If the tachycardia cannot be controlled, referral for ablation of the focus or accessory pathway using intracardiac mapping is indicated.

Atrial flutter can be a difficult arrhythmia to manage and frequently develops into atrial fibrillation. Rate response can be achieved as for atrial fibrillation but if this proves difficult, the patient can be shocked under general anesthesia back into sinus rhythm. The decision whether to go for rate or rhythm control may depend on the presence of structural heart disease, that is, large atria, and the degree to which cardiac output is dependent on atrial filling.

Atrial fibrillation is one of the most common arrhythmias encountered in clinical practice. The classic signs include a tachycardia with an irregularly irregular rhythm, narrow complex and lack of P waves. There can be exceptions, for example, the Irish Wolfhound with slow AF that can mimic sinus arrhythmia or a dog with a concomitant bundle branch block that has a wide complex tachycardia which can be mistaken for ventricular tachycardia but is irregular. As the disease is usually associated with atrial enlargement and DC cardioversion usually reverts to AF after a short period, most dogs are treated with negative chronotropes. These include:

- *Beta blockers:* Effective and the dose can be titrated upwards to give adequate rate control. Unfortunately the negative inotropic action limits their use
- *Calcium channel blockers:* Diltiazem is frequently used. While it has some negative inotropic action, this is not as marked as

beta blockers. It may potentiate digoxin and dose reduction may be required when it is introduced. It should be given three times daily but the sustained release version may be administered twice daily.

- *Digoxin:* Because of the long half-life, this drug can take up to 5–7 days to become effective and reach steady state. As its action is vagally mediated, it is used in combination with diltiazem and the combination reduces heart rate more effectively than either drug alone. Hopefully this translates into increased long-term survival but this has yet to be demonstrated. The drug has a narrow therapeutic window so owners need to be aware of the toxic side effects which if they occur will be towards the end of the first week or beyond. These include:
    o GI signs: Vomiting, diarrhea, anorexia.
    o Arrhythmias: Almost any arrhythmia may be cause by digoxin
    o Neurological signs: Dogs often appear very "depressed" according to their owners.
- Blood samples should be collected after 7 days for serum levels and most laboratories suggest a trough level at 8 hours post pill.

This raises that question of what is adequate rate control. This is poorly defined in the veterinary world and no studies exist to confirm actual numbers. It is evident that dogs presented in the clinic with controlled AF will have higher heart rates than those monitored with a Holter device. In the clinic, rates of 140–160 bpm are probably adequate, while using Holter monitors, an average rate of 120–140 bpm should be the target. If the rate is not adequately controlled and the digoxin level is low, the dose could be increased. However, if the dose is adequate, the dose of diltiazem should be increased.

Treatment of ventricular arrhythmias is a subject of ongoing debate among cardiologists especially since the CAST study that showed an increased in sudden cardiac death associated with the use of the class 1 agents, encainide and flecainide. As a result in humans, there has been a move towards the use of intracardiac defibrillators which detect VT and deliver a shock to convert the rhythm to sinus. To date these require further refinement in dogs as the current algorhythms cannot differentiate an excited dog from one in VT.

Treatment of acute symptomatic VT involves the use of lidocaine. Typically boluses of 2 mg/kg are given intravenously with a pause between each administration to see if the rhythm converts. When the total dose reaches 6 mg/kg (third bolus), the patient is observed for signs of nausea (licking lips, etc.) or tremoring, If either of these is seen, the final bolus should not be given as convulsions are likely to occur. If they do occur, they are usually short lived because of the short half-life of lidocaine in the blood stream. If lidocaine is unsuccessful, a review of whether this is truly VT should be considered. The most common rhythm abnormality that causes confusion is wide complex AF but this is usually irregular while VT is usually regular. Other agents that could be considered would include:

- Other class 1 agents: Procainamide. The failure of one class 1 agent does not necessarily mean that all class 1 agents will be unsuccessful
- Beta blockers: Esmolol is used as it is very short acting so if it is unsuccessful, other agents can be considered
- Class 3 agents: Sotalol or amiodarone. Intravenous amiodarone can cause histamine release due to the agent polysorbate 80 which increases solubility of amiodarone. Pretreatment with anti-histamine is recommended.
- Magnesium: While hypomagnesemia is recognized as a cause of ventricular arrhythmias, the serum levels may not represent actual tissue levels. Often this is tried when common anti-arrhythmic agents have failed and it should be given by slow intravenous injection.

Once VT has been controlled with lidocaine, the patient is continued on a CRI while oral medication is commenced. When the arrhythmia is adequately controlled on oral medication, the patient can be discharged.

Doberman Pinschers and Boxers have frequent ventricular arrhythmias as part of their DCM/ARVC. It has been shown that the combination of a class 1 agent and a beta blocker give better control than either agent individually. Practically, this translates into starting the patient on sotalol and repeating a Holter monitor after one month as all anti-arrhythmic medications have the potential to be pro-arrhythmic. If adequate control is not achieved, the dose can be increased or mexiletine can be added. Again, after every dose change or medication introduction, the Holter monitor should be repeated. As the daily variation in VPC count can be up to 85%, a greater than 85% reduction in VPCs is considered a success.

While the treatment of VT is necessary, there is further debate on the treatment of VPCs and short runs of VT detected on a Holter monitor. Overall, the owner should be aware that there is no evidence that anti-arrhythmic medication reduces the risk of sudden cardiac death, although it may reduce syncopal episodes. A normal dog may have occasional VPCs on a 24 hour Holter monitor and the number increases with age. If ventricular arrhythmias are detected on a Holter monitor, the decision to treat may depend on:

- The number of VPCs: If there are many thousands, treatment is more likely to be recommended
- Speed of ventricular couplets: A ventricular couplet represents two VPCs together and is never found in a normal dog. The coupling interval is important and should be reported from a Holter monitor. Although there is no published evidence, many cardiologists use a rate over 250 bpm as a guide to starting treatment.
- R on T phenomenon: This also represents a coupling interval whether between a couplet or a normal complex and a VPC. It suggests depolarization occurs during the

repolarization which a dangerous substrate for ventricular fibrillation and would warrant treatment.

- History of syncope: This suggests that the ventricular arrhythmias are hemodynamically significant, that is, they are fast or sustained enough to reduce blood pressure. The actual cause of syncope can be difficult to document on a Holter monitor. The application of a Holter monitor may alter the dog's behavior so the episode does not occur. Indeed, many cardiologists believe that a Holter monitor is a good therapeutic tool to use in collapsing dogs!
- Runs of VT: Again these are not found in a normal dog and unless slow would suggest that treatment is indicated.

Quality of Life with Euthanasia Decision

If the ventricular arrhythmias can be well controlled, then the prognosis is reasonable given the underlying cause, for example, ARVC may be progressive. According to the Harpster classification of ARVC in Boxers, Boxers with VPCs and no evidence of systolic dysfunction have the best prognosis and have mean survival times of 2 years. However, the owner should always be counselled regarding the risk of sudden death.

Treatment of ventricular arrhythmias is never straightforward and the owner must understand that one drug will not work in all cases so they need to be engage as the clinician embarks on treatment, trying drugs to find one that is appropriate and not becoming frustrated when drugs are not successful. Clearly, the most commonly effective drugs with the least side effects are tried first but on occasions these will not control the arrhythmia and others must be tried. It is unlikely that medication will stop all the arrhythmias but if they can reduce the hemodynamically significant ones, signs should resolve.

In some dogs, it may prove impossible to stop syncopal episodes and the owner must understand that these are effectively aborted sudden death. If these episodes are frequent and distress the dog and/or owner, euthanasia must be considered. In addition, most disease causing ventricular arrhythmias are incurable and progressive, so if the signs are initially well controlled, ultimately they may escape that control.

Systemic Hypertension

Blood pressure is the result of cardiac output and systemic vascular resistance and cardiac output is the result of heart rate and stroke volume. Hence anything that raises heart rate, stroke volume or vascular resistance can cause hypertension. Chronically elevated blood pressure can result in a variety of end-organ damage and so should be identified and controlled. Primary hypertension is rare in dogs and cats and so diagnosis should prompt the search for an underlying cause.

Brief Review of Diagnostics

Diagnosis is by the detection of a persistently elevated blood pressure using a sphygmomanometer and Doppler technique or the oscillometric technique. Both have been validated in dogs and cats but many find the Doppler technique more reliable in small dogs and cats. The cuff should be about 40% of the diameter of the limb. The measurement is repeated until consistent results are achieved. This technique gives the systolic pressure while the oscillometric gives systolic, diastolic, and mean pressures. A blood pressure of less than 150/95 mmHg is normal while greater than 160/100 mmHg is now regarded as abnormal in dogs and cats and further diagnostics or treatment may be warranted. An ECG, echocardiogram, or chest radiograph may show left ventricular hypertrophy.

Therapeutics Acute, Chronic, and Expected Outcome

An ACVIM consensus statement has defined the risk categories for systemic hypertension:

- *Mild risk (BP = 150–159/95–99):* This is an equivocal level and is commonly seen in stressed cats ("white coat" hypertension).

Underlying causes of hypertension may increase susceptibility to end-organ damage. No treatment is recommended but continue to monitor blood pressure
- *Moderate risk (BP = 160–179/100–119):* If confirmed by repeated measurements, begin search for underlying cause and begin anti-hypertensive treatment if end-organ damage or clinical signs
- *Severe risk (BP > 180/120):* Confirm and begin anti-hypertensive treatment even if no end-organ damage or clinical signs present.

Many diseases are found in association with systemic hypertension and the relationship can be causal:

- *Renal disease:* This is the most common underlying cause in dogs and cats and 20–30% of cats with renal disease have hypertension. The severity of renal injury is associated with a degree of hypertension. Often it is unclear whether this is a cause or effect of the hypertension
- *Adrenocortical disease:* Hyperadrenocorticism is a common cause in dogs while primary hyperaldosteronism is rarely seen
- *Diabetes mellitus:* Hypertension is seen in diabetic dogs, but has not been reported in cats. However, they should be screened if proteinuria is present
- *Hyperthyroidism:* This is a common cause in cats with 10–30% of hyperthyroid cats having hypertension
- *Pheochromocytoma:* This catecholamine producing tumor can produce severe hypertension episodically
- *Polycythemia:* The increased blood viscosity increases peripheral vascular resistance
- *Acromegaly:* This is recognized in cats.

Consequences

Many hypertensive patients are asymptomatic. Most vascular beds may autoregulate blood flow with vasomotor tone over a wide range of blood pressure. However, once the upper limit of blood pressure is exceeded, the elevated blood pressure is transmitted to the small arteries and capillaries leading to tissue damage:

- *Cardiovascular:* Concentric hypertrophy of the left ventricle rarely develops into congestive heart failure. Arteriosclerosis and hemorrhage, such as epistaxis, may be seen.
- *Renal:* Renal disease causes hypertension, but hypertension also worsens renal disease. The glomerulus, nephron, and interstitium may all be damaged by exposure to increased blood pressure leading to progression of renal disease. Glomerular damage can lead to proteinuria and the degree of proteinuria is prognostic in cats.
- *Ocular:* Hypertensive retinopathy with tortuous retinal vessels and papilledema can be seen. Retinal edema, hemorrhage, and detachment may cause acute blindness especially in cats which may be permanent.
- *Central nervous system:* CNS signs may be evident especially if hypertension is over 180 mmHg. Signs include hypertensive encephalopathy due to cerebral edema, cerebrovascular accidents (stroke) from rupture of small arteries and local ischemia but these are rare in dogs and cats These manifest as behavior alterations such as depression, ataxia, focal neurologic deficits, stupor, coma, seizures, and death.

Treatment

The rationale for treatment is to eliminate clinical signs and prevent or potentially reverse end-organ damage. Therefore, the decision to treat should be based on the presence or relative risk of end-organ damage and clinical signs. Hypertension in dogs is often more difficult to control than in cats. Since hypertension is most often secondary, underlying causes must be diagnosed and managed. In most cases though, anti-hypertensive therapy is continued indefinitely.

Treatment is usually started with one therapy and titrated to effect. Two or more drugs may be combined if initial response is inadequate:

Salt restriction: The goal is to decrease total body sodium and extracellular fluid volume but this alone does not reduce blood pressure, except in some cases of essential hypertension. Salt restriction may actually activate the renin-angiotensin-aldosterone system to increase peripheral vascular resistance and can worsen cardiovascular and renal consequences. As a result, salt restriction is not recommended, but high salt intake should be avoided.

ACE inhibitors: These act by blocking the conversion of angiotensin I to angiotensin II as well as decreasing breakdown of bradykinin and hence causing vasodilation. They also reduce secretion of aldosterone and antidiuretic hormone to cause sodium and water excretion. They are renoprotective as they reduced glomerular pressure and proteinuria. However, they also decrease glomerular filtraction rate and may cause azotemia and hyperkalemia. As single agents, they are unlikely to provide sufficient blood pressure control alone but may help in cats with renal insufficiency and proteinuria. Decreases in blood pressure of 5–10 mmHg can be expected so they can be combined with other drugs (e.g., calcium channel blockers) in both dogs and cats. Enalapril and benazepril are the most commonly used but benazepril may be preferred as it is 50% cleared by the liver.

Calcium channel blockers: These decrease calcium influx into vascular smooth muscle cells to cause vasodilation but this may activate the renin-angiotensin-aldosterone system. Often used in combination with ACE inhibitors, the most commonly used drug is amlodipine which has almost exclusive vascular effects. Amlodipine is the first-line anti-hypertensive drug in cats and may be in dogs. It may cause preferential vasodilation of afferent renal arterioles and increase intraglomerular pressure which can promote glomerular damage hence combining with an ACE inhibitor may be beneficial. As with any drug that lowers blood pressure, it can cause a reflex tachycardia in dogs.

Adrenergic blockers: Beta-blockers decrease heart rate and contractility to reduce cardiac output. They are the treatment of choice for hypertension due to hyperthyroidism, combined with amlodipine. Some cats remain hypertensive and require therapy even when their hyperthyroidism is controlled. They should not be used for pheochromocytomas before adequate alpha-blockage. The two commonly used beta blockers are propranolol which is a nonspecific beta-blocker and atenolol which is a cardio-selective β_1-blocker. α_1-blockers cause peripheral vasodilation and are the treatment of choice for pheochromocytomas, for example, phenoxybenzamine and prazosin which are non-specific alpha- and beta-blockers that decrease cardiac output and cause vasodilation.

Hydralazine: This causes direct vasodilation by an unknown mechanism and is a potent vasodilator with rapid onset of action. Reflex tachycardia is a significant and dose-limiting side effect.

Nitroprusside: This is a nitric oxide donor which is a potent vasodilator. It has a very rapid onset of action and very short half-life but must be administered by a constant rate infusion. High doses or prolonged treatment may lead to cyanide toxicity. While it may be needed in the emergency treatment of congestive heart failure, it has no role in chronic treatment.

Quality of Life with Euthanasia Decision

Control of blood pressure can usually be achieved although there may be exceptions. In many cases, it is the progression of the underlying disease that is the deciding factor in the decisions regarding quality of life. While some patients can cope well with acute onset blindness, others become very depressed and show marked behavior changes with poor quality of life.

Pulmonary Hypertension

Similar to systemic blood pressure, pulmonary pressures are the product of the blood flow, vascular resistance, and pulmonary venous pressure. An increase in any of these can result in pulmonary hypertension. The pulmonary vasculature is a low resistance, high capacitance circuit with a normal systolic pressure of 25 mmHg. Hypoxia leads to vasoconstriction regionally so that perfusion is matched to circulation. Vascular tone is maintained by a balance between vasodilating and vasoconstricting factors with the endothelium playing a key role locally.

Vasodilating factors derived from the endothelium include:

- Nitric oxide
- Prostacyclin (PGI$_2$)

While vasoconstricting factors include:

- Thromboxane and serotonin derived from platelets
- Endothelin 1 from the endothelium
- Angiotensin II both systemically and locally derived

Brief Review of Diagnostics

Clinical signs are usually non-specific including lethargy and anorexia although respiratory signs including tachypnea and a cough can be seen. The patients may be cyanotic on exercise and may become syncopal. In chronic cases, right heart failure with ascites may be documented. On physical examination, abnormal lungs sounds, cyanosis, and evidence of right heart failure may be found. A split S2 heart sound is suggestive and a right apical systolic murmur of tricuspid regurgitation may be auscultated.

Direct measurement of pulmonary artery pressures would require cardiac catheterization so this is not usually performed. Thoracic radiographs may show evidence of right heart enlargement and/or respiratory disease. The main pulmonary arteries are dilated in chronic disease with a bulge at the 1–2 o'clock position on the DV. The pulmonary arteries may be tortuous or rapidly tapering. An ECG may show evidence of right heart enlargement (tall P wave, deep negative S wave and right axis deviation). Echocardiography can demonstrate the right ventricular concentric hypertrophy with right atrial enlargement. The pulmonary artery is usually larger than the aorta. If tricuspid regurgitation is present, spectral Doppler can be used to estimate the pulmonary artery pressures by the modified Bernoulli equation (pressure gradient in mmHg = $4 \times V^2$ in m/s). Pulmonic regurgitation may be used to estimate pulmonary diastolic pressure. Systolic pressures under 50 mmHg suggest mild disease, 50–80 moderate and over 80 severe (Figure 5.22).

Causes are usually divided into pre-capillary, capillary, and post-capillary. As for systemic hypertension, primary pulmonary hypertension is rare in dogs and cats. Pre-capillary causes include heartworm disease, pulmonary thromboembolism, congenital cardiac shunts (e.g., uncorrected PDA). Capillary hypertension is caused by lung disease such as chronic bronchitis or interstitial pulmonary fibrosis. Post-capillary causes refer to disease associated with chronically elevated pulmonary venous pressure, for example, myxomatous mitral valve disease

and DCM. Heartworm disease or myxomatous mitral valve disease are the most common causes depending on which part of the world you live.

Therapeutics Acute, Chronic, and Expected Outcome

Specific treatment for pulmonary hypertension is usually unsuccessful as the pulmonary vasculature is already irreversibly damaged. However, clinical signs can be improved. Control of left heart failure can be beneficial and addressing heartworm infection will stop ongoing damage although the disease may show acute deterioration when the worms are killed. Treatment options include oxygen which is a potent vasodilator but not a long-term solution and nitric oxide which also must be inhaled.

For chronic disease, calcium channel blockers, for example, diltiazem is used in humans but has not been studied in dogs and cats. ACE inhibitors have little effect on pulmonary artery pressure but may help delay pulmonary vascular remodeling. Phosphodiesterase 5 inhibitors are the most widely used agents, for example, sildenafil and tadalafil. Although the reduction in pulmonary artery pressure is modest and sometimes hard to document,

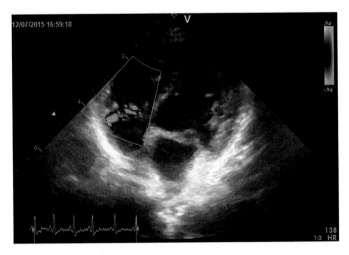

Figure 5.22 Left parasternal long axis cranial systolic frame showing the right ventricle, right atrium, and tricuspid valve. There is a green turbulent jet of tricuspid regurgitation and the velocity can be measured. Using the modified Bernoulli principle, the pressure in the right ventricle and hence pulmonary artery can be estimated. This can be used to asses for pulmonary hypertension non-invasively.

clinical signs can improve significantly. However, they can increase left heart preload and precipitate congestive heart failure so in cases of advanced left-sided disease, they should be introduced at a low dose and titrated upwards. Pimobendan is a phosphodiesterase 3 inhibitor and may have some action on the pulmonary vascular tone. Endothelin antagonists, for example, bosentan, are effective but their costs prohibit their use in most cases.

Quality of Life with Euthanasia Decision

The prognosis depends on the underlying disease. In dogs with degenerative valve disease, a pulmonary artery pressure over 55 mmHg suggests a poorer prognosis and may warrant treatment. Dogs with shunts such as a PDA cannot have the PDA closed as this leads to acute death but their polycythemia can be chronically managed. Heartworm disease should be treated as per the American Heartworm Association guidelines but the pulmonary hypertension does not usually resolve. If right heart failure develops, it should be treated as described previously.

Pericardial Effusion

As fluid in the pericardium accumulates, the pressure rises. Initially there are no clinical signs until the pressure starts to exceed the pressure in the lowest pressure chamber, the right atrium. Cardiac tamponade describes the clinical syndrome of right heart failure secondary to a pericardial effusion.

While heart failure is usually treated with diuretics, this is the exception as diuretics will decrease systemic venous pressure which is responsible for filling the right heart. In the short term, intravenous fluids may be used to augment cardiac output although unless the patient is critical, these are often not needed. Causes include:

- Idiopathic: Seen in younger dogs especially St Bernards
- Neoplastic: Hemangiosarcomas are common in older dogs especially Golden Retrievers

and German Shepherd Dogs, Heart base tumors (chemodectomas) are seen in brachycephalic breeds such as Boxers. Other tumors are occasionally recognized including mesothelioma, ectopic thyroid carcinomas, and lymphoma
- Left atrial tear secondary to chronic degenerative mitral valve disease
- Infectious causes and secondary causes such as hypoalbuminemia are seen.

Brief Review of Diagnostics

Clinical examination: Muffled heart sounds with a weak rapid pulse may be detected. If right heart failure is present, a distended abdomen with a fluid thrill may be seen. Pulsus paradoxus is present in some cases. The pulse disappears during inspiration but returns during expiration. This is an example of ventricular interdependence.

ECG: Small complexes are seen due to the presence of fluid. In some cases, electrical alternans may be present with alternating heights of the R waves due to changing mean electrical axis as the heart swings in the fluid.

Radiographs: A round globoid "still" cardiac silhouette is seen. The caudal vena cava is enlarged especially if ascites is detected.

Echocardiography: This is the diagnostic test of choice (Figure 5.23). Not only can it confirm the diagnosis showing the dark fluid around the heart and the cardiac tamponade with collapse of the right atrial wall but it can also guide treatment and help detect an underlying cause. Common places for neoplasia include the right auricle and right AV junction for hemangiosarcoma and the great vessels for chemodectomas. Masses are most easily visualized when some fluid is present. But it should be noted that echocardiography is not a good guide to identify tumor type. Echocardiography can also be used to guide treatment.

Therapeutics Acute, Chronic, and Expected Outcome

Acute drainage of the pericardium usually causes rapid resolution of clinical signs. In the short term, intravenous fluid should be

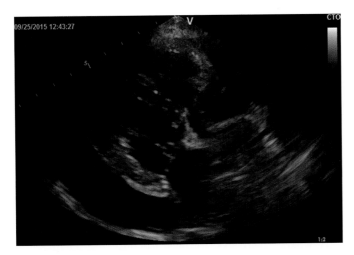

Figure 5.23 Right parasternal long axis echocardiogram from a dog with a pericardial effusion. The dark ring around the heart is the effusion. The collapse of the right atrial free wall can be visualized suggesting cardiac tamponade is present. Detection of a tumor is easier if fluid is still present but once this has been performed, drainage of the fluid is indicated.

given at a high rate to maintain systemic venous pressures and hence right atrial filling. In critical patients, the effusion may need to be drained before a detailed echocardiogram can be performed but in less severely affected dogs, an echocardiographic search for a neoplastic cause should be completed.

Pericardiocentesis is usually preformed from the right side with the patient in left lateral recumbency under mild sedation. Echocardiography is used to image a window such that the depth of fluid is maximized and the needle is likely to impinge on the pericardium at 90° hence there is less chance it will glance off into the surrounding lung tissue. (Figure 5.24) The needle is then advanced along the same line and angle as the echocardiographic probe while negative pressure is applied to the syringe. A variety of pericardiocentesis catheters are available but many use 14 G catheters with extra holes cut. An ECG should be attached to document any arrhythmias that may indicate the right ventricle has been touched with the needle. Once fluid starts to return, the catheter is advanced off the needle and a drainage system attached. The fluid should be retained as it does not usually clot unless the hemorrhage is acute. In addition, the supernatent will differ from serum if spun down in a

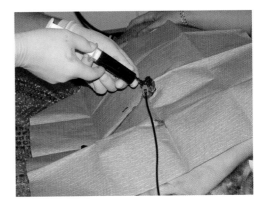

Figure 5.24 Image of a dog undergoing drainage of a pericardial effusion. The dog has been sedated with an opiate and a local anesthetic was used in the chest wall. Having obtained an echocardiographic image maximizing the depth of pericardial effusion, a fenestrated catheter is advanced under suction along the probe line until fluid returns. The catheter is then fed off the needle and a three-way tap attached. Echocardiography can be repeated to assess the amount of fluid remaining.

centrifuge. Once the drainage starts to decrease, echocardiography should be performed. The right heart should re-expand and the pericardial effusion be reduced significantly. The volume of the effusion can vary up to 2 liters depending on the size of the patient and speed of development. The ascites usually resolves in 24–48 hours and diuretics are not needed although the ascites will resolve faster if they are used.

Although the pericardial effusion should be submitted for cytology, it is rarely helpful. It is rarely possible to differentiate reactive mesothelial cells from mesothelioma. However on occasions the fluid is not a modified transudate or lymphoma cells are seen. The common neoplasia do not exfoliate.

Reevaluation depends on the underlying cause. For idiopathic effusion, they can re-effuse after very variable intervals so repeat echocardiography may not be helpful. Instead, the owner should be vigilant for the clinical signs and return if they recur. Owners should be warned that there is a 50% chance of recurrence. However, if the effusion recurs, the owner should be advised that pericardectomy should be performed as repeated drainage increases the risk of constrictive pericardial disease. Pericardectomy should be curative in these cases. Neoplastic causes are likely to have more rapid recurrence of clinical signs but again, treatment would only be performed if the effusion was causing clinical signs. Pericardectomy may be offered for control although this depends on tumor type. For chemodectomas which are relatively benign and slow growing, pericardectomy can offer prolonged survival times of up to 3 years. Surgical resection of the tumor is not usually possible. Hemangiosarcomas have a poorer prognosis and surgical resection may not prolong life although survival times of 7–8 months with resection and chemotherapy have been reported. The owner should be warned that an acute bleed into the pleural cavity after pericardectomy may result in sudden death. In cases of mesothelioma, pericardiocentesis will cause tumor cells to spread to the pleural cavity allowing a pleural effusion to develop. Chemotherapy may improve survival time up to 10 months.

Pericardectomy: Sub-total pericardectomy may be performed with a lateral or sternal thoracotomy. While the sternal approach allows better visualization to look for any masses, recovery is slower with more complications. This is the treatment of choice in constrictive pericardial disease but the surgery is associated with high morbidity and mortality as the thickened fibrotic pericardium is stripped from the heart with significant hemorrhage. Thorascopic pericardectomy can be performed but this often results in a window being cut in the pericardium which may seal with time causing recurrence of clinical signs. Balloon dilation of the pericardium to tear a window has been described but is not widely performed.

Quality of Life with Euthanasia Decision
Many dogs can be managed with repeated drainage of their pericardium. However, if the frequency increases, there needs to be consideration as to whether the periods that are symptom free justify continued treatment. For patients with neoplastic effusion, sudden death can occur or a pleural effusion may prompt a discussion regarding quality of life.

Further Reading

Bonagura JD, Twedt DC Kirk's current veterinary therapy XV. Elsevier. 2014: 720–838.

Cote E, MacDonald KA. Feline cardiology. Wiley-Blackwell. 2011

Ettinger SJ, Feldman EC. Textbook of veterinary internal medicine, 7th Ed. Saunders/Elsevier. 2010: 1143–1394.

Luis Fuentes V, Johnson RL, Dennis S. BSAVA manual of canine and feline cardiorespiratory medicine, 2nd Ed. Quedgeley: British Small Animal Veterinary Association. 2010.

Smith FWK, Oyama MA, Tilley LP, Sleeper MM. Manual of canine and feline cardiology, 5th Ed. Elsevier. 2016.

Ware WA. Cardiovascular disease in small animal medicine. The Veterinary Press. 2011.

6

Canine Cognitive Dysfunction

Sheila Carrera-Justiz

Introduction

Canine Cognitive Dysfunction (CCD), also known as canine dementia, is an age-related neurobehavioral syndrome. It is common in geriatric dogs, typically at least 12 years of age, but it is commonly underdiagnosed. Estimates place the prevalence of this disorder anywhere from 14–60% with increasing age. The disorder is characterized by deficits in learning, memory, and spatial awareness. Changes in social interactions and sleeping patterns are also common.

There are many characteristic changes associated with CCD, but four key clinical signs are most obvious: sleeping during the day and restlessness at night, decreased interaction, disorientation at home, and anxiety. The Canine Dementia Scale (CADES) is an example of one scoring method for assessing CCD (Table 6.1).

Diagnosis

Index of Suspicion

It is important to question owners of geriatric dogs about the characteristic behavior changes. Many owners do not notice or report these behaviors and take it for granted that this "is just normal aging." I ask owners about sleep-wake cycles by asking if the dog sleeps through the night or is waking them up. I ask about urination and bowel habits and if the dog is having accidents in the house. If so, then I try to determine if it is incontinence or inappropriate urination and defecation. I also ask about social interactions and behaviors such as tricks and following commands. Some owners are very astute and note changes like the dog going to the wrong side of the door to be let out.

Diagnostics

As, these patients are geriatric, other diseases may be present in the same patient. There are many systemic disorders that can make a patient with mild brain dysfunction decompensate and clinically look much worse. I highly recommend screening these patients with a complete blood count, serum chemistry profile, urinalysis, and blood pressure measurement. Inappropriate urination and loss of house training are often seen with CCD, but it is important to culture a sterilely collected urine sample to rule out a bacterial cystitis or pyelonephritis that could induce or worsen these behaviors. Disorders like hypertension, hyperadrenocorticism, anemia, and many others can induce behavior changes or exacerbate preexisting anxiety.

Thoracic radiographs and an abdominal ultrasound are my next steps. With these tests I am looking for significant concurrent

Chronic Disease Management for Small Animals, First Edition. Edited by W. Dunbar Gram, Rowan J. Milner and Remo Lobetti.

Table 6.1 *Canine* Dementia Scale (CADES) Frequency: 0 points - abnormal behavior of the dog was never observed, 2 points – abnormal behavior of the dog was detected at least once in the last 6 months, 3 points – abnormal behavior appeared at least once per month, 4 points – abnormal behavior was seen 2–4 times per month, 5 points - abnormal behavior was observed several times a week. Source: Table adapted from Madari *et al.* 2015, p. 140. Reproduced with permission of Elsevier.

Domain/items

A. Spatial orientation	**B. Social interaction**
1, disorientation in a familiar environment (inside/outside)	6, changes in interaction a man/dog, dog/other dog (playing, petting, welcoming)
2, to recognise familiar people and animals inside or outside the house/apartment	7, changes in individual behaviour of dog (exploration behaviour, play, performance)
3, abnormally respond to familiar objects (a chair, a wastebasket)	8, response to commands and ability to learn new task
4, aimlessly wandering (motorically restless during day)	9, irritable
5, a reduced ability to do previously learned task	10, expression of aggression
SCORE (0–25)	SCORE (0–25)
C. Sleep-wake cycles	**D. House soiling**
11, abnormally responds in night (wandering, vocalization, motorically restless)	13, eliminate at home at random locations
12, switch over from insomnia to hypersomnia	14, eliminate in its kennel or sleeping area
Score × 2(0–20)	15, changes in signalisation for elimination activity
	16, eliminate indoors after a recent walk outside
	17, eliminate at uncommon locations (grass, concrete)
	SCORE(0–25)

Total score(A + B + C + D)(0–95).
Clinical stage: Normal ageing (Score 0–7), Mild cognitive impairment (8–23), Moderate cognitive impairment (24–44), Severe cognitive impairment (45–95).

Box 6.1

Common signs of CCD include: sleeping during the day and restlessness at night, decreased interaction, disorientation at home, and anxiety.

disease that could explain current signs or significantly alter my treatment and management recommendations.

Definitive diagnosis of CCD is difficult. It is really a diagnosis of exclusion, though there are multiple typical characteristics. Physical examination findings can vary from patient to patient. Neurological examination and behavioral evaluation are more helpful. Dogs with CCD are not mentally appropriate, ranging from mildly obtunded to demented. They are generally prone to be compulsive and anxious in a foreign environment like an examination room. They also tend to get very anxious and mentally inappropriate when restrained. They also often exhibit inappropriate vocalization. The neurologic examination is generally symmetrical with no overt deficits other than mentation changes and compulsion. If you note lateralizing, asymmetrical abnormalities, then you should be more concerned about an active process.

Imaging of the brain by magnetic resonance imaging (MRI) is the most definitive diagnostic test to support your clinical diagnosis as it will rule out a brain tumor, which is your main differential diagnosis. MRI can also show the characteristic imaging changes of canine cognitive dysfunction, which are generalized brain atrophy, enlarged ventricles, and reduced thickness of the interthalamic adhesion. The other supportive test for CCD is to have the owner complete a validated questionnaire for CCD. Table 6.2 shows an example utilizing another scoring method used to help make the diagnosis. This patient's score utilizing the Canine Cognitive Dysfunction Rating Scale (CCDR) exceeded the threshold of 50 points.

Differentials

The main differential diagnosis for a geriatric dog with progressive behavior changes is a brain tumor. Because of this, consultation with a veterinary neurologist and an MRI of the brain should be offered to the owner. A brain tumor is not yet truly curable, but can be managed so as to ensure a good quality of life.

Therapeutics

Unfortunately, there is no rapidly acting treatment to improve clinical signs, nor is there any treatment that can reverse or even halt this process. However, management of anxiety can make a significant impact on the quality of life of both the patient and the family. There are multiple options for managing anxiety in dogs. Alprazolam is my first choice as it is very safe and does not interfere with most concurrent diseases. It can be administered at 0.01–0.1 mg/kg once to twice daily or as needed an hour before bed to aid in sleep. It is a benzodiazepine, so there is the potential for a paradoxical reaction. Trazodone can also be used as an anxiolytic at 2–5 mg/kg two to three times daily. Trazodone and tramadol can be administered together with care – dose adjustments must be made as higher doses of both in combination can

induce serotonin syndrome. Oral acepromazine is another option, but oral absorption is erratic and unreliable in the dog, so you must carefully titrate the dose to effect; overdoses of acepromazine can also cause significant hypotension. I never recommend using phenobarbital for sedation as it can have significant side effects including hepatopathies and blood dyscrasias.

Chronic therapeutic options include pharmaceuticals and neutraceuticals. Selegiline (Anipryl), is a monoamine oxidase B inhibitor that should be administered at 0.5–1 mg/kg once daily in the morning. Selegiline should not be combined with tricyclic antidepressants or selective serotonin reuptake inhibitors, and should be used cautiously with other drugs that can enhance serotonin function (like tramadol and trazodone) due to the potential for serotonin syndrome. S-adenosylmethionine (SAMe) has also been shown to reduce age-related mental decline in dogs; it should be administered at 18 mg/kg for at least 2 months. L-Carnitine and omega-3 fatty acids have also been used in dogs with CCD. There is also some evidence for vitamins E and C and antioxidants in the diet. None of these therapies can halt the progression of disease nor can they make clinical signs go away completely. These treatments also are slow to act. They all need to be administered for at least one month, ideally two, before any clinical effect is seen.

There is no one therapy that has significant benefits over another, though multiple therapies can be initiated at once.

Rescue or relapse therapies for CCD mainly focus on preventing or treating anxiety. This can be done preemptively, when a known stressful scenario is coming and the owners can pre-treat. A good example of this would be houseguests visiting and disrupting the normal schedule of the household. This kind of aberration often induces marked anxiety in CCD patients, so a short-acting anxiolytic drug like alprazolam or trazodone can be used to effect. The same drugs can be used if there is an unforeseen event that causes a crisis. In this scenario, a benzodiazepine is more

Table 6.2 Canine cognitive dysfunction rating scale with example data for a dog over the threshold (P50) for query diagnosis.

	(1) Never	(2) Once a month	(3) Once a week	(4) Once a day	(5) >Once a day	Score
How often does your dog pace up and down, walk in circles and/or wander with no direction or purpose?				X		4
How often does your dog stare blankly at the walls or floor?			X			3
How often does your dog get stuck behind objects and is unable to get around?	X					1
How often does your dog fail to recognise familiar people or pets?				X		4
How often does your dog walk into walls or doors?		X				2
How often does your dog walk away while, or avoid, being patted?			X			3
	Never	1–30% of times	31–60% of times	61–99% of times	Always	
How often does your dog have difficulty finding food dropped on the floor?				X		4
	Much less	Slightly less	The same	Slightly more	Much more	
Compared with 6 months ago, does your dog now pace up and down, walk in circles and/or wander with no direction or purpose					X	5
Compared with 6 months ago, does your dog now stare blankly at the walls or floor			X			3
Compared with 6 months ago, does your dog urinate or defecate in an area it has previously kept clean (if your dog has never house-soiled, tick 'the same')				X		4
Compared with 6 months ago, does your dog have difficulty finding food dropped on the floor				X		x2 8
Compare with 6 months ago, does your dog fail to recognise familiar people or pets					X	x3 15
	Much more	Slightly more	The same	Slightly less	Much less	
Compared with 6 months ago, is the amount of time your dog spends active				X		4
					Total	60

Source: Salvin *et al.* 2011, p. 334. Reproduced with permission of Elsevier.

effective as it is more rapid-acting. Unfortunately, there is no true rescue therapy as there is nothing that has been shown to reverse the disease process.

All of the above-listed drug therapies have been shown to have some effect, but they do not all work in every case! Generally, any one therapy will work in about 50% of dogs, but they will take at least a month to show any effect. If no intervention is performed, the condition will simply progress in its natural course.

Any of the therapies listed will have a greater effect if started earlier in the clinical disease process. The later in the disease, and the more severely affected the animal, the less likely you are to get a great clinical effect from any medication.

As a clinician, it is important to have objective measurements for the patient. Here, you can use serial neurological examinations and behavioral assessments to monitor progression of the disease. The CADES or CCDR scales are also very useful as monitoring tools as they will give you a number and not just an opinion. Because quality of life means different things to different people, the objectivity of validated scales can be very helpful. Pain is not typically a component of CCD, but geriatric dogs often suffer from degenerative joint disease or chronic spinal cord disease and may show discomfort as a result of that; if there is any question of pain, it should be treated. The inappropriate vocalizations often exhibited by patients affected with CCD may represent disorientation, anxiety, or pain. These patients exhibit progressive loss of mental function and will eventually end up totally unaware of their surroundings. This progression can occur over months to years, depending on how early signs are noted. As the disease progresses, there will be loss of function manifested in deterioration

---

Box 6.2

A pet's chronic progressive loss of function and ability to perform normal activities can be devastating to clients.

---

of mental abilities, less and less recognition of the owner and familiars, loss of house training, and decreased interaction.

A caregiver's expectations, ability, and quality of life are also considerations with regards to the care of a pet with CCD. Client ability to provide care or accept patient's status must be taken into account. Considerations such as medication regime, emotional, financial, and physical ability of a client to care for the patient should be discussed. To make the unknown less intimidating, it is important to inform the owners that this is a progressive and incurable condition. Whatever treatments are chosen are meant to be palliative and will only help slow the progression; they will not cure the disease. In some circumstances, hospice care (see chapter 36) could be helpful to the client.

End of Life

Canine cognitive dysfunction is not itself a terminal disease, but it will progress and eventually compromise quality of life for both the pet and the owner to such a point that euthanasia is the best option for all parties involved. Patients with CCD are generally euthanized due to concerns over quality of life. The CADES or CCDR questionnaire scales can provide an objective measure to help clients decide not only when to initiate treatment, but to point out when there has been significant decline and aid in the decision to euthanize.

Further Reading

Fast R, Schutt T, Toft N, Moller A, Berendt M. An observational study with long-term

follow-up of canine cognitive dysfunction: clinical characteristics, survival, and risk factors. Journal of Veterinary Internal Medicine. 2013; 27: 822–829.

Landsberg GM, DePorter T, Araujo JA. Clinical signs and management of anxiety, sleeplessness, and cognitive dysfunction in the senior pet. Veterinary Clinics of North America: Small Animal Practice. 2011; 41(3): 565–590.

Madari A, Farbakova J, Katina S et al. Assessment of severity and progression of canine cognitive dysfunction syndrome using the CAnine DEmentia Scale (CADES). Applied Animal Behaviour Science. 2015; 171: 138–145.

Salvin HE, McGreevy PD, Sachdev PS, Valenzuela MJ. The canine cognitive dysfunction rating scale (CCDR): A data-driven and ecologically relevant assessment tool. The Veterinary Journal. 2011; 188(3): 331–336.

7

Vestibular Syndromes

Sheila Carrera-Justiz

Introduction

The vestibular system is responsible for balance, coordination, and maintenance of posture in the face of gravity. It is a bilateral system that is always on; the receptors in the inner ear send information to nuclei in the brainstem that project to higher centers in the brain and down to the spinal cord. It is the balance of inputs from both left and right inner ears that allows for us to be upright. If there is dysfunction anywhere along this system, there can be abnormalities in head or body posture, balance, and ambulation.

Diagnosis

Hallmark clinical signs of vestibular disease include a head tilt, abnormal resting nystagmus, and vestibular ataxia. However, a complete neurological examination is necessary to be able to make a neurolocalization and appropriate list of differential diagnoses. The first, critical step with vestibular disease is to distinguish a central from a peripheral lesion.

Box 7.1

Differentiation of a central lesion from a peripheral lesion is the first critical step in determining the cause of vestibular symptoms

---

Diagnostic testing will give you the information necessary to make a more definitive diagnosis and appropriately determine prognosis. Watchful monitoring is really only a good option in the mildly affected patient. Medical management of the moderate to severely vestibular patient is labor intensive and difficult.

Diagnostic testing is of crucial importance in central vestibular cases. Once your list of differential diagnoses has been made, it is important to consider advanced imaging to determine prognosis. Magnetic resonance imaging (MRI) is the test of choice for diseases affecting the caudal fossa (brainstem and cerebellum). Computed tomography (CT) does not allow for good visualization of the brainstem and cerebellum due to artifact (beam hardening) from all the bone in the area. If you believe the disease to truly be peripheral, then CT is a very good test for visualization of the ear canals and tympanic bullae. If you have any concern that there may be central involvement, then MRI is your test of choice (Figure 7.1).

Peripheral Vestibular Structures

The peripheral vestibular structures include the receptors, the ganglion, and the peripheral axons of the vestibular portion of CN VIII. Dysfunction of the peripheral vestibular system can cause loss of balance, vestibular ataxia, head tilt toward the affected side,

Chronic Disease Management for Small Animals, First Edition. Edited by W. Dunbar Gram, Rowan J. Milner and Remo Lobetti.
© 2018 John Wiley & Sons, Inc. Published 2018 by John Wiley & Sons, Inc.

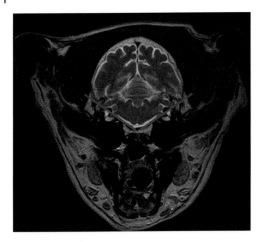

Figure 7.1 Magnetic resonance image of a brain with lines. Inside the lines is central vestibular (brainstem and cerebellum) while outside are peripheral vestibular structures (ear canals, tympanum, tympanic bulla and CN VIII).

horizontal or rotary nystagmus, and positional strabismus. Typically, dogs with peripheral vestibular dysfunction have more rapid nystagmus (>60 beats per second) than dogs with central disease. Both Horner's syndrome and facial nerve paralysis can be seen with peripheral vestibular disease as those nerves travel in the vicinity of the tympanic bulla.

Central Vestibular Structures

The central vestibular structures include the nuclei in the medulla of the brainstem and their projections to the cerebellum, spinal cord, and rostral brainstem. Animals with central vestibular dysfunction can show all the clinical signs of those with peripheral vestibular dysfunction as well as many others. Important findings to definitively localize a vestibular lesion as central are proprioceptive deficits and paresis (motor deficits) – if deficits are noted, the lesion is located centrally, in the brainstem. This is because the lesion is affecting those ascending sensory or descending motor tracts. However, the converse is not always true; a lack of proprioceptive deficits does not rule out a central lesion. Other signs, including vertical nystagmus, nystagmus for which the fast phase changes

direction, cerebellar signs (hypermetria), altered mental status, spinal ataxia, dysmetria, upper motor neuron paresis, intention tremors, and any cranial nerve deficit other than VII, are consistent with central vestibular disease.

Paradoxical Vestibular Disease

Paradoxical vestibular disease is always central! In this case, the head usually tilts away from the side of the lesion while all the other abnormalities (nystagmus, falling, proprioceptive deficits, hypermetria) are on the affected side.

The lists of differential diagnoses are vastly different for central and peripheral lesions, so it is very important to make this distinction. Generally speaking, peripheral diseases have a better prognosis and are easier to definitively diagnose than central disorders. Central vestibular disorders can have a more guarded prognosis and require more advanced and expensive diagnostic tests.

Box 7.2

Peripheral vestibular disorders tend to have a better prognosis and are easier to definitively diagnose than central disorders

---

Peripheral Vestibular Disease

Differentials include idiopathic geriatric vestibular disease, otitis media/interna, inflammatory polyps, cholesteatomas, aural neoplasia, toxicosis, hypothyroidism, and polyneuropathy. Idiopathic geriatric vestibular disease, "old dog vestibular disease," typically occurs in geriatric large breed dogs, though any breed can be affected.

A note about bilateral peripheral disease. There is the scenario where you have disease affecting both left and right inner ears. Because both receptors are non-functional, you lose ALL perception of gravity and movement. This means physiologic nystagmus is lost and animals' gait typically becomes very low, crouched and wide-based.

Central Vestibular Disease

Differentials include CNS neoplasia, inflammatory CNS disease, otogenic intracranial infections, trauma, toxicoses, vascular and infectious disease. Dogs with central vestibular lesions are more likely to be non-ambulatory than those with peripheral dysfunction. Primary CNS neoplasia typically has a chronic, progressive history, though metastatic lesions can have a peracute onset. Inflammatory, immune-mediated CNS disease is very common and mostly affects young to middle-aged small-breed terrier and toy breed dogs. Otogenic intracranial infections, expansion of otitis media/interna into the cranial vault, are rare. They typically occur in dogs with a history of chronic ear disease, though it is possible to have disease in the bulla without disease in the ear canals.

Metronidazole Toxicity

Metronidazole can cause central vestibular dysfunction at doses of 60 mg/kg/day in as little as 3 days. The clinical signs will improve once the medication is discontinued, and diazepam at 1 mg/kg PO TID in dogs can be used to hasten recovery.

Diagnostic Conundrum

It's too vestibular to tell! Occasionally, the animal can be so severely affected, for example, alligator rolling, that you cannot determine if the lesion is central or peripheral. In this situation there are two choices: you can medically manage the patient for 24 hours and monitor for improvement or refer for workup. If this is a geriatric large-breed dog, the chances are good this is idiopathic geriatric vestibular disease and you will see improvement in 24–48 hours.

Therapy

There are multiple potential therapeutic targets in the acutely vestibular patient. The first thing to consider is nausea. It is always recommended to use veterinary labelled drugs when available. Maropitant is an effective anti-emetic and is convenient at once daily dosing. Other options include meclizine at 25 mg/dog/day, but this only exists as a capsule.

Another therapeutic target in the severely affected vestibular patient is anxiety. These patients often benefit from some form of anxiolytic therapy. Benzodiazepines (diazepam, midazolam) and phenothiazines (acepromazine, chlorpromazine) can be administered IV for rapid effect in the very anxious, nauseated patient.

Cats should never be administered diazepam PO as an anxiolytic or appetite stimulant. They can develop idiosyncratic hepatic necrosis with enteral administration, but parenteral administration of diazepam is safe.

Box 7.3

Cats should never be administered diazepam PO due to the potential of idiosyncratic hepatic necrosis.

These patients often also require fluid therapy in the acute phase due to ptyalism, vomiting, panting, and lack of intake.

There is no non-specific maintenance therapy for vestibular dysfunction. Treatments are either symptomatic (for nausea or anxiety) or targeted to the specific cause. The only over-the-counter rescue therapy for any vestibular symptom is meclizine. Meclizine will help with nausea associated with vestibular dysfunction, but will not hasten the course of the disease. It is only available in an oral formulation which can be difficult, if not impossible, to administer to a nauseated patient. The majority of anti-anxiety and anti-emetic medications are prescription-only at this time.

Surgical intervention is only an option for a few vestibular lesions. Namely, chronic, severe otitis media/interna can warrant a total ear canal ablation and/or bulla osteotomy, especially when the ear is no longer responsive to medical management. Otogenic intracranial infections are ideally treated with surgical drainage by bulla osteotomies along with targeted antimicrobial and anti-inflammatory therapy and these have a good prognosis with treatment.

Prognosis is truly extremely variable and dependent on the underlying disease process.

Quality of Life for Patient and Caregiver

Vestibular dysfunction can cause deficits ranging from mild to severe. Dogs and cats with peripheral vestibular head tilts can live normal lives with no compromise in quality of life. Severely vestibular animals, whether central or peripheral, are often non-ambulatory and require significant nursing care for an unknown period of time.

Objective measurements for patient quality-of-life assessment can include things like mobility and appetite. If these are chronically compromised and do not respond to medical management, quality of life should be reevaluated.

End-of-Life Decisions

Severely affected vestibular animals are of the most difficult to care for. They pose a significant challenge in nursing care as they are generally nauseated, vomiting, and unwilling to eat on their own. In addition, they can be non-ambulatory and will fall or roll uncontrollably. This combination of signs makes for a high risk of aspiration pneumonia, urinary tract infections, and all the cutaneous complications that come with recumbency. Death of the patient with vestibular disease can come from the primary disease, such as progression of the brain tumor or inflammatory brain disease, or from related complications such as aspiration pneumonia. Vestibular patients that do not improve or progress in the face of treatment should be reevaluated for other confounding factors or signs of progressive disease. Quality of life should be evaluated in those cases and discussed with the owners; progression to non-ambulatory status and intractable nausea causing anorexia are generally considered end points for this condition.

Further Reading

Kent M, Platt SR, Schatzberg SJ. The neurology of balance: Function and dysfunction of the vestibular system in dogs and cats. The Veterinary Journal. 2010; 185: 247–258.

Rossmeisl JH. Vestibular disease in dogs and cats. The Veterinary Clinics of North America: Small Animal Practice. 2010; 24(1): 81–100.

Troxel MT, Drobatz KJ, Vite CH. Signs of neurologic dysfunction in dogs with central versus peripheral vestibular disease. Journal of the American Medical Association. 2005; 227(4): 570–574.

8

Seizure Disorders

Sheila Carrera-Justiz

Introduction

A seizure is a transient event due to abnormal and excessive neuronal activity in the brain, specifically the forebrain (cerebrum and diencephalon). Characteristics of seizures include autonomic signs (salivation, urination, defecation, pupillary dilation), tonic or tonic-clonic movements, and rhythmic contractions of facial or appendicular muscles. Generally, mentation is not normal during a seizure, and there is often a post-seizure phase with abnormal behavior and mentation.

Seizures can be characterized by type and pattern. Seizures are often classified as generalized, partial, and complex partial or psychomotor. A generalized seizure, also known as "grand mal," shows bilateral clinical signs and involves both cerebral hemispheres. A partial seizure has clinical signs that reflect restriction to one cerebral hemisphere; therefore only one area of the body is affected. A complex partial seizure, also known as a limbic or psychomotor seizure, involves abnormal mentation and some kind of repetitive motor activity like lip smacking. These seizures typically have a significant emotional component, a distinct lack of awareness (no loss of consciousness), and may manifest as aggression, fear, vocalization, or hysterical running. Most seizures occur as single, discrete events. More than one seizure in a 24-hour period is considered

a cluster event. Status epilepticus is often defined as continuous seizure activity for a certain minimum duration (>5–30 minutes) or more than two seizures without regaining full consciousness between episodes.

The terminology for seizure disorders is changing. Epilepsy, in essence, means recurrent seizures. Currently, what was previously known as idiopathic epilepsy is now called either genetic epilepsy (known genetic defect) or unknown epilepsy (unidentified genetic defect). Structural epilepsy encompasses symptomatic epilepsy, meaning seizures secondary to things like tumors, trauma, or meningitis. Cats with seizures and a normal neurologic examination but no diagnostic tests and survive more than 2 years are considered to have presumptive unknown epilepsy.

Diagnosis

Seizures are often diagnosed based on the history supplied by the owner rather than on the clinician witnessing the event. Because of this, it is important to ask appropriate questions to confirm that the episode was in fact a seizure and not something else. In the modern age of smart phones, it is commonplace for clients to supply videos of episodes at home which can be critical for diagnosis. If the owners' description is not convincing, asking for the owner to supply a video of the episode is a very helpful tool.

Chronic Disease Management for Small Animals, First Edition. Edited by W. Dunbar Gram, Rowan J. Milner and Remo Lobetti.
© 2018 John Wiley & Sons, Inc. Published 2018 by John Wiley & Sons, Inc.

A history and general physical examination are very important, followed by a neurologic examination. Though we generally treat all seizures the same way, it is of critical importance to know what is causing the seizures, both for appropriate long-term treatment and accurate prognosis. We must first determine if seizures are due to extra-cranial or intra-cranial disease. This is where the minimum database is crucial: a complete blood count, serum chemistry profile and urinalysis can reveal many abnormalities. A blood pressure measurement, a thyroid measurement in cats, and thoracic radiographs are also helpful in many cases. Animals with extra-cranial causes of seizures do not often require anti-seizure medications once the underlying disease is treated. Major systemic abnormalities to consider include hypoglycemia, hypocalcemia, and hepatopathies, including portosystemic shunts. Common intracranial causes of seizures include idiopathic processes, inflammatory diseases, neoplasia, and malformations. Less common causes include infectious diseases, vascular events, and inborn errors of metabolism.

Animals with genetic or unknown (idiopathic) epilepsy, by definition, will have a normal neurologic examination between seizures. If there is an abnormal neurological examination, there is a 16.5 times greater chance that there is a structural lesion causing seizures. This is an important consideration as the results of the neurologic examination will heavily impact your diagnostic recommendations.

Approximately 80% of dogs over 7 years of age with a new onset of seizures will have a structural reason; the remaining 20% will be cryptogenic epilepsy (having a late-onset seizure disorder with a grossly structurally normal brain). Many dogs with a structural intracranial lesion will have a normal neurologic examination because there are silent areas in the brain.

Cats are a bit different. In domestic felines, symptomatic epilepsy is most common, accounting for 40–50% of seizure cases. Presumptive idiopathic and reactive epilepsies are about tied for the second and third causes of seizures, between 25% and 50% each. Cardiac syncope comes in as the fourth most common cause of "seizures," though these are truly cats with severe arrhythmias, such as a third-degree AV block or sick sinus syndrome. In cats, focal and generalized seizures appear with even frequency. A generalized seizure in a cat will be similar to that of a dog; there will be ptyalism, tonic-clonic muscular activity, urination, defecation, but cats may vocalize during the seizure. Cats can also have seizure episodes with minimal overt motor activity; there may be twitching of part of the face and ptyalism, but a key finding in these cases is hyperthermia. Epilepsy of unknown cause in cats has a higher survival rate than in dogs with an approximately 45% remission rate. Basically, we do see epileptic cats, and they tend to do much better than dogs.

Differential diagnosis lists for intracranial causes of seizures will vary based on age and breed, but the following list is a guide:

- < 1 year: Metabolic (hypoglycemia), Congenital (hydrocephalus), Infectious
- 1–5 years: Genetic/Idiopathic, Inflammatory, Neoplastic
- >6 years: Neoplastic, Inflammatory, Cryptogenic
- Geriatric: Neoplastic, Vascular, Cryptogenic

Breed should also be considered when thinking about seizures. A young, large-breed dog is most likely to have a genetic or unknown epilepsy while a young to adult terrier or toy-breed dog is more likely to have an inflammatory meningoencephalitis. A middle-aged brachycephalic breed with a new onset of seizures should raise concern for intracranial neoplasia – a glial tumor in particular. Geriatric large-breed dolichocephalic dogs, in contrast, are at higher risk of meningiomas.

Box 8.1

Common intracranial etiologies of seizures
  Age first seizure noted: Common Causes
  <1 year: Metabolic (hypoglycemia), Congenital (hydrocephalus), Infectious
  1–5 years: Genetic/Idiopathic, Inflammatory, Neoplastic
  >6 years: Neoplastic, Inflammatory, Cryptogenic
  Geriatric: Neoplastic, Vascular, Cryptogenic

Therapy

Seizures can generally all be treated the same way. The goals of treatment are to reduce the frequency and severity of seizures; it is very unlikely that seizures will be completely eliminated with medication, and this is a critical concept to transmit to the owners. It is important that the owners' expectations are on par with your working diagnosis and prognosis.

In the emergency scenario, injectable diazepam or midazolam are the treatment of choice. An injection of 0.5 mg/kg IV should stop an active seizure. If IV access is not available, 1–2 mg/kg of diazepam can be given rectally or intranasally to stop the current seizure. Diazepam will only exert anticonvulsant effects for about 15 minutes – long enough to place an IV catheter and get preliminary blood work such as a packed cell volume, total solids, and a blood glucose measurement. During this time, someone should get a brief history from the owners to begin to determine the underlying cause of the seizures to help direct treatment. For example, there is no reason to start a known diabetic, hypoglycemic cat on phenobarbital if it has been inadvertently over dosed with glargine. Conversely, a geriatric dog who has had multiple seizures over the last few months is likely going to require initiation of a maintenance anti-seizure medication.

Cluster seizures and status epilepticus are emergency situations. Prolonged seizure activity can lead to neuronal damage, hyperthermia, disseminated intravascular coagulation (DIC), and death.

Boluses of diazepam can be repeated as needed, but if repeat dosing (more than two or three times) is necessary, a long-term maintenance anti-seizure medication should be considered. There are multiple long-term therapeutic options for seizure control. Traditionally, long-term treatment is considered effective if there is at least a 50% reduction in the number of seizures during a given time. Treatment is a balance between seizure control and side effects of the medications.

Box 8.2

Medical intervention with anticonvulsants is meant to prevent a crisis scenario from occurring. Treatment of seizure disorders is a balance between seizure control and the side-effects of the medications.

Phenobarbital (PB) is generally dosed at ≥2.2 mg/kg PO BID in the dog as maintenance therapy and it must be dosed at the same amount twice daily. It can be loaded at 16–20 mg/kg IV once to be followed by maintenance dosing 12 hours later. This loading dose should be reduced in geriatric or compromised patients by 25–50% so as to not induce marked sedation and paresis. Serum phenobarbital levels should be kept between 20 and 30 ug/mL; a serum level over 30 ug/mL will not confer better seizure control and will make a hepatopathy more likely. Cats often require a lower dose of PB to reach therapeutic levels. PB is metabolized by the liver and induces its own metabolism and the inducible insoenzyme of alkaline phosphatase (ALP), so ALP levels are *expected* to go up in dogs on phenobarbital. Hepatotoxicity due to phenobarbital is associated with chronically high serum levels, generally over 40 ug/mL for over 6 months. In those cases, alanine aminotransaminase (ALT) is generally higher than ALP. For therapeutic drug monitoring, sampling is not time-sensitive. It is recommended to check a serum biochemical profile and a serum drug level every 6 months. Phenobarbital will also interfere with thyroid hormone testing; dogs will show a low total T4 and fT4, but will not be truly hypothyroid. Once an animal is on PB, thyroid testing is not recommended as the results cannot be reliably interpreted.

Levetiracetam (Keppra) is a newer anti-seizure medication that is safe for use in dogs and cats. It is dosed starting at 20 mg/kg TID for the regular formulation and starting at 30 mg/kg PO BID for the extended release formulation. Extended release tablets can *not* be split! Levetiracetam is available in injectable parenteral, liquid, and tablet formulations. Levetiracetam has not been shown to cause any significant pathology and can cause some mild sedation, especially when added into a protocol with other anti-seizure medications. Safety studies have shown doses up to 100 mg/kg to have minimal side effects. If a starting dose does not achieve the desired effect, the dose should be increased by 25–50%. In the author's experience, if an adequate response is not seen at a dose of 80 mg/kg, the drug is considered ineffective and discontinued. The half-life of levetiracetam is so short that there is no need for weaning, but tapering is also acceptable.

Zonisamide is a sulfonamide anti-seizure medication that is safe for use in dogs and cats. It is generally dosed at 5 mg/kg PO BID, but must be increased to 10 mg/kg PO BID in dogs concurrently receiving phenobarbital. Zonisamide comes in 25 mg, 50 mg, and 100 mg capsules and can be compounded into a suspension. Similar to the sulfonamide antibiotics, it is hepatically metabolized and can induce hepatopathies. There are also scattered reports of suspected idiosyncratic reactions including hepatopathies and dermatologic disorders associated with zonisamide administration. Rare, unpublished reports of neutropenia exist, but more

common side effects include sedation, ataxia, vomiting, and inappetance.

Bromide is a halide salt that is an effective anti-seizure medication in the dog; it has recently been shown that it is not as effective nor as well tolerated as phenobarbital. It is not recommended for use in the cat due to life-threatening respiratory side effects and poor efficacy. It is typically dosed at 40 mg/kg/day, and it is sometimes possible to use a lower dose of 20–30 mg/kg/day when combined with phenobarbital. The target therapeutic seerum range is from 1–3 mg/mL. Bromide doses can be given SID or divided in half and administered BID to reduce gastrointenstinal upset. Bromide is not metabolized and is excreted unchanged by the kidneys; avoidance is recommended in animals with renal dysfunction. Because of renal excretion, bromide levels are very sensitive to diet, and dogs on bromide must be fed a constant, moderate- to low-salt diet. The inadvertent or accidental ingestion or administration of a large amount of chloride (generally as sodium chloride), can cause a rapid increase in renal excretion of bromide and a precipitous drop in the serum level, thereby reducing the seizure threshold and allowing for seizures. Bromide has a very long half-life, so steady state is not reached for approximately 3 months. Loading can be performed to reach therapeutic levels more quickly; this can be done orally with KBr or IV with NaBr. Because of the lack of metabolism of bromide, this is a good choice in animals with significant hepatic disease where phenobarbital and zonisamide should be avoided. Common side-effects include sedation, ataxia, paraparesis, polydipsia and polyuria, and polyphagia. Bromide toxicity, known as bromism, is generally associated with a higher serum level of bromide, and dogs can show show mentation changes, mydriasis, blindness, ataxia, paresis, decreased segmental reflexes, dysphagia, and muscle pain. Suspected idiosyncratic reactions to bromide include behavior changes and aggression, erythematous dermatitis and pruritus, cough, and pancreatitis. Because of the long half-life of bromide, therapeutic drug monitoring is not time sensitive.

Drugs Not Recommended for Maintenance Use

Diazepam is not an effective long-term anti-seizure medication in the dog and cat. In the cat, oral diazepam can cause an idiosyncratic hepatic necrosis and is therefore not recommended. Dogs develop tolerance to oral diazepam as early as 5 days after maintenance therapy, and it is then no longer effective. Gabapentin is a poor anticonvulsant and so not generally recommended for primary seizure control. Phenytoin is no longer used as it is not truly effective in the dog. Primidone is also no longer used as it is predominantly metabolized to phenobarbital, which has a longer half-life.

Absolute Indications for Anti-seizure Medications

Absolute indications for anti-seizure medications include cluster seizures, structural intracranial disease, an abnormal neurologic examination, and aggression pre- or post-seizure. Another very important indication for medication is a progressively shortening interictal interval – if seizures are getting closer together, then anti-seizure medications are highly recommended.

Drug Selection: Which Drug and When

When choosing an anti-seizure medication, it is important to consider how quickly you need seizure control, for how long you will need it, comorbid conditions and, if it's a maintenance medication, the owners' limitations for medication administration frequency.

Levetiracetam provides seizure control immediately if given IV and within 24 hours if started at maintenance orally. Phenobarbital provides seizure control within minutes if loaded IV and levels become therapeutic in about one week and stable by 10–14 days if started at maintenance doses. Zonisamide

becomes effective after 3–5 days and reaches steady state by 7–10 days. Bromide can reach therapeutic levels within hours if NaBr is loaded IV or within a week if KBr is loaded PO, though it may not be effective for up to a month at maintenance doses and will not reach steady state for 3 months.

No one anticonvulsant is definitively better than another, but the positive and negative effects and interactions of each drug may affect how attractive an individual drug is for a specific case. Both phenobarbital and zonisamide are metabolized by the liver and so both should be avoided in patients with significant hepatopathies.

Bromide is very slow to effect, so it is not recommended for short-term seizure control within 2 months. It is also very sensitive to diet, so it is not a good choice in families with small children that throw food on the floor, or dogs that swim in salt water.

In geriatric dogs with significant degenerative joint disease and compromised mobility, it is advisable to avoid sedation. A good consideration would be levetiracetam, as it does not cause any sedation or paresis and therefore does not compromise mobility. Phenobarbital, zonisamide and bromide can all contribute to paresis and ataxia.

Rescue/Relapse Therapies

If a dog or cat is known to have single seizures, there is no need for a rescue therapy at home. Giving additional medications in that scenario can prolong recovery and is not likely to have any benefit. Animals that are known to have clusters of seizures are different. Depending on the pattern of seizures, a rescue therapy at home may be indicated. If the seizures are minutes apart, and the animal does not recover enough to be able to swallow, then rectal diazepam is likely the best option. This presents multiple difficulties: it is a controlled drug with the potential for abuse and it is most rapidly absorbed when given in its liquid state (the injectable form). This requires the owner to draw up the diazepam into a syringe, remove the needle, then place a tomcat catheter or similar device to allow placement of the drug into the rectum – many owners are overwhelmed by this. Diazepam should not be left in clear plastic containers (like syringes) as it is light sensitive and will gradually be adsorbed by the plastic and lose efficacy. Suppositories are not recommended in this scenario as they, by definition, must melt and work slowly. A different option is to use levetiracetam at home. In the scenario described above, the injectable form of levetiracetam can be administered IM or per rectum for seizure control. If the patient recovers enough between seizures in a cluster to be able to swallow, then oral levetiracetam can be administered with the aim of breaking the cycle of the cluster seizures.

Medical intervention with anticonvulsants is meant to prevent a crisis scenario from occurring. More definitive treatments, such as surgery or radiation, may or may not be an option for intracranial tumors. In this scenario, consultation with a veterinary neurologist is strongly recommended. Watchful monitoring is not often recommended in a dog or cat with seizures unless they are single seizures that are very far apart (months) chronologically.

Quality of Life

Quality of life is a major concern when managing a patient with a seizure disorder. It can be very difficult to balance seizure control with side effects from the medications. When side effects begin to compromise quality of life, or when seizure frequency increases despite changes in medication protocols, then the goals need to be reevaluated.

Patient

One of the more objective measurements for patient quality of life is seizure frequency. It is helpful to have owners keep track of seizure episodes so that therapy and progression of disease can be objectively measured. This can also help the owners objectively see when a seizure disorder is progressing despite treatment. Another consideration is ease of medication administration.

Client

There are many client considerations to think about. With a seizure disorder, medication regime is at the top of the list. Some seizure disorders will progress despite treatment and may require multiple anticonvulsant drugs to be used at once to attain adequate seizure control. An animal on multiple anti-seizure medications will have to be administered many pills multiple times of day; this is not practical or feasible for some working owners. Daily schedule adjustments play into end-of-life decisions for some families. Some owners cannot emotionally handle their pet having a seizure; in this case, there is *nothing* we can do to reliably prevent all seizures from happening. Financial limitations often come into play in managing a pet with a seizure disorder as there is significant cost associated with multiple anti-seizure medications and the recommended monitoring and blood work.

Medical management of seizures associated with brain tumors will only help for a certain amount of time, though that time is variable. Here, anti-seizure medication therapy is meant to prevent a crisis, though progression is inevitable. Some cats with meningiomas can live years with anticonvulsants and short courses of prednisone (as needed), while others will be so severely affected that a decision for intervention versus euthanasia has to be made more precipitously. Although we do not have extensive data on the natural course of disease with meningiomas or gliomas in dogs, survival times with medical management can vary significantly based on tumor type, location within the brain, and growth rate of the tumor.

Quality of Life

Of genetic epileptic patients, 20–60% will suffer at least one episode of status epilepticus and about half of all epileptic patients will have cluster seizures. Mean life span is affected by status epilepticus: pets that have suffered status epilepticus have an average lifespan of 8 years versus over 11 years in those without status epilepticus. Because of the physiologic derangements that can occur with status epilepticus (DIC, organ failure), this scenario is often a pivotal point for owners. Many owners simply realize that their pet's quality of life is simply too compromised, either by the side effects of medications or by the increased seizure frequency. When owners come to that realization, other therapeutic options may be available, but rate of response to anti-seizure medications decreases with each additional medication, humane euthanasia is often the best option.

Further Reading

Pakozdy A, Halasz P, Klang A. Epilepsy in cats: Theory and practice. Journal of Internal Veterinary Medicine. 2014; 28(2): 255–263.

Podell M. Antiepileptic drug therapy and monitoring. Topics in Companion Animal Medicine. 2013; 28(2): 59–66.

Wahle AM, Brühschwein A, Matiasek K, et al. Clinical characterization of epilepsy of unknown cause in cats. Journal of Internal Veterinary Medicine. 2014; 28(1): 182–188.

Wessmann A, Volk HA, Parkin T, et al. Evaluation of quality of life in dogs with idiopathic epilepsy. Journal of Internal Veterinary Medicine. 2014; 28(2): 510–514.

9

Feline Hyperthyroidism

Sylvie Daminet and Kate Hill

Introduction

Hyperthyroidism in geriatric cats is a life-threatening disease requiring prompt veterinary attention. Euthyroidism can be achieved by: pharmacological therapy, nutritional therapy, thyroidectomy, or radioiodine therapy. All four options have advantages and disadvantages and which treatment is selected depends on a number of factors including: concurrent disease, age of the cat, cost, surgical skill, availability of nuclear medicine facilities, and the owner's informed opinion.

Diagnosis

Typical clinical signs are polyuria, polydipsia, weight loss, vomiting, and one or more palpable thyroid nodule(s) (Figure 9.1). Diagnosis is confirmed with total thyroxine (TT4) serum measurement. Weight loss or presence of a palpable thyroid nodule (or nodules) justifies investigation for hyperthyroidism in a geriatric cat. Complete blood count, biochemistry, and urinalysis are essential to eliminate concurrent diseases. A mild to moderate increase in liver enzyme activity is observed in most hyperthyroid patients. An increased serum TT4 is the biochemical hallmark of feline hyperthyroidism and will be observed in most cats (Peterson, Melian, and Nicholls 2001). Measurement of free T4 after equilibrium dialysis (FT4ED) should be used prudently in cats because of its poor specificity in this species.

Management

Hyperthyroid cats can be managed using anti-thyroid medication (oral or topical), iodine restricted diet, thyroidectomy, or radioactive iodine (I^{131}). All four options have advantages and disadvantages (summarized in Table 9.1). Surgery and I^{131} are considered definitive treatment options. Anti-thyroid medication and diet are reversible options. An initial reversible treatment allows counteracting cardiac and metabolic consequences of hyperthyroidism before a definitive treatment is considered. This is especially important before surgery. It is important to underline that pharmacologic and dietary options, do not address the cause of the disease (thyroid hyperplasia/neoplasia) but 'only' block thyroid hormone synthesis. Some authors have suggested that after several years of medical therapy, thyroid tissue can become malignant (Peterson and Broome, 2012). Reported survival times are longer for cats treated with I^{131} (Milner *et al.*, 2006). When selecting a treatment option for cats with hyperthyroidism all treatment options need to be discussed and the pros and cons for each evaluated for the cat and its owner.

Chronic Disease Management for Small Animals, First Edition. Edited by W. Dunbar Gram,
Rowan J. Milner and Remo Lobetti.
© 2018 John Wiley & Sons, Inc. Published 2018 by John Wiley & Sons, Inc.

Pharmacological Treatment

Oral or topical methimazole and carbimazole inhibit thyroid hormones synthesis. Anti-thyroid drugs can be used short-term to stabilize the patient prior to a definitive treatment or as a long-term medical management. The recommended initial dose of methimazole is 2.5 mg PO BID. In cases where compliance is an issue, 5 mg PO once a day can be used. A starting dosage of slow release carbimazole tablets of 15 mg SID and 10 mg SID if TT4 values are only mildly increased is recommended.

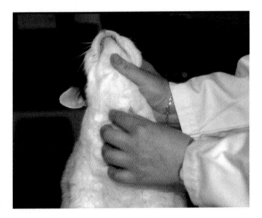

Figure 9.1 Technique for palpation of thyroid glands.

Adverse reactions are less likely to occur when the dosage of anti-thyroid drugs is started low and gradually increased to effect. If the owner does not observe adverse reactions, physical examination reveals no new problems, results of a complete blood count are within reference limits, and serum T_4 concentration is "normal/high" after 2 weeks of therapy, the dose is increased. Reevaluation is performed again 2 weeks later. The dosage should continue to be increased every 2 weeks by 2.5 mg/day adjustments until TT_4 concentration is "normal/low" or until adverse reactions develop.

Adverse reactions to methimazole typically occur within the first 4 to 8 weeks of therapy. Side effects most commonly observed (<10% of cats) are anorexia, vomiting, and lethargy. These side effects are most often transient and do not necessitate discontinuation of methimazole. Side effects that are more serious are also reported and often necessitate cessation of treatment: facial excoriations (Figure 9.2), hepatopathy, hematological abnormalities (thrombocytopenia, leucopenia, eosinophilia, hemolytic anemia) (Peterson, Kintzer, and Hurvitz 1988; Daminet *et al.* 2014).

Methimazole prepared in Pluronic® lecithin organogel (PLO) gel and applied to the inner pinna of cats has been shown to be a

Table 9.1 Advantages and disadvantages of different treatment options for feline hyperthyroidism.

Treatment	Advantages	Disadvantages
Methimazole Carbimazole	Efficient Reversible No anesthesia	Side effects common Lifelong treatment Requires monitoring
Iodine restricted diet	Ease for the owner Reversible	Requires monitoring Lifelong daily treatment Needs to eat diet strictly Long-term studies required
Thyroidectomy	Efficient In principle definitive	Requires anesthesia Complications Recurrence possible
Radioactive iodine	Efficient In principle definitive Few complications No anesthesia Addresses the underlying disease	Requires a specialized center Hospitalization Use of radioactive products

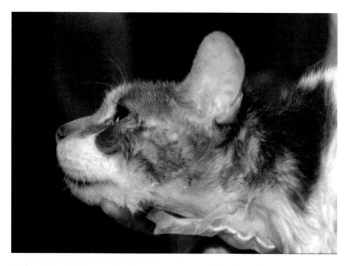

Figure 9.2 Facial excoriations in a cat treated with methimazole.

safe option for the long term therapy of hyperthyroid cats, however the dose of methimazole may need to be increased over time (Boretti *et al.* 2014). Owners should wear gloves to administer this topical cream and should use each ear alternatively. Gastrointestinal side effects are observed less commonly than with the oral tablets. Some cats will have crusting and erythema of the pinnae. This preparation can definitively be of benefit in cats that are difficult to "pill." A lipophilic transdermal formulation for once-daily dosing (Hill *et al.* 2011) has recently become commercially available in some parts of the world (e.g., New Zealand).

The beta-blocking agents propanolol and atenolol have no direct effect on the thyroid gland but can be useful in certain cases to control polypnea, hypertension, hyperexcitability, tachycardia and eventual arrhythmias related to the hyperthyroidism. Propanolol (ß1ß2: 2.5–5 mg 2 to 3 times daily) and atenolol (ß1: 6.25 mg 1 to 2 times daily).

Adequate monitoring during pharmacological and nutritional therapy is essential. An expert panel recently recommended that practitioners should aim at obtaining a TT4 in the lower half of the reference range (Daminet *et al.* 2014). Overzealous therapy also needs to be avoided (see iatrogenic hypothyroidism).

Nutritional Therapy

The major advantage of this dietary option is the ease of administration. After feeding the diet for approximately 8 weeks, between 40–75% of cats will have a TT4 concentration within reference range (van der Kooij *et al.* 2014; Hui *et al.* 2015). Nutritional management is not a good option for outdoor cats with access to other iodine sources, for cats that find the food unpalatable or for cats that have other concurrent diseases that require specific diets. One study has reported poor owner compliance or palatability issues in 25% of cats (van der Kooij *et al.* 2014). The combination of the low iodine diet and antithyroid drugs is not recommended.

As with pharmacologic therapy, adequate monitoring is important. The clinician should not be satisfied with a cat that improves somewhat clinically and has TT4 values just above or just within normal range.

Radioactive iodine therapy

Radioactive iodine therapy is a simple, effective, safe and in principle definitive treatment for hyperthyroidism. Iodine[131] is taken up by the thyroid gland, the radiation emitted by iodine[131] destroys primarily the abnormal thyroid tissue. Atrophied thyroid tissue is spared, precluding the development of hypothyroidism in most cats. Often, a single dose of I^{131} is sufficient to restore a euthyroid state. After treatment with I^{131}, more than 80% of cats become euthyroid within 3 months, most within 2 weeks. More than 95% of treated cats are euthyroid at 6 months. Less than 5% of cats require a second treatment with I^{131}. A recurrence of hyperthyroidism after some years is also possible. Hypothyroidism can develop, especially in cats with large and bilaterally affected thyroid glands. The major disadvantages of ^{131}I is that there are special licensing requirements required to administer and house the cats after treatment to ensure radiation exposure to humans is minimized. These requirements limit the availability of this treatment.

Surgery

Surgical removal of the thyroid glands is an effective and relatively quick treatment for hyperthyroidism. However it must be remembered that 70% of cats with hyperthyroidism have bilateral disease (Peterson and Broome, 2015), so surgical cure may not be permanent if a unilateral thyroidectomy is performed. Unilateral thyroidectomy is safe and effective, although recurrence of clinical signs occurs in around 5% of cases. Serum thyroid concentrations should be measured after surgery, to ensure the cat does not develop iatrogenic hypothyroidism, as asymptomatic hypothyroidism can progress chronic kidney disease in cats (Williams *et al.* 2010).

Renal Function and Hyperthyroidism

Renal function is profoundly influenced by thyroid status (van Hoek and Daminet, 2009). Through their ino- and chronotropic effects, excessive thyroid hormone concentrations can lead to an increased cardiac output. Further, hyperthyroidism diminishes peripheral vascular resistance by dilating arterioles

of the peripheral circulation. The increased glomerular filtration rate (GFR) associated with hyperthyroid states is thought to result from the increased cardiac output and intra-renal vasodilatation and leads to a decline in blood-urea-nitrogen (BUN) and serum creatinine concentrations. With effective treatment, a marked decline of renal function has been reported (van Hoek *et al.* 2009), which is "normalization" of renal function rather than a "decline."

Chronic kidney disease (CKD) and hyperthyroidism are both frequently encountered diseases in geriatric cats and thus finding both diseases in one cat is common. As renal function can decline ("normalize") after treatment of hyperthyroidism, this can unmask renal disease in some cats. Decreased muscle mass associated with emaciation and therefore decreased production of creatinine can contribute to the declined serum creatinine concentrations observed in untreated hyperthyroid cats. The presence of a hyperthyroid state could contribute to the development or progression of CKD. Systemic hypertension can lead to intra-glomerular hypertension, hyper-filtration and contribute to the development of glomerulosclerosis.

Pre-existing Azotemia *in a* Newly Diagnosed Hyperthyroid Cat

In such a case, the diagnosis of hyperthyroidism can be somewhat complicated by a decline in thyroid hormones (euthyroid sickness) within the reference range and given the further decline in GFR to be expected after resolution of the hyperthyroid state, it is important to start an azotemic hyperthyroid cat with a reversible anti-thyroid therapy. This allows assessing the impact of anti-thyroid therapy on renal function. These patients should be monitored every 2 weeks. Dosage adjustments should be made prudently. In such cases, a compromise between improved renal function and persistence of hyperthyroidism may be required to optimize quality of life.

Development of Azotemia *after* Treatment *of* Hyperthyroidism

Resolution of the hyperthyroid state can unmask CKD. Excess thyroid hormones increase GFR and treatment of hyperthyroidism will decrease GFR, leading to an increase in BUN and creatinine values. Up to 30% of the patients, develop overt azotemia after treatment of hyperthyroidism. Post-treatment development of azotemia does not seem to decrease the survival of hyperthyroid cats after treatment. The appearance of mild stable azotemia should not affect treatment advice for hyperthyroidism given to clients. As long as TT4 and renal parameters are monitored closely, there is no reason to stop or reduce anti-thyroid drug treatment in azotemic cats in order to normalize creatinine concentration. However, as these cats carry a similar prognosis to cats not developing post-treatment azotemia and are unlikely to increase more than one IRIS stage, a recent "consensus panel" did not recommend routine use of a therapeutic trial in non-azotemic hyperthyroid cat to assess effect on renal function (Daminet *et al.* 2014).

Iatrogenic Hypothyroidism

Excessive treatment leading to iatrogenic hypothyroidism should be avoided as iatrogenic hypothyroidism can contribute to development of azotemia and shorten survival of azotemic cats (Williams *et al.* 2010). However, diagnosis of iatrogenic hypothyroidism is not always straightforward in cats. Cats affected present lethargy, anorexia, weight gain, and dermatologic signs. A decrease in TT4 is not specific. Therefore, measurement of an increased TSH (with canine kit) can help confirming the diagnosis (Aldridge *et al.*, 2015).

In conclusion, early detection is important and in most cats, diagnosis can be confirmed with TT4 measurement. Treatment with anti-thyroid drugs or diet is the cornerstone of medical management (either short term or long term). While monitoring TT4 is essential to detect under-treatment, overtreatment should be avoided too. Radioactive iodine therapy is the treatment of choice in many cats as it addresses the underlying disease and is noninvasive.

References

Aldridge C, Behrend EN, Martin LG, Refsal K, Kemppainen RJ, Lee HP, Chciuk K. Evaluation of thyroid-stimulating hormone, total thyroxine, and free thyroxine concentrations in hyperthyroid cats receiving methimazole treatment. Journal of Veterinary Internal Medicine. 2015; 29: 862–868. DOI: 10.1111/jvim.12575

Boretti FS, Sieber-Ruckstuhl NS, Schaefer S, Gerber B, Baumgartner C, Riond B, Hofmann-Lehmann R, Reusch CE. Transdermal application of methimazole in hyperthyroid cats: a long-term follow-up study. Journal of Feline Medicine and Surgery. 2014; 16: 453–459. DOI: 10.1177/1098612x13509808

Daminet S, Kooistra HS, Fracassi F, Graham PA, Hibbert A, Lloret A, Mooney CT, Neiger R, Rosenberg D, Syme HM, Villard I,

Williams G. Best practice for the pharmacological management of hyperthyroid cats with antithyroid drugs. Journal of Small Animal Practice. 2014; 55: 4–13. DOI: 10.1111/jsap.12157

Hill KE, Gieseg MA, Kingsbury D, Lopez-Villalobos N, Bridges J, Chambers P. The efficacy and safety of a novel lipophilic formulation of methimazole for the once daily transdermal treatment of cats with hyperthyroidism. Journal of Veterinary Internal Medicine. 2011; 25(6): 1357–1365. DOI: 10.1111/j.1939-1676.2011.00799.x

Hui TY, Bruyette DS, Moore GE, Scott-Moncrieff JC. Effect of feeding an iodine-restricted diet in cats with spontaneous hyperthyroidism. Journal of Veterinary Internal Medicine. 2015; 29: 1063–1068. DOI: 10.1111/jvim.13368

Milner RJ, Channell CD, Levy JK, Schaer M. Survival times for cats with hyperthyroidism treated with iodine 131, methimazole, or both: 167 cases (1996–2003). Journal of the American Veterinary Medical Association. 2006; 228(4): 559–563.

Peterson M, Broome M. Hyperthyroid cats on long-term medical treatment show a progressive increase in the prevalence of large thyroid tumors, intrathoracic thyroid masses, and suspected thyroid carcinoma. Journal of Veterinary Internal Medicine. Abstract from 22nd ECVIM-CA Congress. 2012; 26: 1523.

Peterson ME, Broome MR. Thyroid scintigraphy findings in 2096 cats with hyperthyroidism. Veterinary Radiology & Ultrasound. 2015; 56(1): 84–95 DOI: 10.1111/vru.12165

Peterson ME, Kintzer PP, Hurvitz AI. Methimazole treatment of 262 cats with hyperthyroidism. Journal of Veterinary Internal Medicine. 1988; 2: 150–157.

Peterson ME, Melian C, Nichols, R. Measurement of serum concentrations of free thyroxine, total thyroxine, and total triiodothyronine in cats with hyperthyroidism and cats with nonthyroidal disease. Journal of the American Veterinary Medical Association. 2001; 218: 529–536.

van der Kooij M, Becvarova I, Meye HP, Teske E, Kooistra HS. Effects of an iodine-restricted food on client-owned cats with hyperthyroidism. Journal of Feline Medicine and Surgery. 2014; 16: 491–498. DOI: 10.1177/1098612x13512627

van Hoek I, Daminet S. Interactions between thyroid and kidney function in pathological conditions of these organ systems: a review. General and Comparative Endocrinology. 2009; 160: 205–215.

van Hoek I, Lefebvre H, Peremans K, Meyer E, Croubels S, Vandermeulen E, Kooistra H, Saunders J, Binst D, Daminet S. Short-and long-term follow-up of glomerular and tubular renal markers of kidney function in hyperthyroid cats after treatment with radioiodine. Domestic Animal Endocrinology. 2009; 36: 45–56.

Williams TL, Peak KJ, Brodbelt D, Elliott J, Syme HM. Survival and the development of azotemia after treatment of hyperthyroid cats. Journal of Veterinary Internal Medicine. 2010; 24: 863–869. DOI: 10.1111/j.1939-1676.2010.0550.x

10

Hypoadrenocorticism in Dogs

Sylvie Daminet

Introduction

Primary hypoadrenocorticism (Addison's disease) is more common and can lead to both mineralocorticoid and glucocorticoid deficiency. A few cases present with evidence of glucocorticoid deficiency alone and do not have the typical hyponatremia and hyperkalemia (atypical Addison). With time, these patients may progress to mineralocorticoid deficiency and develop electrolyte imbalances. In secondary hypoadrenocorticism, a deficiency of adrenocorticotropic hormone (ACTH) results in glucocorticoid insufficiency only. These patients do not develop mineralocorticoid deficiency.

Clinical Presentation and Diagnosis

Owners sometimes describe a "waxing and waning" illness. Anorexia (total or partial), lethargy, and weight loss are the most common recognized clinical signs, followed by intermittent gastrointestinal signs, and dehydration. If the disease remains unrecognized, the signs typically progressively worsen and some dogs eventually present in an acute addisonian crisis. These dogs can exhibit moderate to severe shock. A shock situation accompanied by an inappropriate bradycardia can be an important clue in the suspicion of the disease. Other possible clinical signs include polyuria/polydipsia, abdominal pain, melena and occasionally hematemesis (Lathan 2015; Scott-Moncrieff 2015; Van Lanen and Sande 2014). Important differentials include acute kidney injury, hepatic and gastrointestinal disease.

Most dogs present with hyperkalemia and hyponatremia with hypochloremia also commonly observed. Besides these electrolyte abnormalities, azotemia, acidosis, and hypoalbuminemia are frequently observed. Less commonly, a mild hypercalcemia, a mild increase in liver enzymes or hypoglycemia can be seen. Although the biochemical hallmark of primary Addison's disease is hyperkalemia, this can be observed with several other diseases such as renal or gastrointestinal disease and pleural effusion (chylothorax). Atypical cases do not present with the typical electrolyte imbalances and are therefore more difficult to recognize.

Lymphocytosis and eosinophilia can sometimes be observed. In a stress situation, these findings should alert the clinician to the possibility of hypoadrenocorticism. Indeed, lymphopenia and eosinopenia are expected in a sick animal and even finding normal values for eosinophils or lymphocytes in a sick animal can be a hint for the diagnosis of hypoadrenocorticism. Hypoadrenocorticism is also frequently associated with mild nonregenerative normocytic normochromic anemia. However, following gastrointestinal hemorrhage, a regenerative anemia may be present.

Chronic Disease Management for Small Animals, First Edition. Edited by W. Dunbar Gram, Rowan J. Milner and Remo Lobetti.
© 2018 John Wiley & Sons, Inc. Published 2018 by John Wiley & Sons, Inc.

Urine specific gravity is often used in clinics to help differentiate prerenal from renal azotemia. However, in cases of hypoadrenocorticism the patient cannot always concentrate its urine even if dehydrated because of the hypoaldosteronism and natriuresis.

Hyperkalemia can cause typical changes in an ECG such as spiked T-waves, shortened Q-T interval, prolongation of the QRS complex, reduction or absence of P-waves and bradycardia. With severe hyperkalemia, ventricular asystole or ventricular fibrillation may also be observed.

Microcardia, small cranial pulmonary artery and caudal vena cava, and occasional mega-esophagus can be observed on survey radiographs. Adrenal ultrasonography can reveal a reduction of size of these glands.

Confirmation of the Diagnosis

No clinical or biochemical abnormalities are pathognomonic for Addison's disease. Basal serum cortisol can be useful as a screening test for hypoadrenocorticism using a cut-off value of ≤2 µg/dl. Hypoadrenocorticism is unlikely if basal cortisol is >2µg/dl (Bovens *et al.* 2014). Diagnosis must be confirmed with an ACTH stimulation test. Several protocols have been described, but most often, synthetic ACTH is administered IV and blood samples for cortisol measurements are taken at T0 and after 1 hour. An inadequate increase in cortisol concentration following ACTH administration confirms the diagnosis.

Most glucocorticoid preparations, except dexamethasone, cross-react with most commonly used commercial cortisol assays and cause falsely increased cortisol values. Dexamethasone sodium phosphate can therefore be used as emergency treatment in a suspected acute hypoadrenocorticoid crisis, while the ACTH stimulation test is being performed.

Endogenous ACTH or aldosterone (pre and post exogenous ACTH administration) serum concentrations can be measured to distinguish primary and atypical cases from secondary hypoadrenocorticism. Endogenous

ACTH is highly labile and strict sample handling precautions must be followed to prevent in vitro degradation following sample collection (use apportioning or dry ice). Until recently, it was assumed that normal aldosterone concentrations were essential to maintain normal electrolyte values (Baumstark *et al.* 2014b; Scott-Moncrieff 2015). However, in a recent study describing aldosterone concentration in dogs with hypoadrenocorticism, several dogs with atypical primary HA, also had very low aldosterone concentrations (Baumstark *et al.* 2014b). These findings suggest that some other mechanism must be involved to maintain normal sodium and potassium serum concentrations in dogs with atypical hypoadrenocorticism.

Treatment

Emergency Treatment

Rapid institution of treatment is vital for the dog presented in an acute Addisonian crisis. Initial treatment is directed at correcting hypovolemia and electrolyte/acid-base abnormalities, and at glucocorticoid supplementation.

Adequate intravenous fluid therapy is the most important part of the treatment. Traditionally NaCl 0.9% has been recommended as the fluid of choice because of its high sodium concentration and lack of potassium. A lactated Ringer's solution is also adequate as it might correct the acidosis more rapidly and its potassium content is low. Fluid therapy is usually required for only a few days and can be withdrawn when the dog is eating well and major laboratory abnormalities are corrected. Electrolyte abnormalities usually resolve after adequate fluid therapy has been instituted. With life threatening hyperkalemia (K > 9 mEq/L and/or ECG abnormalities) further specific therapy is needed. Hypoglycemia can be addressed by adding dextrose to the isotonic fluid bag in order to make a 2.5 or 5% solution. If clinical signs related to hypoglycemia are present boluses of 25% dextrose solution, 1 mL/kg in 0.9% saline may be administered (Lathan 2015).

Administration of glucocorticoids should also be started without delay if a patient is highly suspected of Addison's. Ideally dexamethasone sodium phosphate is used as it will not interfere with the cortisol measurement performed with the ACTH stimulation test and therefore does not delay performing the diagnostic test. Initial recommended dosages vary from 0.1 to 2 mg/kg IV once and is followed by 0.05–0.1 mg/kg q12 h (Scott-Moncrieff 2015). Alternatively prednisone sodium succinate can be used but only after finalising the ACTH stimulation test.

Urine production, electrolytes, and glycemia should be monitored closely – shortly after initiating therapy and thereafter q 8–12 hours, until these parameters normalize. The clinical response to emergency therapy in a dog presenting in an acute hypoadrenal crisis is usually excellent and maintenance oral therapy with mineralocorticoid and glucocorticoid supplementation should be started as soon as tolerated by the patient (usually when starting to eat).

Maintenance Therapy

Mineralocorticoid supplementation is possible with oral fludrocortisone acetate or with injectable desoxycorticosterone pivalate (DOCP). The choice between both mineralocorticoids is mainly based on product availability, cost price, and personal preference of both veterinarian and owner. Some studies suggest that DOCP leads to a better suppression of plasma renin activity and therefore could be the mineralocorticoid of choice when both are available (Baumstark *et al.* 2014a).

Fludrocortisone Acetate (Florinef®)
Oral fludrocortisone acetate should be started at 0.01 mg/kg twice daily. Initially, serum sodium and potassium concentrations should be monitored every 1 to 2 weeks and the fludrocortisone dosage adjusted as needed. The dosage of fludrocortisone required typically increases during the initial 6–18 months. Therefore, monitoring is important and once stable, twice-yearly evaluation of the patient and electrolytes is essential. Fludrocortisone possesses a small degree of glucocorticoid activity, therefore over time; many dogs do not require extra glucocorticoid supplementation except in periods of stress. Besides traditional electrolyte monitoring, plasma renin activity seems a reliable tool to monitor treatment of hypoadrenocorticism (Baumstark *et al.* 2014a).

Desoxycorticosterone Pivalate (DOCP, Percorten®)
DOCP is administered SQ or IM at an initial dosage of approximately 1.5 mg/kg and this provides mineralocorticoid activity for an average of 28 days. Traditionally monitoring is also based on blood electrolyte measurements performed 14 and 28 days after the injection. If hyperkalemia and hyponatremia are observed on day 14, the next dosage should be increased by 5–10%. If electrolytes are within normal range at day 14 but are abnormal at day 28, the dosing interval should be shortened by 48 hours. Once the injection schedule is stable, owners can be instructed to administer DOCP at home.

Oral glucocorticoid therapy should also be instituted as soon as the patient has been stabilized. Initial therapy with prednisolone is initiated at 0.25–0.5 mg/kg q 12 h, however, this dosage should be tapered to 0.1–0.25 mg/kg q 24 h. Adjustments in the dose should be based on clinical response and the presence of side effects. In half of the dogs administered fludrocortisone, the prednisolone therapy can eventually be stopped except at times of stress. However, some dogs will permanently require a low maintenance dose. Dogs treated with DOCP always require daily oral glucocorticoid supplementation.

Other
In situations of stress, (sickness, travelling, surgery, boarding) it is recommended to administer prednisolone at a supra-physiologic

dosage (2 to 5 times physiologic dose). Therefore, owners should have prednisolone available at home.

Salt supplementation can occasionally be helpful in maintaining serum sodium concentrations when high dosages of fludrocortisone are needed to obtain normal or almost normal sodium concentrations.

Treatment of 'Atypical' Hypoadrenocorticism

Currently oral glucocorticoid therapy is probably the only drug required to treat secondary and atypical cases. Further studies should clarify if dogs with atypical primary hypoadrenocorticism would benefit from mineralo-

corticoid therapy. Anyways, monitoring is advised with atypical cases as mineralocorticoid deficiency may also develop with time.

Quality of Life

With adequate treatment and monitoring prognosis is excellent and dogs can have a normal life expectancy with excellent quality of life. Owners should be instructed that daily lifelong therapy is mandatory. Supplementation with mineralocorticoids can be expensive leading to euthanasia of some dogs. Nonchalant compliance can lead to death. The most important cause of insufficient response to therapy is inadequate mineralocorticoid dosage or glucocorticoid side effects.

References

Baumstark ME, Nussberger J, Boretti, FS, Baumstark MW, Riond B, Reusch CE., Sieber-Ruckstuhl NS. Use of plasma renin activity to monitor mineralocorticoid treatment in dogs with primary hypoadrenocorticism: desoxycorticosterone versus fludrocortisone. Journal of Veterinary Internal Medicine. 2014a; 28(5): 1471–1478.

Baumstark ME, Sieber-Ruckstuhl NS, Müller C, Wenger M, Boretti, FS, 2014a. Evaluation of aldosterone concentrations in dogs with hypoadrenocorticism. Journal of Veterinary Internal Medicine. 2014b; 28(1): 154–159.

Bovens C, Tennant K, Reeve J, Murphy KF. Basal serum cortisol concentration as a

screening test for hypoadrenocorticism in dogs. Journal of Veterinary Internal Medicine. 2014; 28(5): 1541–1545.

Lathan P. Canine hypoadrenocorticism. In: E Côté, Ed. Clinical veterinary advisor – dogs and cats, 3rd edn. Elsevier. 2015: 525–527.

Scott-Moncrieff JCR. Hypoadrenocorticism. In: EC Feldman, RW Nelson, CE Reusch, JCR Scott-Moncrieff and EN Behrend, Eds. Canine and feline endocrinology, 4th edn. Elsevier Saunders. 2015: 485–520.

Van Lanen K, Sande A. Canine hypoadrenocorticism: pathogenesis, diagnosis, and treatment. Topics in Companion Animal Medicine. 2014; 29: 88–95.

Further Reading

Boretti FS, Meyer F, Burkhardt WA, Riond B, Hofmann-Lehmann R, Reusch CE, Sieber-Ruckstuhl NS. 2015. Evaluation of the cortisol-to-ACTH ratio in dogs with

hypoadrenocorticism, dogs with diseases mimicking hypoadrenocorticism and in healthy dogs. Journal of Veterinary Internal Medicine. 2015; 29(5): 1335–1341.

11

Canine Hypothyroidism

Sylvie Daminet

Introduction

The vague and non-specific clinical signs of hypothyroidism and the fact that numerous factors can influence thyroid function-test results are major contributors to the difficulty in diagnosing this disease. Treatment is usually considered straight forward but follow-up can be optimized by paying attention to timing of sampling for TT4 measurement and administration of food.

Diagnosis

A thorough physical examination of the patient, knowledge of the advantages and limitations of all available tests, and knowledge of the factors that can influence the results, will allow the veterinarian to correctly diagnose the disease. Laboratory results should be interpreted in light of history and physical examination findings with the diagnosis confirmed through specific evaluation of the thyroid gland. Table 11.1 contains the main presenting complaints and clinical signs. Table 11.2 contains a summary of the advantages and limitations of the most commonly used thyroid tests in dogs. The presence of typical clinical signs in combination with a decreased total thyroxine (TT4)

and increased thyrotropin (TSH) serum concentration is diagnostic and will allow to accurately diagnose approximately 75% of the patients with hypothyroidism. The addition of free T4 (after equilibrium dialysis) and/or measurement of thyroglobulin antibodies can offer additional information. Some cases will require further diagnostic tests, such as thyroid scintigraphy or recombinant human TSH (rhTSH) stimulation test, to make a reliable diagnosis (Daminet *et al.* 2007; Shiel *et al.* 2012).

Main Influences on Thyroid Function Tests

Physiologic Influences

Certain breeds such as sight hounds and performance dogs such as racing sled dogs have TT4 serum concentrations physiologically lower (up to half) than established laboratory reference intervals (Lee *et al.* 2004; van Geffen *et al.* 2006; Pinilla *et al.* 2009). This can complicate the diagnosis of hypothyroidism, especially if only serum TT4 is measured. Often free T4 (after equilibrium dialysis) is less different compared to other breeds. Serum TT4 concentrations tend to mildly decrease with age and intense exercise in sled dogs (Lee *et al.* 2004).

Table 11.1 Summary of the most common clinical signs observed in dogs with hypothyroidism.

Frequent	Less frequent	Doubtful relationship
Lethargy/weakness	Neuropathy, vestibular syndrome	Male infertility
Obesity	Female infertility	Larynx paralysis
Alopecia/hypotrichosis	Myxoedema	Mega-esophagus
Seborrhea	Lipid keratopathy	Behavioral changes (aggressive)
Pyoderma or recurrent otitis		

Table 11.2 Advantages and limitations of the most commonly used thyroid tests.

Test	Advantages	Disadvantages
TT4	Readily available, not expensive Normal values often allow "exclusion" of hypothyroidism	↓ with systemic disease (euthyroid sick syndrome) ↓ after administration of certain drugs A ↓ T4 alone does not allow a reliable diagnosis of hypothyroidism (low specificity)
TSH	Readily available, not expensive	1/4 of hypothyroid dogs have TSH values within the reference interval (low sensitivity) Always use in combination with T4
FT4	Is less influenced by systemic disease or drug administration than TT4	The only reliable method includes equilibrium dialysis Not readily available in all countries
Anti-thyroglobulin Ab	Testing for thyroid autoimmunity	Not routinely available in all countries Does not reflect thyroid *function* Positive in approximately 50% of hypothyroid dogs
Scintigraphy (^{99m}Tc04-)	Reliable, considered as a gold standard	Limited availability Use of radio nuclides Sometimes need for sedation
Thyroid ultrasonography	Theoretically interesting	Very operator- and machine dependent
TSH stimulation test	Reliable, considered as a gold standard (use rhTSH)	rhTSH* is expensive (less if aliquoted) 6 hours lasting test Anaphylactic reactions were described with bovine TSH (not yet with rhTSH)

* rhTSH: recombinant human TSH: Dosages ranging from 50–100 µg have been used, however, in the presence of concurrent disease or drug administration, a dosage of 150 µg is recommended (De Roover *et al.* 2006; Daminet *et al.* 2007; Boretti *et al.* 2009).

Iatrogenic Influence: Effect of Medication

The influence of certain drugs on thyroid function tests has long been underestimated in dogs (Daminet and Ferguson 2003). Table 11.3 gives a summary of the influence of drugs on canine thyroid function tests. Measurement of serum TT4 or TSH should preferably be performed when the patient is not receiving any medication except if it has been demonstrated that no effect is to be expected as with imepitoin (Bossens *et al.* 2016).

Table 11.3 Effects of drugs on canine thyroid results.

Drugs	TT4	FT4	TSH	TSH stimulation test
Glucocorticoids (immunosuppressive)	↓	= or ↓	=	Blunted at high doses and durations
Potassium bromide	=	=	=	=
Phenobarbital	↓	= or ↓	= or ↑	
Sulfonamides*	↓	↓	↑	↓
Carprofen	= or ↓	= (↓)	= or ↓	Not studied
Aspirin	↓	=	=	Not studied
Meloxicam	=	=	=	Not studied
Ketoprofen	=	=	=	Not studied
Clomipramine	↓	↓	=	Not studied
Anesthesia (and surgery)	↓	↑	Not studied	Not studied
Imepitoine	=	=	=	Not studied

* Sulfonamide-induced hypothyroid crisis has been reported.
Source: Daminet 2003. American College of Veterinary Internal Medicine.

Pathologic Influences: Euthyroid Sick Syndrome

The presence of a systemic non-thyroidal disease, such as diabetes mellitus, liver disease, hyperadrenocorticism and renal- or heart failure, is a frequent cause for decreased thyroid hormone concentrations. This phenomenon is referred to as the "euthyroid sick syndrome" (Scott-Moncrieff 2010). These changes probably reflect a physiological adaptation of the organism leading to a decrease in tissue energy requirements. The administration of synthetic thyroid hormones to these patients is not recommended.

Treatment

Treatment of hypothyroidism consists in lifelong administration of synthetic levothyroxine. Initial treatment dosages varies from 10–22 µg/kg SID-BID according to the author and the formulation used, with a maximum of 0.8 mg/dog BID. Use of a veterinary preparation is important as bioavailability of generic forms vary (Scott-Moncrieff 2010; Daminet 2015).

In most countries, two veterinary preparations are available: Forthyron© (tablets) and Leventa© (liquid preparation). Registered starting dosages (based on optimal body weight) are 20 µg/kg SID and 10 µg/kg BID (Dixon, Reed, and Mooney 2002; Van Dijl *et al.* 2014; Daminet 2015).

The patient is reevaluated 1–2 months after initiating therapy and dosage is adjusted based on clinical response, and results of serum TT4. Once euthyroidism is achieved, monitoring every 6 months is advised. Lethargy should improve within 1–2 weeks. Hair regrowth will be more gradual and may take up to 1–4 months. With neurological signs the improvement will be gradual and may take months before resolution. When interpreting the result of TT4, time of sampling compared to the administration of the medication, and the effect of a meal, should be taken into consideration. First, if blood sample is drawn just before administration of the medication, it is especially the duration of action of the medication that is evaluated (pre-pill test). Most commonly, blood is taken 3–6 hours after the last medication is administered (post-tablet test) and peak concentrations are measured. In this case, TT4 is expected to be within the reference range (upper half limit), and a TT4 value just above the reference range is accepted. In most patients, follow-up of TSH does not offer a significant advantage over a measurement of T4 solely (Dixon, Reed, and Mooney 2002; Le Traon *et al.* 2009). Second, administration of a meal does decrease absorption of L-thyroxine. Therefore, it is recommended to administer L-thyroxine 2–3 hours before a meal. For many owners this is not feasible and therefore it is important to follow the daily routine of the owner also on the day of blood sampling, which may mean that the patient is not fasted.

If major clinical improvement is not observed within 3 months despite adequate thyroid hormone supplementation (verified by TT4 serum concentrations), an erroneous diagnosis or presence of unidentified concurrent disease should be suspected. As the hypo-thalamic-pituitary-thyroid axis has been inhibited by thyroid hormone supplementation, if the practitioner doubts the diagnosis and would like to investigate thyroid function again, treatment has to be ceased for a minimum period of 4–8 weeks. With concurrent hypoadrenocorticism, chronic kidney disease, liver failure, or diabetes, the initial dosage should be decreased by 25–50% and gradually increased over a 1–2 months period.

Quality of Life

The difficulty in management of hypothyroidism lies in its diagnosis. Treatment is usually straightforward and improvement should be spectacular, thus negating the need for euthanasia as a hypothyroid dog can lead a normal life if it is treated with thyroid hormone supplementation.

References

Boretti FS, Sieber-Ruckstuhl NS, Wenger-Riggenbach B, Gerber B, Lutz H, Hofmann-Lehmann R, Reusch CE. Comparison of 2 doses of recombinant human thyrotropin for thyroid function testing in healthy and suspected hypothyroid dogs. Journal of Veterinary Internal Medicine. 2009; 23: 856–861.

Bossens K, Daminet S, Duchateau L, Rick M, Van Ham L, Bhatti S. The effect of imepitoin, a recently developed antiepileptic drug, on thyroid function test parameters and fat metabolism in healthy Beagle dogs. Preliminary findings. Veterinary Journal. 2016; 213: 48–52.

Daminet S. Canine hypothyroidism In: E Côté, Ed. Clinical Veterinary Advisor - Dogs and Cats, 3rd edn. Mosby Elsevier, 2015: 536–538.

Daminet S, Ferguson DC. Influence of drugs on thyroid function in dogs. Journal of Veterinary Internal Medicine. 2003; 17: 463–472.

Daminet S, Fifle L, Paradis M, Duchateau L, Moreau M. Use of recombinant human thyroid-stimulating hormone for thyrotropin stimulation test in healthy, hypothyroid and euthyroid sick dogs. Canadian Veterinary Journal. 2007; 48: 1273–1279.

De Roover K, Duchateau L, Carmichael N, Geffen C, Daminet S. Effect of storage of reconstituted recombinant human thyroid-stimulating hormone (rhTSH) on thyroid-stimulating hormone (TSH) response testing in euthyroid dogs. Journal of Veterinary Internal Medicine. 2006; 20: 812–817.

Dixon, R.M, Reid SWJ, Mooney CT. Treatment and therapeutic monitoring of canine hypothyroidism. Journal of Small Animal Practice. 2002; 43: 334–340.

Le Traon G, Brennan SF, Burgaud S, Daminet S, Gommeren K, Horspool LJI, Rosenberg D. et al. Clinical evaluation of a novel liquid formulation of L-thyroxine for once daily treatment of dogs with hypothyroidism.

Journal of Veterinary Internal Medicine. 2009; 23: 43–49.

Lee J.A., Hinchcliff KW, Piercy RJ, Schmidt KE, Nelson S. Effects of racing and non-training on plasma thyroid hormone concentrations in sled dogs. Journal of the American Veterinary Medical Association. 2004; 224: 226–231.

Pinilla M, Shiel RE, Brennan SF, McAllister H, Mooney CT. Quantitative thyroid scintigraphy in greyhounds suspected of primary hypothyroidism. Veterinary Radiology & Ultrasound. 2009; 50: 224–229.

Scott-Moncrieff JCR. Hypothyroidism In: SJ. Ettinger and EC. Feldman, Eds. Textbook of veterinary internal medicine, 7th edn. Elsevier. 2010: 1751–1761.

Shiel RE, Pinilla M, McAllister H, Mooney CT. Assessment of the value of quantitative thyroid scintigraphy for determination of thyroid function in dogs. Journal of Small Animal Practice. 2012; 53: 278–285.

Van Dijl IC, Le Traon G, van de Meulengraaf BD, Burgaud S, Horspool LJ, Kooistra HS. Pharmacokinetics of total thyroxine after repeated oral administration of levothyroxine solution and its clinical efficacy in hypothyroid dogs Journal of Veterinary Internal Medicine. 2014; 28: 1229–1234.

van Geffen C, Bavegems V, Duchateau L, De Roover K, Daminet S. Serum thyroid hormone concentrations and thyroglobulin autoantibodies in trained and non-trained healthy whippets. Veterinary Journal. 2006; 172: 135–140.

12

Hyperadrenocorticism in Dogs and Cats

Eric Zini and Michele Berlanda

Introduction

Clinical and Diagnostic Aspects

Hyperadrenocorticism (HAC) can either be pituitary dependent (PDH) due to hypersecretion of corticotropin (ACTH) by the pituitary gland, adrenal dependent (ADH) due to functional adrenocortical tumors, or iatrogenic from the administration of corticosteroids. HAC is rare in cats.

In dogs, the most common clinical signs are polyuria and polydipsia, polyphagia, alopecia, pendulous abdomen, hepatomegaly, panting, and muscular atrophy (Arenas, Melián, and Pérez-Alenza 2013). In cats, the clinical signs are less obvious since HAC is associated with diabetes mellitus in 90% of cases (Mellett, Bruyette, and Stanley 2013); the most characteristic abnormality is thinning and extreme skin fragility (Figure 12.1). Systemic hypertension is more frequent in dogs than cats.

The initial approach to an animal suspected with HAC includes complete blood count, serum biochemistry, and urinalysis. The most common findings are stress leukogram (dogs), moderate thrombocytosis (dogs), variable increase in ALP (dogs and cats), ALT (dogs and cats), cholesterol, and triglycerides (dogs and cats), hyperglycemia (more common in cats), frequent isosthenuria or hyposthenuria (dogs), and proteinuria (dogs and cats). In both species, diagnosis of naturally acquired HAC will be confirmed through dexamethasone suppression and/or ACTH stimulation test; the latter is also useful to diagnose the iatrogenic form and monitor treatment. The urine cortisol:creatinine ratio may not be helpful as a screening test for HAC because of its variable sensitivity and low specificity. Ultrasound evaluation of the adrenal glands and endogenous ACTH measurement are useful for distinguishing PDH from ADH, and CT and MRI can be used to characterize the pituitary gland.

Therapy

The choice of treatment depends on the underlying cause of HAC. Therefore, it is important to differentiate between PDH and ADH, after excluding the iatrogenic form.

Chronic Disease Management for Small Animals, First Edition. Edited by W. Dunbar Gram, Rowan J. Milner and Remo Lobetti.

(a)

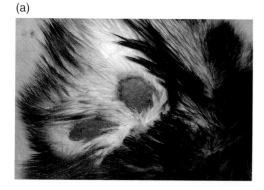

(b)

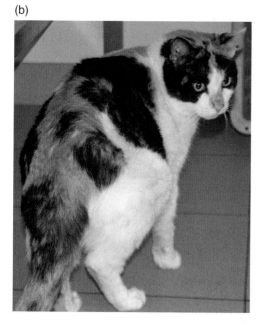

Figure 12.1 Cat (11 years old, spayed female, domestic shorthair) with pituitary-dependent hyperadrenocorticism. Skin tears are observed on the dorsal aspect of the thorax due to increased cutaneous fragility (Figure 12.1a). Trilostane treatment allowed healing of lesions (Figure 12.1b). At diagnosis the cat was not diabetic. Diabetes mellitus developed after approximately 1 year of trilostane administration, despite improvement of hyperadrenocorticism.

Medical and surgical options are available to treat both PDH and ADH. Treatment of HAC quickly improves polyuria and polydipsia, as well as polyphagia, whereas a few months may be necessary for improvement of dermatologic and muscular signs. Reduction of cortisol, however, can unveil clinical signs related to arthropathy or an allergic disorder. Regarding biochemical parameters, these can take weeks to improve and resolve; persistence of alterations may indicate that the treatment is not sufficient or that there is concurrent disease.

Medical Therapy for Pituitary Dependent Hyperadrenocorticism

Trilostane

This is an inhibitor of β-3 hydroxysteroid dehydrogenase in adrenal glands and is currently the drug most frequently used and recommended in dogs and cats due to the high rate of improvement of clinical signs and few side effects. In dogs, the dosages administered orally are 0.2–1.1 mg/kg, twice daily, with larger breeds requiring lesser quantity; some dogs require daily administration (with higher dosages) (Feldman and Kass 2012; Arenas, Melián, and Pérez-Alenza 2013). In the cat, dosages vary from 1 mg/kg 3 times a day, up to 13 mg/kg once daily (Mellett, Bruyette, and Stanley 2013). It is worth noting that trilostane is absorbed better when given with food (Figure 12.2).

The correct dosage of trilostane is initially checked after 10–15 days and the goal, in dogs, is to reach a cortisol post-ACTH stimulation ranging between 1.5 and 5 µg/dL. Recent studies have reassessed the utility of basal cortisol only: values ≥1.3 µg/dL exclude excessive suppression, while values < 2.9 µg/dL exclude inadequate control. Because clinical benefits can be observed only after about 30 days, at first control the dosage should not be increased, but rather reduced if cortisol is low. Later, modifications of the dosages in dogs are based both on clinical response and cortisol concentrations post-ACTH stimulation:

- If <1.5 µg/dL and clinical signs are improving or absent, the administration of trilostane should be discontinued for 3–7 days and restarted at a lower dosage; if anorexia, vomiting, tremors, and weakness are present, the administration should be

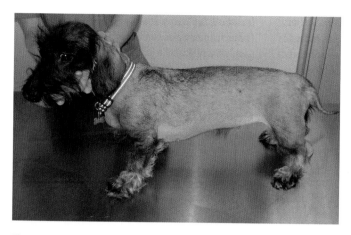

Figure 12.2 Dog (6 years old, intact female, Dachshund) with pituitary dependent hyperadrenocorticism. The dog received trilostane treatment (2 mg/kg, twice daily) without food and showed polyuria, polydipsia, and alopecia; cortisol post-ACTH stimulation was 23.6 µg/dL. To ameliorate trilostane absorption the dog received it with food and, after one month, had improved polyuria and polydipsia and cortisol post-ACTH stimulation dropped to 10.5 µg/dL.

interrupted for one month and integration with glucocorticoid and mineralocorticoid may be necessary;

- If between 1.5 and 5 µg/dL, the dosage should not be changed;
- If between 5 and 9 µg/dL, the dosage can remain unchanged if clinical signs are well controlled, otherwise it should be increased.

The ACTH stimulation test should be repeated 10–15 days after any change in the dosage of trilostane and any increase or reduction in dosage should be 25%. It is underlined that the ACTH stimulation test should be performed about 4 hours after the administration of trilostane, either for once or twice daily administration.

Side-effects of trilostane are usually mild and include lethargy, weakness, anorexia, vomiting, and diarrhea. An uncommon side effect is acute necrosis of the adrenal cortex leading to temporary or permanent hypoadrenocorticism (with or without electrolyte abnormalities). This side effect is more likely in dogs that receive higher dosages. The ACTH stimulation test and ultrasound of the adrenal glands are important to confirm this complication. Sudden death of dogs on

trilostane treatment has been described. Median survival of dogs with PDH treated with trilostane varies from 549–900 days; 70% survive >1 year and 29% >3 years (Clemente *et al.* 2007). The number of cats treated is still too limited to provide accurate information on maintenance therapy and survival.

Mitotane

Mitotane (o, p'-DDD) has cytotoxic action primarily on the area fasciculata and reticularis of the adrenal cortex. For years it was the main drug used for HAC treatment in dogs, while in cats it is not recommended due to its low efficacy. Mitotane in dogs provides good improvement of clinical signs, but can cause serious side effects (hypoadrenocorticism in 6–10%, often irreversible) and relapses are common (50–60% in the first year) (Kintzer and Peterson 1991).

Therapy with mitotane includes two phases:

Initiation phase: 30–50 mg/kg of oral mitotane, preferably divided in two daily administrations, with food. Dogs undergoing treatment should have a good appetite. The initiation phase is interrupted if the owner observes a major decrease in appetite, thirst, vomiting, or diarrhea. After 8–10 days, or at any time before if a dog shows these clinical signs, the ACTH stimulation test should be repeated. Cortisol post-ACTH should be 1–4 µg/dL to start maintenance therapy; if >4 µg/dL, a second course of therapy can be repeated. In case of severe clinical signs of hypoadrenocorticism or if cortisol decreases to <1 µg/dL, the administration of corticosteroids and mineralocorticoid is recommended.

Maintenance therapy: 25–50 mg/kg of mitotane per week, divided in several administrations. Monitoring with ACTH stimulation test should be repeated every 3–6 months. If post-ACTH cortisol is >4 µg/dL, it is recommended to restart the loading phase. Median survival of dogs treated with mitotane is approximately 2 years; according to one study, treatment with trilostane is associated with longer survival than mitotane (Clemente *et al.* 2007).

Ketoconazole

This is an inhibitor of the 11 β-hydroxylase in the adrenal glands but is not frequently used in dogs. The initial dosage is 5 mg/kg twice daily, which may be gradually increased to 20–30 mg/kg, according to clinical signs. The efficacy of treatment is assessed using the ACTH stimulation test. On occasion, the treatment is not effective or may cause liver damage. Median survival of treated dogs is 25 months (Lien & Huang 2008). Ketoconazole is not recommended in cats to treat HAC.

Other Drugs

Bromocriptine, cyproheptadine, selegiline, retinoic acid, metyrapone, and aminoglutethimide are not currently recommended in dogs and cats.

Surgical Therapy for Pituitary Dependent Hyperadrenocorticism

Transsphenoidal hypophysectomy is a good therapeutic option in dogs, especially for tumors of limited size. The most frequent postoperative complications are central diabetes insipidus and hypernatremia, especially if the tumor is large, as well as secondary hypothyroidism and keratoconjunctivitis sicca. Dogs undergoing surgery may experience recurrence in 28% of cases, with a median disease-free period of 896 days (Hanson *et al.* 2005). The number of cats treated by transsphenoidal hypophysectomy is still limited.

Radiation Therapy for Pituitary Dependent Hyperadrenocorticism

This may be considered for pituitary tumors that cause neurological signs. In dogs, radiation therapy can significantly reduce tumor size. However, despite the benefit, in the case of tumors of considerable size neurological signs may persist. Medical treatment of HAC is not discontinued, despite radiation therapy. The number of cats treated with radiation therapy is still limited.

Surgical Therapy for Adrenal Dependent Hyperadrenocorticism

Adrenalectomy is the treatment of choice for dogs with ADH, after careful assessment of risks and benefits. Vascular infiltration, the presence of tumors >5 cm and metastases are adverse prognostic factors. Metastases are observed in 6–18% of cases by radiography, ultrasound, or CT. Intraoperative and perioperative mortality is variable, but can exceed 25%; animals that survive, however, have excellent life expectancy, from 1 to over 4 years. To stabilize the dog before surgery, it is important to administer medical therapy (preferably trilostane) for 3–4 weeks. Intraoperative and postoperative complications are intraperitoneal bleeding, hypoadrenocorticism, pancreatitis, and acute renal failure (Massari *et al.* 2011). In cats, experience is still limited.

Medical Therapy for Adrenal Dependent Hyperadrenocorticism

Trilostane is also effective to treat dogs with ADH, although sometimes with a slightly lower dosage than that used for PDH. Median life expectancy ranges from 12–14 months. Mitotane can be used for medical therapy of dogs with ADH, although the effective dosages are 50–100% higher compared to those used for PDH, for both the initiation phase and maintenance therapy. Median survival of dogs with ADH treated with trilostane or mitotane is comparable (Helm *et al.* 2011).

Other Therapies

Because HAC can lead to hypertension, it is necessary to assess whether this is present and treat it with anti-hypertensive drugs. Furthermore, HAC in dogs often causes glomerulopathy and proteinuria, which may require anti-proteinuric treatment. Dogs, and especially cats, can have concurrent diabetes mellitus. Treatment for HAC improves glycemic control in many cats, but not always in the dog. Finally, since HAC in dogs may promote a hypercoagulable state and thromboembolism, antiplatelet agents may be necessary (Park *et al.* 2013).

Quality of Life

The quality of life of most dogs and cats affected by HAC that are correctly treated is excellent; therefore, medical or surgical treatment is always recommended. In some cases, inadequate control with medical treatment and growth of the pituitary or adrenal gland tumor can cause persistence or appearance of new clinical signs. In such cases the owner may decide for euthanasia.

References

Arenas C, Melián C, Pérez-Alenza MD. Evaluation of 2 trilostane protocols for the treatment of canine pituitary-dependent hyperadrenocorticism: twice daily versus once daily. Journal of Veterinary Internal Medicine. 2013; 27: 1478–1485.

Clemente M, De Andrés PJ, Arenas C, et al. Comparison of non-selective adrenocorticolysis with mitotane or trilostane for the treatment of dogs with pituitary-dependent hyperadrenocorticism. Veterinary Record. 2007; 161: 805–809.

Feldman EC, Kass PH. Trilostane dose versus body weight in the treatment of naturally occurring pituitary-dependent hyperadrenocorticism in dogs. Journal of Veterinary Internal Medicine. 2012; 26: 1078–1080.

Hanson JM, van't HM, Voorhout G, et al. Efficacy of transsphenoidal hypophysectomy in treatment of dogs with pituitary-dependent hyperadrenocorticism. Journal of Veterinary Internal Medicine. 2005; 19: 687–694.

Helm JR, McLauchlan G, Boden LA, et al. A comparison of factors that influence survival in dogs with adrenal-dependent hyperadrenocorticism treated with mitotane or trilostane. Journal of Veterinary Internal Medicine. 2011; 25: 251–260.

Kintzer PP, Peterson ME. Mitotane (o,p'-DDD) treatment of 200 dogs with pituitary-dependent hyperadrenocorticism. Journal of Veterinary Internal Medicine. 1991; 5: 182–190.

Lien YH, Huang HP. Use of ketoconazole to treat dogs with pituitary-dependent hyperadrenocorticism: 48 cases (1994–2007). Journal of the American Veterinary Medical Association. 2008; 233: 1896–1901.

Massari F, Nicoli S, Romanelli G, et al. Adrenalectomy in dogs with adrenal gland tumors: 52 cases (2002–2008). Journal of the American Veterinary Medical Association. 2011; 239: 216–221.

Mellett KAM, Bruyette D, Stanley S. Trilostane therapy for treatment of spontaneous hyperadrenocorticism in cats: 15 cases (2004-2012). Journal of Veterinary Internal Medicine. 2013; 27: 1471–1477.

Park FM, Blois SL, Abrams-Ogg AC, et al. Hypercoagulability and ACTH-dependent hyperadrenocorticism in dogs. Journal of Veterinary Internal Medicine. 2013; 27: 1136–1142.

13

Diabetes Mellitus

Eric Zini and Michele Berlanda

Introduction

Diabetes mellitus (DM) is a common endocrinopathy of dogs and cats that is due to an absolute or relative deficiency of insulin by pancreatic β-cells. Most dogs have a type I-like DM, generally caused by the development of autoimmunity against pancreatic islets. DM can also be associated with pancreatitis, hyperadrenocorticism, and administration of corticosteroids; diestrus and pregnancy may be predisposing factors in bitches. Samoyed, Miniature Schnauzer, and Poodle are at increased risk for DM.

The majority of cats (80%) present with type II-like DM, characterized by decreased production of insulin and insulin resistance. Depositions of pancreatic amyloid and glucose toxicity are among the mechanisms that contribute to destruction of β-cells. Obesity and inflammatory conditions promote insulin resistance by secreting pro-inflammatory cytokines. Pancreatitis and pancreatic tumors in cats can also damage β-cells and lead to DM. Burmese cats are predisposed to DM (Nelson and Reusch 2014).

Diagnosis

DM in dogs and cats is suspected in the presence of clinical signs such as polyuria, polydipsia, polyphagia, and weight loss. Other clinical signs caused by DM are visual impairment secondary to diabetic cataract (dogs), plantigrade stance and generalized weakness due to diabetic polyneuropathy (cats), systemic hypertension (dogs), vomiting and lethargy induced by diabetic ketoacidosis, and pollakiuria and stranguria for cystitis.

Hyperglycemia, glycosuria, and increased serum fructosamine are used to diagnose DM. Fructosamines are irreversibly glycosylated proteins that are increased in dogs and cats with DM and are the expression of average blood glucose of the previous 1–3 weeks. It is important to remember that hyperglycemia and glycosuria may be induced by stress in cats. In these cases, fructosamine concentrations will be normal. Other laboratory abnormalities in diabetic dogs and cats are hypertriglyceridemia, hypercholesterolemia, and increased ALT and ALP activity (less likely in cats). It is recommended that the initial assessment of diabetic dogs and cats is as complete as possible in order to identify any complications and concomitant or predisposing diseases.

Therapy

The cornerstones of treatment in diabetic dogs and cats are administration of insulin and a specific diet (Rucinsky *et al.* 2010; Sparkes *et al.* 2015). Treatment goals are

Chronic Disease Management for Small Animals, First Edition. Edited by W. Dunbar Gram, Rowan J. Milner and Remo Lobetti.

resolution of clinical signs, control of body weight, and prevention of diabetic complications and episodes of hypoglycemia. In addition, in all diabetic cats and bitches with DM associated with diestrus and pregnancy, treatment should be aimed at achieving remission of disease.

Insulin

Short-acting insulin is preferred in animals with diabetic ketoacidosis or hyperosmolar syndrome, while insulins with an intermediate or long duration are administered in uncomplicated cases. The most widely used insulins and recommended for uncomplicated DM include:

- *Porcine insulin zinc suspension.* Duration of effect 8–14 hours in dogs, 6–12 hours in cats. First choice in dogs, with an initial dosage of 0.25 UI/kg, twice daily. Not first choice in cats, because it can have a short duration.
- *Human recombinant protamine zinc insulin.* Duration of effect 10–16 hours in dogs, 10–14 hours in cats. First choice in cats with a starting dosage of 0.25 UI/kg, twice daily, without exceeding the dosage of 2 UI/cat for each administration. Not available in some countries.
- *Insulin glargine (recombinant human insulin analogue).* Duration of effect 8–16 hours in cats (Gilor *et al.* 2010). First choice in this species (like the above) with an initial dosage of 0.5 UI/cat for weight <2 kg, 1 UI/cat if ≤4 kg, and 1.5 UI/cat if >4 kg. Do not exceed 1 UI/cat if the initial glucose concentration is <350 mg/dL. In dogs, it is less beneficial than other insulins. It is not currently registered for dogs or cats.

Care must be taken with the use of insulins for human because they have concentrations of 100 UI/mL, while those registered for dogs and cats have concentrations of 40 UI/mL; it is therefore advisable to use the correct syringes for each type of insulin or make the correct conversion. Furthermore, it is suggested to administer insulin under the skin of the lateral chest and switch sides at each administration; this decreases the chances of local inflammation that in turn reduces insulin absorption.

Oral Antidiabetic Drugs

Oral hypoglycemic drugs are not commonly used in diabetic dogs and cats. In cats, glipizide (sulfonylurea) stimulates insulin secretion by the β-cells. Glipizide is ineffective in diabetic dogs because they have almost a complete absence of β-cells. In cats, glipizide is used orally at an initial dosage of 2.5 mg/cat, twice daily; the dosage may be increased up to 5 mg/cat, twice daily, but vomiting and hepatocellular damage may occur. Glipizide is effective in approximately 30% of cats and promotes the deposition of amyloid. It may be used in cats that do not tolerate injections or with poor owner compliance (Feldman *et al.* 1997).

Diet

Diets for diabetic dogs and cats should have good palatability, reduced amounts of easily digestible sugars (complex carbohydrates are preferred), and high quality proteins. Fiber-rich diets may be less palatable and reduce the absorption of nutrients leading to a decrease in body weight. While these diets are useful in overweight animals, they should be used with caution in others because they can cause malnourishment. In the cat, it is preferable to favor diets rich in protein and with very small amounts of carbohydrates (Figure 13.1). In both species, wet diets are preferred because they have lower caloric density and carbohydrates. In animals that easily eat, it is advisable to provide two equal meals associated with the administration of insulin every 12 hours. In those used to eat freely throughout the day, it is possible to provide a half meal in the morning along with the dosage of insulin, and allow free access to the remaining diet; the second dosage of insulin should be given 8 hours after the previous meal. In animals that are overweight, a reduction in body weight of 1–2%

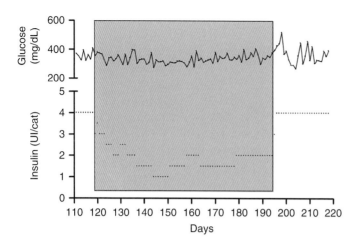

Figure 13.1 Diabetic cat treated with insulin glargine switched to a diet with very low content of carbohydrates from day 119 to 194 (grey box). The dose of insulin was decreased in order to maintain stable glycemia, clinical signs and fructosamine concentrations. The cat was a 10 years old, neutered male, domestic short-hair with body weight of 6 kg. The graph shows the insulin dose administered with each injection (bottom) and the morning glucose concentration (top).

per week is suggested. In addition, promoting physical activity is recommended because it increases the absorption of glucose in muscles through an insulin-independent mechanism (Elliott *et al.* 2012).

Despite the essential role of diabetic diets, the presence of concomitant diseases can make other types of diet more important; for example, in a diabetic animal with chronic kidney failure it is necessary to give priority to a renal diet.

Monitoring

Diabetic dogs and cats under treatment should be monitored regularly to identify the most appropriate dosage of insulin. The dosage is adjusted according to the clinical conditions, serum fructosamine, and serial glucose curves. Monitoring is recommended 1, 2–3, 4–6, 8–12, and 24 weeks after diagnosis, and then every 3–6 months. The frequency, however, would vary according to individual needs. The disappearance of the clinical signs, fructosamine <400–450 mg/dL, and blood glucose between 90 and 250 mg/dL suggest good metabolic control of DM in both species.

If fructosamine levels are normal or low; it is necessary to ensure that the animal does not have episodes of hypoglycemia. It is important to remember that cats, unlike dogs, often do not show clinical signs of hypoglycemia, such as restlessness and seizures, and some cats present only weakness. Fructosamine concentrations >600 mg/dL are typically seen in diabetic dogs and cats with inadequate metabolic control.

Blood glucose curves can be performed at home by the owner or by the veterinarian after hospitalization (Casella *et al.* 2003). The former prevents the stress associated with hospitalization and may be preferable in cats, with 70% of owners able to perform glucose monitoring at home. Additionally, since hospitalization can lead the animal to not eat, it is preferable to administer food and insulin at home before reaching the veterinarian. The glucose curve is generated with capillary blood sampling (preferably from the inner pinna) every 1–2 hours for 12 hours; a longer duration may be required if a rebound hyperglycemia (Somogyi effect) is suspected. Blood sugar levels are measured with portable glucose meters for veterinary or human use and validated for dogs and cats. The ideal blood glucose curve has a nadir (lowest value of glucose) between 80 and 140 mg/dL and a duration of action of insulin that is approximately 12 hours. In case of hypoglycemia, the insulin dosage should be reduced by 25–50% and insulin should be resumed only when blood glucose is >180 mg/dL. In case of poor metabolic control, the insulin dose should be increased in cats by increments of 0.5 UI and in dogs by 1–5 UI (depending on weight). Finally, it is emphasized that blood glucose curves can vary from one day to the next (Fleeman and Rand 2003). Therefore, treatment decisions should always be made also considering clinical conditions and concentrations of fructosamine.

Remission

Remission of DM occurs in about 50% of diabetic cats and is defined as the disappearance of clinical signs for at least 4 weeks along with normalization of blood glucose despite discontinuation of insulin therapy. Remission occurs in the first 3–6 months after first diagnosis and is more likely if cats are elderly, have no polyneuropathy, have recently been treated with corticosteroids, and if strict glycemic control is initially provided (Zini *et al.* 2010). Even cats with ketoacidosis can achieve remission. In dogs, remission is rare with the exception of bitches in diestrus or pregnancy. Remission in these cases is more likely if spaying is performed within 4 weeks from onset of clinical signs or if hyperglycemia at diagnosis is not very high.

Quality of Life

In diabetic dogs, the median survival is 24 months and 33% of animals live >3 years. In the cat, median survival after initial diagnosis is 17 months. Cats that achieve remission have longer survival, whereas kidney failure is a negative prognostic factor; ketoacidosis is not associated with survival (Callegari *et al.* 2013). The quality of life of dogs and cats with DM is good if treatment is tightly administered. The need for injections can sometimes make the lives of owners less simple, although the greater care required can tighten the bond between the owner and the animal.

References

Callegari C, Mercuriali E, Hafner M, et al. Survival time and prognostic factors in cats with newly diagnosed diabetes mellitus: 114 cases (2000–2009). Journal of the American Veterinary Medical Association. 2013; 243: 91–95.

Casella M, Wess G, Hässig M, Reusch CE. Home monitoring of blood glucose concentration by owners of diabetic dogs. Journal of Small Animal Practice. 2003; 44: 298–305.

Elliott KF, Rand JS, Fleeman LM, et al. A diet lower in digestible carbohydrate results in lower postprandial glucose concentrations compared with a traditional canine diabetes diet and an adult maintenance diet in healthy dogs. Research in Veterinary Science. 2012; 93(1): 288–295.

Feldman EC, Nelson RW, Feldman MS. Intensive 50-week evaluation of glipizide administration in 50 cats with previously untreated diabetes mellitus. Journal of the American Veterinary Medical Association. 1997; 210: 772–777.

Fleeman LM, Rand JS. Evaluation of day-to-day variability of serial blood glucose concentration curves in diabetic dogs. Journal of the American Veterinary Medical Association. 2003; 222: 317–321.

Gilor C, Ridge TK, Attermeier KJ, Graves TK. Pharmacodynamics of insulin detemir and insulin glargine assessed by an isoglycemic clamp method in healthy cats. Journal of Veterinary Internal Medicine. 2010; 2(4): 870–874.

Nelson RW, Reusch CE. Animal models of disease: classification and etiology of diabetes in dogs and cats. Journal of Endocrinology. 2014; 222(3): T1–9.

Rucinsky R, Cook A, Haley S, et al. AAHA diabetes management guidelines. Journal of the American Animal Hospital Association. 2010; 46(3): 215–224.

Sparkes AH, Cannon M, Church D, et al. ISFM consensus guidelines on the practical management of diabetes mellitus in cats. Journal of Feline Medicine and Surgery. 2015; 17(3): 235–250.

Zini E, Hafner M, Osto M, et al. Predictors of clinical remission in cats with diabetes mellitus. Journal of Veterinary Internal Medicine. 2010; 24(6): 1314–1321.

14

Chronic Pancreatitis
Penny Watson

Introduction

Pancreatitis describes sterile pancreatic inflammation due to unregulated trypsin release within the pancreatic parenchyma. Chronic pancreatitis (CP) describes lymphoplasmacytic inflammation and fibrosis of the pancreas, leading to progressive loss of pancreatic exocrine and endocrine function. This differentiates it from truly acute pancreatitis where there is neutrophilic inflammation with varying amounts of pancreatic edema and necrosis, but the pancreas returns to normal functionally and histologically if the animal recovers from the acute bout. The definitions of acute and chronic pancreatitis are functional and histological rather than clinical, because some cases present acutely in spite of underlying chronic disease. The relationship between acute and chronic pancreatitis is a complex one involving an interaction between an animal's genetic make-up and environmental triggers. For a more detailed discussion see Watson (2015).

The prevalence of CP in dogs and cats is difficult to estimate since most animals do not have histological confirmation of disease, however, it does appear to be a common disease in both species. Historically, CP was considered a relatively rare disease in dogs and more common in cats, but recent canine studies have confirmed its importance in this species also.

Most cases in cats and dog remain idiopathic. The causes of CP are poorly understood with possible triggers including high fat diets, hypertriglyceridemia, hypothyroidism, diabetes mellitus, hyperadrenocorticism, and certain drugs (azathioprine, potassium bromide, phenobarbitone; organophosphates, asparaginase, sulphonamides, zinc, clomipramine). It is important to recognize potential triggers of disease in susceptible dogs because these should be addressed during treatment and long-term management

Increased prevalence in certain breeds of dog such as cavalier King Charles spaniels (CKCS), Boxers, Collies and English Cocker Spaniels (ECS) suggest some genetic predispositions but these are likely to interact with environmental triggers and risk factors to produce disease.

Diagnosis

Recent clinical studies in both dogs (Bostrom *et al.* 2013; Watson *et al.* 2007) and cats have confirmed CP as a clinically relevant disease, causing intermittent and/or on-going recurrent gastrointestinal signs and epigastric pain in a large number of affected animals. The gastrointestinal signs of CP are typically low grade, waxing and waning anorexia and vomiting. Diarrhea is not a prominent feature

Chronic Disease Management for Small Animals, First Edition. Edited by W. Dunbar Gram, Rowan J. Milner and Remo Lobetti.
© 2018 John Wiley & Sons, Inc. Published 2018 by John Wiley & Sons, Inc.

until the development of exocrine pancreatic insufficiency (EPI) in the end stage of disease. However, animals with CP will often have large-bowel type diarrhea with some fresh blood a day or two after an episode, presumably due to irritation of the transverse colon as it passes close to the left limb of the pancreas.

Some dogs with CP will present for the first time with an acute-on-chronic bout of pancreatitis, which looks clinically identical to classic acute pancreatitis, with sudden onset acute vomiting and severe abdominal pain. Some animals have recurrent acute flare-ups, often with no apparent trigger; others are presented during an acute exacerbation of disease with acute onset icterus due to extrahepatic biliary obstruction. Affected cats can also be icteric, although in cats this is more often due to concurrent cholangitis than to extrahepatic biliary obstruction.

Pain is a consistent and clinically important feature of CP. Chronic pancreatic pain is notoriously difficult to recognize and treat. Owners may be more aware of this pain than their veterinary surgeon, particularly in cats, which are very good at hiding pain in the consulting room. It is therefore very important for clinicians to be alert for signs of postprandial pain in the history and to work in partnership with owners for effective identification and treatment. The pain is not to be under-estimated: in humans, the pain of CP is often so severe that it leads to chronic opiate addiction or even total pancreatectomy. Clinical signs suggestive of pain in dogs or cats with CP can include stretching or pacing around after eating; listlessness; discomfort when picked up, particularly around the abdomen; snappiness with owner and other animals when approached; and/or acquired food aversions particularly to high fat foods.

Pain is particularly difficult to assess in cats but tends to present as similar behavior changes and a reduction in previous activity level. The pain of CP in humans can sometimes be referred to the lumbar spine, which has been described in dogs. However, some breeds affected with CP, such as the ECS, are

also at increased risk of intervertebral disc disease so it is important to differentiate this from CP.

On clinical examination in dogs, the low-grade pain of CP is more difficult to recognize than the pain of acute disease. In the latter, palpation of any part of the abdomen usually elicits pain whereas with CP, the pain is only elicited over the pancreas. Dogs will usually show a pain response whereas cats rarely show pain on clinical examination even in the face of severe acute exacerbations of chronic disease.

Dogs and cats with CP may also show clinical signs consistent with chronic small intestinal maldigestion, with polyphagia, weight loss and dry coat. Some animals also have chronic steatorrhea with foul-smelling, voluminous feces although this does not appear to be a prominent feature in many animals developing EPI as an end stage of CP.

Confirmation of diagnosis of CP is challenging. Pancreatic histopathology is the most sensitive and specific test but pancreatic biopsies are not usually indicated because they are invasive and do not change the treatment. Diagnosis therefore has to rely on a combination of clinical signs, transcutaneous ultrasonography and pancreas specific blood tests such as lipase and canine- and feline-specific pancreatic lipase immunoreactivity. CP is therefore likely to be under-recognized because of the difficulty in obtaining a non-invasive diagnosis. Affected animals also usually show clinicopathological evidence of a systemic inflammatory response often with neutrophilia and pre-renal azotemia. Some animals will show evidence of diabetes mellitus. It is also important to measure serum trypsin-like immunoreactivity (TLI) and cobalamin in affected animals to assess for development of EPI. Cobalamin deficiency is common in dogs and cats with EPI because the pancreas is the only significant source of intrinsic factor, which is required for the absorption of cobalamin in the ileum. Dogs produce some intrinsic factor in their stomach, but the pancreas is the only source in cats. The sensitivity of a reduced TLI to diagnosis EPI in dogs and cats with CP is less than in dogs with pancreatic acinar atrophy. This is because ongoing pancreatic inflammation can increase the TLI back in to the normal range even in cases with clinically significant exocrine insufficiency.

It is very important to undertake some form of diagnostic imaging in affected animals to rule out serious concurrent diseases such as gastrointestinal or biliary tract obstructions. It is not uncommon for pancreas-specific blood tests to be positive in animals with a concurrent more clinically significant disease such as gastrointestinal neoplasia or obstruction (Haworth et al. 2014).

Treatment

Treatment of CP is largely symptomatic as in most cases there is no specific treatment, with the possible exception of the ECS. However, supportive treatment remains very important because it can make a real difference to the quality of life of the affected dog and can be life-saving in acute exacerbations of underlying chronic disease. The most challenging aspect of long-term management is dealing with the chronic pain, but addressing functional loss is also important. In addition, acute exacerbations of disease should be addressed with intensive management in the same way as truly acute pancreatitis cases.

Treatment of Ongoing Chronic Pancreatitis

CP in dogs and cats is usually a low grade, progressive, on-going disease that slowly destroys the pancreatic parenchyma, like a smoldering fire. It is important that the pain, progressive loss of endocrine and exocrine function, and concurrent signs are managed.

In some cases of CP, the disease will eventually 'burn itself out' when the entire pancreas has been destroyed. These cases will have functional loss (diabetes mellitus and EPI) but will no longer suffer from bouts of pain and acute exacerbations of disease. This is in many ways the "ideal" because the exocrine and endocrine insufficiencies can be treated whereas the pain of on-going CP can be very difficult to control. It is impossible to predict in animals, as in humans, which cases of end-stage CP will "burn themselves out" in the animal's life time and which cases will continue to suffer from recurrent bouts of acute flare-ups of disease in spite of functional loss.

Pain can be particularly marked postprandially is often under-recognized by owners and clinicians, particularly in cats. Because of this, all animals with CP should be assumed to be suffering from pain until proven otherwise. Use of effective analgesics often results in behavior changes such as increased activity and playfulness. In most cases, the pain can be controlled long term but in a small number of dogs and cats, it may prove impossible to provide effective long-term analgesia and this may lead to end-of-life decisions based on quality of life.

The pain of CP is similar to other chronic pain conditions in that it appears to cause up-regulation of central pain pathways with resultant hyperesthesia. There are many studies on the mechanisms and treatment of chronic pain in human CP but very little information in dogs and cats. The author has observed lymphocytic infiltrates within nerve sheaths on histology of the pancreas of affected dogs strongly suggesting that neurogenic pain is also important in small animals with CP. Treatment recommendations are thus currently extrapolated from humans. The use of a 'Pain Ladder' is the most helpful, starting with non-steroidals and then adding additional drugs until pain is effectively controlled (Figure 14.1). Traditional non-steroidals are often avoided because of the risk of GI ulceration and the frequency with which animals with CP have concurrent renal compromise, particularly during acute exacerbations of disease. Consideration could be give to their use longer term when the animal is stabilized, with careful monitoring of renal

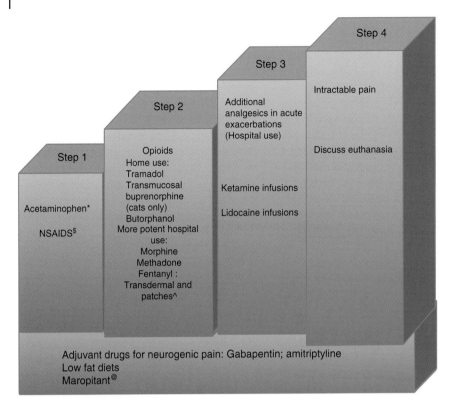

Figure 14.1 Analgesic ladder for dogs and cats with chronic pancreatitis, based on the human analgesic ladder in Sebastiano et al. (2005), which is based on the World Health Organization analgesic ladder for cancer pain. Note each step in the ladder can be added to the previous step for multimodal analgesia. *Preferred non-opioid drug in dogs, provided liver function is normal. Not to be used in cats. $Non-steroidal anti-inflammatories – higher risk of GI side effects in pancreatitis and only to be used when renal function is normal. ^Animals can be sent home with Fentanyl patches but great care must be taken about human contact particularly with children. @ Substance P has been implicated in the neuropathic pain of chronic pancreatitis so maropitant has a role in multimodal analgesia.

function. Acetaminophen is a useful first line drug in dogs, as in humans, but should never be used in dogs with decreased liver function or in cats. Feeding a low-fat diet is likely also to contribute to effective analgesia in dogs and cats with CP. In humans, high-fat diets increase postprandial pain and anecdotally the same is true in small animals.

The loss of exocrine function, together with recurrent bouts of anorexia, means that many affected dogs and cats can suffer from mild or more severe protein-calorie malnutrition, which should be recognized and addressed. Clinicians should be proactive in supplementing pancreatic enzymes in these cases. In addition, it may be necessary to

supplement cobalamin in dogs and particularly cats with EPI. This is traditionally given parenterally, but a recent study suggests oral supplementation may also be efficacious.

Comorbidities are common in canine and feline CP. Affected animals are often elderly, so some may be etiologically unrelated additional diseases of ageing dogs and cats, which may impact on control of the CP. For example, hyperadrenocorticism in dogs appears to increase the risk of acute bouts of pancreatitis. In cats, cholangitis and inflammatory bowel disease are common co-morbidities and their etiological relationship to CP is unclear. Clinicians should treat all co-morbidities as effectively as possible, while considering the potential for any treatments or dietary interventions to worsen the pancreatitis.

CP in ECS may respond to immunosuppression with corticosteroids or systemic cyclosporine. Ideally, diagnosis should be confirmed histologically in either pancreas or kidney prior to medication, but their use could be considered in an animal with convincing diagnostic imaging and clinic-pathological changes. Monitoring efficacy of treatment is currently challenging, as there are no validated blood tests for serial measurement, so animals should be monitored by clinical response.

Corticosteroids may also be indicated in cats with CP, predominantly to treat concurrent inflammatory bowel disease and/or lymphocytic cholangitis. The underlying cause of these diseases in cats remains an area of active research and bacteria have also been implicated, so the concurrent use of antibiotics is logical in cats until the diseases are better understood. A more complete discussion of the potential etiologies of CP and cholangitis in cats can be found in Simpson (2015)

Treatment of Low-Grade Recurrent Flare-ups

Dogs and cats with CP commonly present with stable ongoing chronic disease punctuated by episodes of acute exacerbation (like a smoldering fire which recurrently flares up). Severe acute episodes will require hospitalization and treatment. The owner at home can manage milder episodes, as long as the animal is not dehydrated or anorexic for a prolonged period of time. Mild acute episodes should be managed with an increase in analgesic use and a day or two of fasting. Early enteral feeding is very important in the context of severe acute pancreatitis but in mild disease, a few days fasting is not injurious and will reduce the pain associated with the episode. The author has also observed that some dogs respond to a course of metronidazole (10 mg/kg BID) after an acute bout of disease, particularly CKCS. This is likely to be due to development of secondary antibiotic responsive diarrhea due to secondary small intestinal ileus and malabsorption.

Treatment of Acute Flare-ups

Acute exacerbations of disease may also be very severe. Cases presenting clinically as severe acute pancreatitis should be treated in the same way as truly acute pancreatitis with intensive supportive care. The pillars of treatment of acute pancreatitis, and acute flare-ups of chronic disease, are: fluid therapy, analgesia, anti-emetics, and early enteral feeding.

Quality-of-Life and End-of-Life Assessments

It is important for owners and clinicians to understand that CP in dogs and cats is a lifelong, incurable disease, which never goes away and in fact is progressive. Clinical signs can usually be controlled but triggers for acute exacerbations should be avoided on a daily basis. Owners therefore have to be very careful about diet changes or tit bits, avoiding high fat foods. Clinicians should be mindful of potential drug triggers and avoid these as much as possible. Owners should also learn to recognize when their animal is in pain and understand the potential for and clinical signs of functional impairment so that they can recognize these when they begin to develop and present their animal to a vet. Management of the diabetic pet with CP can be particularly challenging and owners are assisted in this by understanding the potential for acute flare-ups of disease.

The owner and vet can work effectively together in the long-term management of the dog or cat with CP and these cases can be very rewarding. However, there are some cases where the animal's quality of life remains poor due to severe recurrent acute flare ups and ongoing pain for which control proves impossible and in these cases, it is important to discuss the option of euthanasia for the welfare of the animal. In the author's opinion, these cases are rare but do occur.

Pain is intractable in some dogs in spite of attempts to control it.

References

Bostrom BM, Xenoulis PG, Newman SJ, Pool RR, Fosgate GT, Steiner JM. Chronic pancreatitis in dogs: a retrospective study of clinical, clinicopathological, and histopathological findings in 61 cases. Veterinary Journal. 2013;195(1):73–79.

Haworth MD, Hosgood G, Swindells KL, Mansfield CS. Diagnostic accuracy of the SNAP and Spec canine pancreatic lipase tests for pancreatitis in dogs presenting with clinical signs of acute abdominal disease. Journal of Veterinary Emergency and Critical Care. 2014;24(2):135–143.

Sebastiano PD, Weigand MA, Köninger J, et al (2005) Conservative treatment of pain in chronic pancreatitis: guidelines for clinical routine. In: JE Dominguez-Munoz, Ed.

Clinical Pancreatology for Practising Gastroenterologists and Surgeons. Blackwell Publishing. 2005: 273–279

Simpson KW. Pancreatitis and triaditis in cats: causes and treatment. Journal of Small Animal Practice. 2015;56(1):40–49.

Watson P. Pancreatitis in dogs and cats: definitions and pathophysiology. Journal of Small Animal Practice. 2015;56(1):3–12.

Watson PJ, Roulois AJA, Scase T, Johnston PEJ, Thompson H, Herrtage, ME. Prevalence and breed distribution of chronic pancreatitis at post-mortem examination in first-opinion dogs. Journal of Small Animal Practice. 2007;48(11):609–618.

15

Mega-Esophagus and Esophageal Dysmotility
Liza S. Köster

Introduction

Mega-esophagus and esophageal dysmotility are conditions caused by a number of neuro-muscular, immune-mediated, infectious, neurological, rarely congenital, toxic, and possibly endocrine diseases, but many cases are idiopathic. Mega-esophagus is segmental or global esophageal dilation due to loss of motor function with ineffective peristalsis, whereas esophageal dysmotility is poorly defined and can be clinical or subclinical and possibly a forerunner of mega-esophagus but certainly a complication of esophagitis (Bexfield, Watson, and Herrtage 2006). Clinical signs include regurgitation, dysphagia, and aspiration pneumonia. Breeds that are most commonly affected by mega-esophagus include the German Shepherd Dog (GSD) and the Great Dane, with the GSD, Golden Retriever and Irish Setter breeds having a higher risk factor for developing mega-esophagus (Harvey et al. 1974; Gaynor, Shofer, and Washabau 1997; Strombeck 1978). Breeds affected by dysmotility include Bouvier des Flanders, Shar Pei and young terrier breeds (Peeters and Ubbink 1994; Stickle et al. 1992, and Bexfield et al. 2006). Earlier investigations report females being more commonly represented but later studies did not confirm sex or reproductive status as a risk factor. Supportive care is the mainstay of therapy in this syndrome as despite diagnosing the etiology of the mega-esophagus the clinical signs may be refractory to medical therapy, often requiring life-long treatment and management. Death is most commonly ascribable to complications including aspiration pneumonia or poor quality of life as assessed by the owner.

Congenital diseases associated with mega-esophagus, where clinical signs become apparent shortly after weaning, include idiopathic congenital mega-esophagus or secondary mega-esophagus due to congenital myasthenia gravis (MG), vascular ring anomalies (VRA), esophageal hiatal hernia and pituitary dwarfism. Other diseases that cause mega-esophagus, dysmotility, and regurgitation, include MG, esophagitis, inflammatory myopathies, infectious diseases, caudal esophageal neoplasia, degenerative peripheral neuropathies, endocrinopathies, hereditary myopathies, and toxicities.

When no underlying disease is detected the condition is considered idiopathic. Dogs are spontaneously afflicted between 5–12 years of age (Johnson, Denovo, and Mears 2008). Idiopathic mega-esophagus differs from achalasia in that the lower esophageal sphincter is normal in the former. Esophageal achalasia is the absence of esophageal peristalsis and inadequate lower esophageal relaxation due to functional loss of the myenteric plexus ganglion cells in the distal esophagus (Kempf, Beckmann, and Kook 2014). It has been

Chronic Disease Management for Small Animals, First Edition. Edited by W. Dunbar Gram, Rowan J. Milner and Remo Lobetti.

described as a rare acquired syndrome in dogs (Boria, Webster, and Berg 2003). It can be accompanied by mega-esophagus (Boria *et al.* 2003).

Diagnosis

Regurgitation is the hallmark clinical sign of mega-esophagus and esophageal dysmotility and needs to be distinguished from vomiting. Ideally, visualizing the primary complaint by feeding the dog is the most helpful in defining the clinical problem. However, regurgitation will not necessarily regularly occur in less than 30 minutes postprandial. Survey thoracic radiographs are the first diagnostic procedure that should be performed (Figure 15.1). Mega-esophagus, whether it is segmental or global is easily diagnosed without contrast studies and the added benefit of diagnosing an underlying etiology in the case of thymomas and MG. In the absence of mega-esophagus, esophageal dysmotility needs to be distinguished from pharyngeal or cricopharyngeal dysphagia, by fluoroscopic studies using barium contrast in both dogs and cats (Boria *et al.* 2003; Levine, Pollard, and Marks 2014; German *et al.* 2005). In diagnosing VRA, in addition to segmental mega-esophagus, focal leftward tracheal curvature at the region of the heart on dorsoventral or ventrodorsal view and moderate to marked focal narrowing of the trachea is visible in 100% and 74% of thoracic radiographs respectively (Buchanan, 2004).

Physical examination should include a complete neurological examination and evaluation for signs of muscle atrophy that could indicate peripheral neuropathies and myositis respectively. Minimum database should include screening and testing for endocrinopathies associated with lower motor neuron disease including hypothyroidism, typical and atypical hypoadrenocorticism. If these endocrinopathies are diagnosed; response to treatment should be monitored, as they may be a coincidental finding.

Myasthenia gravis can be screened for by acetylcholine receptor antibodies or rapid response to parenteral cholinesterases (Tensilon test), in the case of the generalized form (Shelton and Comparative Neuromuscular Laboratory 2015). Inflammatory myositis should be considered in a dog with dysphagia, weakness and muscle atrophy. Clinical pathology may have elevated creatinine kinase, aspartate transaminase, and alanine transaminase activities (Evans, Levesque, and Shelton 2004). Electromyography has characteristic positive sharp waves. If myositis is suspected; serology for infectious diseases should be conducted, in addition antibodies to 2 M masticatory muscle fibers, followed by muscle biopsy (Evans *et al.* 2004). Esophagitis with or without stricture should be expected within approximately three weeks of surgery, or in any dog or cat with vomiting and post-pilling of acidic drugs. Esophagoscopy is diagnostic. Diagnosis of caudal esophageal neoplasia requires survey and contrast thoracic radiographs, computed tomography, esophagoscopy, and biopsy for a definitive diagnosis by histopathology.

The gold standard for diagnosing achalasia and dysmotility is high-resolution manometry (Kempf et al. 2014). Cricopharyngeal dysphagia has been described by videofluoroscopy as a significant delay in opening and closing of the cranioesophageal sphincter (Pollard *et al.* 2000).

Therapeutics

Therapeutics can be divided into specific therapies to treat the associated underlying disease condition and supportive care to avoid regurgitation and aspiration pneumonia and ensuring adequate enteral nutrition. Even in those cases with a defined underlying cause, early detection and initiation of supportive care is necessary for a successful outcome.

Myasthenia gravis can be managed with pyridostigmine bromide (1–3 mg/kg, orally

(a)

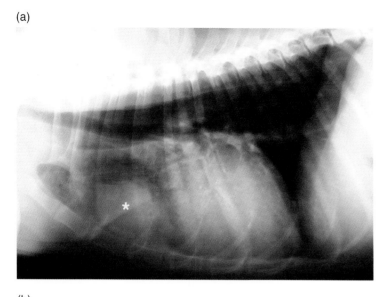

(b)

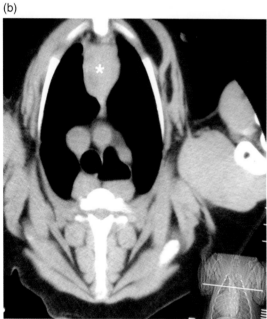

Figure 15.1 Right lateral thoracic radiograph (Figure 15.1a) and transverse computed tomography at the level of the third intercostal space (Figure 15.1b), using a soft tissue window width with the dog in dorsal recumbency, of an 11-year-old, spayed female, Springer Spaniel diagnosed with myasthenia gravis. There is a demarcated, soft tissue opacity visible in the cranial mediastinum (asterisk). A tentative diagnosis of thymoma was made.

BID) (Shelton 2002). Acetyl choline receptor antibody concentration and clinical signs need to be monitored as spontaneous remission can occur (Shelton 2002). Thymectomy is indicated in cats diagnosed with cranial mediastinal mass associated MG. Cats with MG are predominantly managed medically most commonly with a combination of pyridostigmine and steroids, only steroid or pyridostigmine or multiple immunosuppressive agents and pyridostigmine, but it is not possible to make recommendations based on the outcome of these studies (Hague *et al.* 2015). Immune mediated diseases, including MG, and myostis can be managed with immunosuppressive therapy such as glucocorticoids, cyclosporine, mycophenolate mofetil, and intravenous human immunoglobulin. Prokinetics such as metoclopramide and cisapride have been explored with little benefit, as they have no effect on the striated muscle of the canine esophagus (Washabau 2003). Bethanecol will stimulate propagating contractions of the esophagus in some dogs (Washabau 2003).

Surgical interventions are considered in thymomas causing MG, hiatal hernias, VRA, gastro-esophageal intussusception, and caudal esophageal neoplasia.

Calcium channel blockers, Botulinum toxin injections, pneumatic dilatation, esophagomyotomy, and fundic plication have been described in humans with achalasia (Boria *et al.* 2003).

Supportive care in this disease should focus on instituting nutritional support either in the form of postural feeding or enteral feeding devices. Dogs, of various breeds, with idiopathic congenital mega-esophagus provided strict postural feeding was implemented, consistently demonstrated improvement of esophageal motility over 6–9 months when monitored by means of manometry, indicative of delayed neuromuscular junction maturity (Diamant, Szczepanski, and Mui 1974). Meals should be small volume and divided into several portions throughout the day with various consistencies trialed to tailor the diet for the dog (Johnson *et al.* 2008). Solids stimulate peristalsis with less risk of aspiration, liquids have a shorter transit time but higher risk of aspiration (Strombeck 1978). Postural feeding is achieved by using a "Bailey chair"-like feeding platform and keeping the dog uprights for 15 to 20 minutes (*bailey chairs 4 dogs* n.d.). Appropriate feeding needs to address chronic complication like cachexia and hypoalbuminemia (Kang *et al.* 2013).

Oral feeding may not achieve caloric requirements in all dogs in which case gastrostomy tubes are short-term solutions and low-profile gastrostomy tubes are long-term solutions. Gastrostomy tubes can be placed non-invasively by percutaneous endoscopic techniques (PEG). Anesthetic considerations and aspiration pneumonia are important during procedures.

Quality of Life

The overall reported death due to elective euthanasia is 40% and because of a complication is 34% (Harvey *et al.* 1974). Myasthenia gravis is associated with a high rate (58%) of euthanasia in cats and thus mega-esophagus diagnosed in this species has an inherent poor prognosis as MG is highly associated with a diagnosis of a cranial mediastinal mass in this species (Hague *et al.* 2015). Reasons for electing euthanasia are reluctance of owners to pursue surgical removal of the thymoma and/or the difficulty in administering treatment. The knowledge of low rates of spontaneous remission and the continued need to medically manage cats after thymectomy make owners reluctant to consider invasive procedures.

The main considerations for humane euthanasia are assessed by the owner and should specifically consider the dog or cat's pain, appetite, behavior, and ambulatory status. The client needs to be educated to detect signs of aspiration pneumonia. Many conditions associated with mega-esophagus, specifically neuromuscular diseases, inflammatory myopathies are responsible for generalized deterioration and weakness, and the underlying disease very often will cause progressive disease. Other quality-of-life aspects to consider are those that pertain to the person providing care for the dog or cat. Managing a pet with mega-esophagus requires a large amount of contact time for feeding, whether it is with the aid of a "Bailey chair" feeding-platform or via a low-profile gastrostomy tube. Constant worry develops as a result of the strict regime for feeding schedules, concern about travel and leaving the dog under the care of a pet sitter, and the high frequency of veterinary visits for monitoring or treating complications.

Of dogs with mega-esophagus, 26% do not survive discharge from hospital with the most important risk factor identified in all non-survivors being aspiration pneumonia, but large body size and adult age group (>13 months) were also significant, indicative of the poor prognosis of idiopathic acquired mega-esophagus (McBrearty *et al.* 2011). Of patients that did not survive, 42% were euthanized, with 81% of euthanasia cases due to

mega-esophagus or its complication aspiration pneumonia (McBrearty *et al.* 2011). Acquired idiopathic mega-esophagus, or neglected acquired secondary mega-esophagus that has led to severe esophageal distention with irreversible myenteric plexus degeneration, is a disease associated with an unacceptably high mortality rate (Washabau 2003). The reason is due to chronic malnutrition and recurrent aspiration pneumonia. In conclusion, severe mega-esophagus, adult onset, and aspiration pneumonia are all important considerations when making a decision on humane euthanasia when considering long-term outcome.

References

Bailey chairs 4 dogs. Bailey chairs. Online at: https://www.facebook.com/baileychairs4dogs and https://www.baileychairs4dogs. com/(accessed October 4, 2015).

Bexfield NH, Watson PJ, Herrtage ME. 2006. Esophageal dysmotility in young dogs. Journal of Veterinary Internal Medicine. 2006; 20: 1314–1318.

Boria PA, Webster CR, Berg J. Esophageal achalasia and secondary megaesophagus in a dog. The Canadian Veterinary Journal. 2003: 44: 232–234.

Buchanan JW. Tracheal signs and associated vascular anomalies in dogs with persistent right aortic arch. Journal of Veterinary Internal Medicine. 2004; 18: 510–514.

Diamant N, Szczepanski M, Mui H. Idiopathic megaesophagus in the dog: reasons for spontaneous improvement and a possible method of medical therapy. The Canadian Veterinary Journal. 1974; 15: 66.

Evans J, Levesque D, Shelton GD. Canine inflammatory myopathies: a clinicopathologic review of 200 cases. Journal of Veterinary Internal Medicine. 2004; 18: 679–691.

Gaynor AR, Shofer FS, Washabau RJ. Risk factors for acquired megaesophagus in dogs. Journal of the American Veterinary Medical Association. 1997; 211: 1406–1412.

German AJ, Cannon MJ, Dye C, Booth MJ, Pearson GR, Reay CA, Gruffydd-Jones TJ Oesophageal strictures in cats associated with doxycycline therapy. Journal of Feline Medicine and Surgery. 2005; 7: 33–41.

Hague DW, Humphries HD, Mitchell MA, Shelton GD. Risk factors and outcomes in cats with acquired myasthenia gravis (2001–2012). Journal of Veterinary Internal Medicine. 2015; 29: 1307–1312.

Harvey CE, O'Brien JA, Durie VR, Miller DJ, Veenema R. Megaesophagus in the dog: a clinical survey of 79 cases. Journal of the American Veterinary Medical Association. 1974; 165: 443–446.

Johnson BM, Denovo R, Mears E. Canine megaesophagus. In: JD Bonagura and DC Twedt, Eds. Kirk's current veterinary therapy XIV. Saunders Elsevier. 2008: 486–492.

Kang MH, Seung JH, Lee JH, Park HM. Subepidermal blistering disease in a 5-month-old Alaskan Malamute dog with concurrent megaesophagus. Veterinary Quarterly. 2013; 33: 43–46.

Kempf J, Beckmann K, Kook PH. Achalasia-like disease with esophageal pressurization in a myasthenic dog. Journal of Veterinary Internal Medicine. 2014; 28: 661–665.

Levine JS, Pollard RE, Marks SL. Contrast videofluoroscopic assessment of dysphagic cats. Veterinary Radiology & Ultrasound. 2014; 55: 465–471.

McBrearty AR, Ramsey IK, Courcier EA, Mellor DJ, Bell R. Clinical factors associated with death before discharge and overall survival time in dogs with generalized megaesophagus. Journal of the American Veterinary Medical Asociation. 2011; 238: 1622–1628.

Peeters M, Ubbink G. Dysphagia-associated muscular dystrophy: a familial trait in the Bouvier des Flandres. Veterinary Record. 1994; 134: 444–446.

Pollard RE, Marks SL, Davidson A, Hornof WJ. Quantitative videofluoroscopic evaluation of pharyngeal function in the dog. Veterinary Radiology and Ultrasound. 2000; 41: 409–412.

Shelton GD, Comparative Neuromuscular Laboratory. Online at: http:// vetneuromuscular.ucsd.edu/index.html (accessed October 4, 2015).

Shelton GD Myasthenia gravis and disorders of neuromuscular transmission. Veterinary Clinics of North America: Small Animal Practice. 2002; 32: 189–206.

Stickle R, Sparschu G, Love N, Walshaw, R. 1992. Radiographic evaluation of esophageal function in Chinese Shar Pei pups. Journal of the American Veterinary Medical Association, 1992; 201: 81–84.

Strombeck DR Pathophysiology of esophageal motility disorders in the dog and cat. Application to management and prognosis. Veterinary Clinics of North America. 1978; 8: 229–244.

Washabau RJ 2003. Gastrointestinal motility disorders and gastrointestinal prokinetic therapy. Veterinary Clinics of North America: Small Animal Practice. 2003; 33: 1007–1028, vi.

16

Chronic Gastritis

Liza S. Köster

Introduction

The cardinal clinical sign of chronic gastritis is chronic or persistent vomiting in an otherwise healthy animal. The disease is probably underrepresented as many dogs and cats will vomit infrequently and the condition is commonly neglected. Biopsy of the gastric mucosa alone is insufficient to diagnose chronic gastritis as 26% of the healthy population of dogs can have mild gastritis based on endoscopic acquired gastric biopsies (van der Gaag 1988). Gastritis is also associated with chronic enteropathies, for example, chronic antral gastritis is a complication of chronic lymphocytic-plasmacytic enteritis which is thought to be gastrin mediated (Garcia-Sancho *et al.* 2005). The syndrome can be classified into two groups based on etiology, chronic non-specific gastritis also known as idiopathic and thought to be immune-mediated or auto-immune, and secondary gastritis including infectious causes including spiral bacteria like *Helicobacter* spp., parasites including *Ollulanus tricuspis*, and *Physaloptera* spp., reflux gastritis, drug induced, food allergic, toxins, mycosis including gastrointestinal pythiosis, and uremic gastropathy (Guilford and Strombeck 1996). Bilious vomiting syndrome should also be considered as a cause when owners complain that they observe chronic vomiting in their dog first thing in the morning but the dog has normal appetite. This is caused by gastroduodenal reflux, due to motor function of the stomach altering the rate of gastric emptying with bile salts acting as a detergent and inducing gastritis (Webb and Twedt 2003).

It is well established that the presence of large numbers of *Helicobacter*-like organisms, similar to *H. pylori*, is associated with lymphoplasmacytic hyperplasia and glandular degeneration of the junction of the fundus and pylorus (Lee *et al.* 1992). *Helicobacter heilmannii*, *H. felis*, among other species, have been reported and are often referred to as Helicobacter-like organisms (HLO) (Simpson *et al.* 2000). The pathogenic role of HLO has been questioned due to reports of 41–100% and 67–100% prevalence in healthy cats and dogs respectively, with higher prevalence reported in shelter or colony housed animals, less common in younger animals, and 57–100% and 72–90% of chronic vomiting cats and dogs respectively (Simpson *et al.* 2000).

Gastritis has been described in Alaskan racing sled dogs, which is a form of exercise-induced gastritis (Ritchey *et al.* 2011). Complications include gastric ulcers, and hemorrhage and signs can vary from reduced performance to acute death.

Eosinophilic gastro-enterocolitis is a condition in cats that is caused by parasitism, toxoplasmosis, food hypersensitivity,

Chronic Disease Management for Small Animals, First Edition. Edited by W. Dunbar Gram, Rowan J. Milner and Remo Lobetti.
© 2018 John Wiley & Sons, Inc. Published 2018 by John Wiley & Sons, Inc.

hypereosinophilic syndrome, or neoplasia and can be accompanied by peripheral eosinophilia, reported in 20% of cats with this syndrome (Tucker *et al.* 2014). Usually these cats are elderly, with a mean age of 9.2 years (range 1–17 years) and the most commonly affected breeds include domestic shorthair, domestic longhair, and Persian. Two percent of cases will have eosinophilic infiltrates on gastric biopsies despite the most common clinical sign (80%) being chronic vomiting.

Hypertrophic gastropathy with gastritis and gastric outflow obstruction can be caused by a number of diseases such as Zollinger-Ellison syndrome caused by a gastrinoma and acquired antral pyloric hypertrophy and gastritis of older Lhaso Apso, Shih Tzu, Maltese, and Miniature Poodles, more commonly in male dogs (Bellenger *et al.* 1990; Walter and Matthiesen 1993). A severe form of hypertrophic gastritis, Měnětrier's disease, has been rarely described in the dog. It manifests as large gastric folds in the body of the stomach appearing cerebriform, sparing the esophagocardiac area and antrum with hypoalbuminemia and anemia, the sequelae of protein-losing gastropathy (Lecoindre *et al.* 2012).

Breed-specific gastropathies include atrophic gastritis of the Norwegian Lundehund, and hypertrophic gastropathy of the Drentse Patrijshund, and the Basenji. Hypergastrinemia has been documented in many of these dogs and is the most likely cause of the gastritis.

More than 60% of dogs, and 84% of cats with uremia, have clinical signs ascribed to uremic gastropathy, specifically inappetence, weight loss, vomiting, hematemesis, and diarrhea (Peters *et al.* 2005; McLeland *et al.* 2014).

Diagnosis

Vomiting that persists for more than seven days is considered chronic (Twedt 2010). If vomiting manifests in hematemesis then the patient should be triaged, hemoptysis, and coagulopathies are emergent conditions and can be confused with hematemesis from gastric ulceration. Abdominal palpation will help determine if there is an abdominal mass or intestinal obstruction, but ultimately imaging is necessary. The time of vomiting relative to eating can be a clue as to the cause; vomiting more than 8 hours after eating indicates gastric outflow obstruction. Chronic gastritis, among other gastrointestinal diseases, is considered after exclusion of extragastric causes including pancreatitis, hypoadrenocorticism, renal failure, hepatobiliary diseases, and hyperthyroidism in the cat. A minimum database including hematology, biochemistry, urinalysis, and fecal flotation should be conducted. Peripheral eosinophilia could denote an eosinophilic gastritis caused by food allergy, and parasitism or hyperadrenocorticism, and pythiosis.

Most lesions in chronic gastritis are thought to be restricted to the mucosa and submucosa and full thickness biopsies are not usually necessary (van der Gaag 1988). The benefit of endoscopy is that the gross assessment of the gastric mucosa is made (Figure 16.1) and focal lesions can be biopsied. In cats, and a lesser extent dogs, full thickness gastric biopsies are superior due to the distribution of certain diseases, eosinophilic gastroenterocolitis, lymphoma and mast cell tumors infiltrate the submucosal and muscularis propria layers (Kleinschmidt *et al.* 2006; Kleinschmidt *et al.* 2010; Evans *et al.* 2006). Chronic gastritis is classified according to type – simple, hypertrophic, atrophic, or granulomatous – and the distribution of the infiltrate – superficial, diffuse, or follicular gastritis (van der Gaag 1988). In addition the gastritis can also be classified according to the infiltrating inflammatory cell as follows: lymphoplasmacytic, eosinophilic, and granulomatous (Guilford and Strombeck 1996). Of vomiting dogs, 35% will have gastritis on endoscopy (van der Gaag 1988). The most common form of gastritis reported in vomiting dogs is superficial to diffuse gastritis, with atrophy and fibrosis

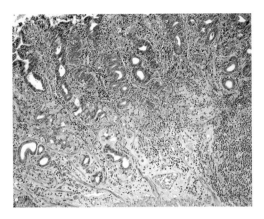

Figure 16.1 Gastric mucosa from a full thickness biopsy collected from the fundus of the stomach of a dog showing severe lymphoplasmacytic gastritis. Lymphocytes and plasma cells are present in severely increased numbers, diffusely and in aggregates, beneath epithelium and between glands, occasionally disrupting glandular architecture. Note mucous neck cell hyperplasia, increase in mucosal fibrous connective tissue, and nested, atrophic or loss of glands. (With permission, Dr Michelle Dennis, Ross University School of Veterinary Medicine).

occurring less commonly, 5% and 4% respectively (van der Gaag 1988). The most common type of gastric infiltrate in dogs with gastric pathology is lymphoplasmacytic (Lidbury, Suchodolski, and Steiner 2009).

Lymphoplasmacytic enteritis inflammatory bowel disease (IBD), manifests clinically with chronic vomiting, and is known to be associated with moderate to severe chronic antral gastritis (Garcia-Sancho *et al.* 2005). Thus IBD should be considered and investigated when this form of gastritis is diagnosed.

Confirming the presence of HLO includes a number of diagnostic tests in the cat or dog including, rapid urease test of biopsies, histopathology, cytobrush touch cytology smears using Gram or Diff quick stain, culture, polymerase chain reaction (PCR), fluorescent in-situ hybridization (FISH) assay, and electron microscopy, with less invasive tests not being readily practical to small animal practice, that is, urea breath test, although this has shown to be helpful in predicting relapse (Neiger and Simpson 2000; Cornetta *et al.*

1998; Simpson *et al.* 1999; Lee *et al.* 1992; Neiger, Seiler, and Schmassmann 1999).

High gastrin concentrations are known to be associated with atrophic gastritis and neoplasia of gastric enterochromaffin cells like gastrinoma and in cases of Měnětrier's disease. Gastrin concentrations are difficult to interpret as they are influenced by prior or current use of proton pump inhibitors, atrophic gastritis, hypochlorhydria, gastric outflow obstruction, small intestinal resection or short bowel syndrome, chronic renal- and liver failure, glucocorticoid excess, and hypercalcemia (Breitschwerdt *et al.* 1984). Acquired antral pyloric hypertrophy is diagnosed by means of ultrasound and endoscopy (Biller *et al.* 1994; Leib *et al.* 1993). Gastric infections with *Pythium insidiosum* should be considered as cause of gastric outflow obstruction in dogs from rural endemic areas.

Therapeutics

Specific therapy is directed at the underlying cause. Bilious vomiting syndrome, is usually managed by feeding the dog late at night and a combination of prokinetics and H_2- blockers (Webb and Twedt 2003). Gastric parasites are treated with tetramisole (2.5% formulation at 5 mg/kg) or fenbendazole (10 mg/kg, orally for two days) for *Ollulanus tricuspis* infections, and pyrantel pamoate (15 mg/kg orally and repeated twice every 2–3 weeks) for *Physaloptera* spp infections. Gastroscopic removal of the adult worm in the case of *Physaloptera* infection is also recommended. Recurrence of Physaloptera-infection is likely if paratenic hosts are ingested. A combination of aggressive surgical resection with 3–4 cm margins and prolonged antifungal therapy (itraconzaole at 10 mg/kg, orally, once daily or terbinafine, 5–10 mg/kg orally once daily) is indicated for treating gastrointestinal pythiosis (Grooters and Foil 2012). Serology can be used to monitor for recurrence, starting at 2–3 months postoperatively.

Supportive care for chronic gastritis includes antacid therapy, including H_2-blockers, proton-pump inhibitors, and the mucosal binder, sucralfate, which are often used empirically. H_2-blockers like famotidine are favored due to ease of dosing, where administering the drug with food improves bioavailability in contrast to omeprazole, which requires dosing on an empty stomach. Omeprazole is, however, considered to be superior. There is strong evidence to demonstrate that sucralfate binds to gastrointestinal mucosa in cats (Clark *et al.* 1987). Whether these drugs should be dosed empirically in gastritis in cats or dogs remains to be elucidated, considering that many forms of chronic gastritis do not manifest in gastric ulceration or erosions and in some instances actually atrophic gastritis is associated with achlorhydria and luminal alkalosis. It is certainly warranted in cases of hematemesis, and ultrasonographic or endoscopic evidence of ulcers.

Most of the therapeutic guidelines for treating HLO in companion animals are extrapolated from the American National Institutes of Health. No therapy is recommended for asymptomatic humans. Treatment in dogs and cats has had mixed success. An uncontrolled treatment trial reported >90% improvement of clinical signs in dogs and cats treated with amoxicillin, metronidazole, and famotidine with confirmed colonization of HLO and 74% of the dogs and cats re-biopsied were free of colonization after treatment (DeNovo and Magne 1995). Amoxicillin, metronidazole, and bismuth subsalicylate, with or without famotidine therapy for 14 days, resolved clinical signs of all dogs that had HLO colonization (Leib, Duncan, and Ward 2007). Eradication of HLO was also associated with improved gastritis on histopathology (Leib *et al.* 2007). There are studies that demonstrate antibiotics suppress colonization but are not effective in long-term elimination (Leib *et al.* 2007; Jergens *et al.* 2009; Simpson *et al.* 1999; Simpson *et al.* 2000).

After exclusion of potential causes of chronic gastritis a diagnosis of idiopathic chronic gastritis is made and immunosuppressive therapy is warranted. Prednisolone, at 1–2 mg/kg dosed orally, BID for 1–2 weeks followed by reducing the doses over 2–3 months. Steroid sparing drugs, or drugs that will substitute steroid use as they are contraindicated for example diabetes mellitus or gastric ulceration include azathioprine in the dog, and chlorambucil in the cat. Azathioprine, which is usually more effective when dosed together with prednisolone, is started at 2 mg/kg, orally, OID, for 7 days then dosed every other day, with hematology and biochemistry to monitor for potential side-effects of neutropenia or hepatotoxicity (Richter 2014). Azathioprine is extremely myelotoxic in cats. Chlorambucil is a good choice for cats and is combined with prednisolone, which is started at a dose at 5–10 mg per cat, OID. The identical chlorambucil protocol used in feline gastrointestinal lymphoma is employed (Richter 2014), dosed either at a high pulse dose at 15 mg/m^2 of body weight, orally daily for 4 days, which is repeated every 3 weeks or 20 mg/m^2 of body weight every 2 weeks or low dose high frequency, at 2 mg per cat daily. Side effects include vomiting, diarrhea, anorexia, and lethargy.

Standard medical therapy for hypertrophic gastritis includes antacids and H_2-blockers and proton-pump inhibitors. Once again, the role of proton pump inhibitors is controversial since it causes hypergastrinemia, which is proposed as part of the etiopathogenesis of acquired antral pyloric hypertrophy and hyperplastic gastritis. Considering the potential complications of Měnětrier's disease (gastric carcinoma), it may be worth considering the use of tyrosine kinase inhibitors in these patients. In medical refractory cases, partial gastrectomy is justified (Lecoindre *et al.* 2012). Most cases of acquired antral pyloric hypertrophy have resolved clinical signs after surgical resection of the outflow obstruction.

Due to the differences in pathology noted between the human and the canine and feline form of uremic gastropathy, often with the lack of identifiable gastric ulceration and hemorrhage in small animal patients, there is no evidence to support the empirical use of antacid therapy. In fact, it is speculated that many of these patients would have increased intragastric pH due to glandular atrophy (Peters *et al.* 2005). Cats, which have fibrosis and mineralization with atrophic non-inflammatory gastropathy therapy should focus on addressing the uremic toxin phosphate, with phosphate binders and phosphate-restricted diet.

Quality of Life

As veterinarians, we cannot solely make recommendations on treatment based on crudely measured outcomes of treatment success such as mean survival time and mortality rates. In a disease like chronic gastritis, with a low mortality rate, these measures of outcome are nonsensical. Quality of life (QOL) is the most important consideration for the pet owner or caregiver. Compassionate care of patients and consideration of the pet and the caregiver's QOL by veterinarians will improve overall compliance and improve successful treatment. Describing achievable goals from the outset will improve compliance; further emphasis on the possibility of long-term management of disease is an inescapable reality the owners must accept. It is important to not only consider QOL but also take steps to initiate change in patient management to improve the human–animal bond and reduce unnecessary suffering.

Chronic gastritis can be considered stressful to both the dog or cat and the owner/caregiver. Due to the chronic nature of the disease, disease improvement needs to be measured as a decrease in frequency of clinical signs rather than immediate resolution of the vomiting. Encouraging owners to keep logs of the vomiting events and review these episodes at rechecks is recommended. A decrease in frequency of vomiting, rather than resolution, may be an objective index in measuring response to treatment, particularly in those cases that vomit infrequently at presentation. This will allow decision making regarding tapering of immunosuppressive medication or in the case of HLO colonization, predicting lack of eradication.

Idiopathic and food responsive chronic gastritis in general have a good prognosis. The reasons for euthanasia in dogs with chronic gastritis are usually due to comorbid diseases and reports include carcinoma, extragastric lymphoid or myeloid tumors, gastric leiomyoma, Zollinger-Ellinson syndrome, and mesothelioma (van der Gaag and Happe, 1989).

Gastro-intestinal pythiosis and familial stomatocytosis-hypertrophic gastritis have a poor prognosis.

References

Bellenger C, Maddison J, Macpherson G, Ilkiw J. Chronic hypertrophic pyloric gastropathy in 14 dogs. Australian Veterinary Journal. 1990; 67: 317–320.

Biller DS, Partington BP, Miyabayashi T, Leveille R. Ultrasonographic appearance of chronic hypertrophic pyloric gastropathy in the dog. Veterinary Radiology and Ultrasound. 1994; 35: 30–33.

Breitschwerdt EB, Ochoa R, Barta M, Barta O, Mcclure J, Waltman C. Clinical and laboratory characterization of Basenjis with immunoproliferative small intestinal disease. American Journal of Veterinary Research. 1984; 45: 267–273.

Clark S, Katz PO, Wu WC, Geisinger KR, Castell DO. Comparison of potential cytoprotective action of sucralfate and cimetidine: Studies with experimental feline esophagitis. The American Journal of Medicine, 1987; 83: 56–60.

Cornetta AM, Simpson KW, Strauss-Ayali D, Mcdonough PL, Gleed RD. Use of a [13C] urea breath test for detection of gastric infection with *Helicobacter* spp in dogs. American Journal of Veterinary Research. 1998; 59: 1364–1369.

DeNovo RC, Magne ML. Current concepts in the management of *Helicobacter* associated gastritis. 13th ACVIM Forum, 1995 Lake Buena Vista, Florida, USA.

Evans SE, Bonczynski JJ, Broussard JD, Han E, Baer KE. Comparison of endoscopic and full-thickness biopsy specimens for diagnosis of inflammatory bowel disease and alimentary tract lymphoma in cats. Journal of the American Veterinary Medical Association. 2006; 229: 1447–1450.

Garcia-Sancho M, Rodriguez-Franco F, Sainz A, Rodriguez A, Silvan G, Illera JC. Serum gastrin in canine chronic lymphocytic-plasmacytic enteritis. Canadian Veterinary Journal. 2005; 46: 630–634.

Grooters AMF, Foil CS. Miscellaneous fungal infections. In: CE Greene, Ed. Infectious Diseases of the Dog and Cat. Saunders Elsevier. 2012: 675–688

Guilford WG, Strombeck R. 1996. Chronic gastric diseases. In: WG Guilford, SA Center, DR Strombeck, DA Williams and DJ Meyer, Eds. Strombeck's Small Animal Gastroenterology. WB Saunders. 1996: 256–260.

Jergens AE, Pressel M, Crandell J, et al. Fluorescence in situ hybridization confirms clearance of visible *Helicobacter* spp. associated with gastritis in dogs and cats. Journal of Veterinary Internal Medicine. 2009; 23: 16–23.

Kleinschmidt S, Harder J, Nolte I, Marsilio S, Hewicker-Trautwein M. Chronic inflammatory and non-inflammatory diseases of the gastrointestinal tract in cats: diagnostic advantages of full-thickness intestinal and extraintestinal biopsies. Journal of Feline Medicine and Surgery. 2010; 12: 97–103.

Kleinschmidt S, Meneses F, Nolte I, Hewicker-Trautwein M. Retrospective study on the diagnostic value of full-thickness biopsies from the stomach and intestines of dogs with chronic gastrointestinal disease symptoms. Veterinary Pathology. 2006; 43: 1000–1003.

Lecoindre P, Bystricka M, Chevallier M, Peyron C. Gastric carcinoma associated with Menetrier's-like disease in a West Highland white terrier. Journal of Small Animal Practice. 2012; 53: 714–718.

Lee A, Krakowka S, Fox J, Otto G, Eaton K, Murphy J. Role of *Helicobacter felis* in chronic canine gastritis. Veterinary Pathology Online. 1992; 29: 487–494.

Leib MS, Duncan RB, Ward DL. Triple antimicrobial therapy and acid suppression in dogs with chronic vomiting and gastric *Helicobacter* spp. Journal of Veterinary Internal Medicine. 2007; 21: 1185–1192.

Leib MS, Saunders GK, Moon ML, et al. Endoscopic diagnosis of chronic hypertrophic pyloric gastropathy in dogs. Journal of Veterinary Internal Medicine. 1993; 7: 335–341.

Lidbury JA, Suchodolski JS, Steiner JM. Gastric histopathologic abnormalities in dogs: 67 cases (2002–2007). Journal of the American Veterinary Medical Association, 2009; 234: 1147–1153.

McLeland SM, Lunn KF, Duncan CG, Refsal KR, Quimby JM. Relationship among serum creatinine, serum gastrin, calcium-phosphorus product, and uremic gastropathy in cats with chronic kidney disease. Journal of Veterinary Internal Medicine. 2014; 28: 827–737.

Neiger R, Seiler G, Schmassmann A. Use of a urea breath test to evaluate short-term treatments for cats naturally infected with Helicobacter heilmannii. American Journal of Veterinary Research. 1999; 60: 880–883.

Neiger R, Simpson KW. *Helicobacter* infection in dogs and cats: facts and fiction. Journal of Veterinary Internal Medicine. 2000; 14: 125–133.

Peters RM, Goldstein RE, Erb HN, Njaa BL. Histopathologic features of canine uremic gastropathy: a retrospective study. Journal of Veterinary Internal Medicine. 2005; 19: 315–320.

Richter KP. Feline gastrointestinal lymphoma. In: JD Bonagura and DC Twedt, Eds. Kirk's current veterinary therapy XV. Elsevier, Saunders. 2014: 545–549.

Ritchey JW, Davis MS, Breshears MA, et al. Gastritis in Alaskan racing sled dogs. Journal of Comparative Pathology. 2011; 145: 68–76.

Simpson K, Neiger R, DeNovo R, Sherding R. The relationship of *Helicobacter* spp. infection to gastric disease in dogs and cats. Journal of Veterinary Internal Medicine. 2000; 14: 223–227.

Simpson KW, Strauss-Ayali D, Mcdonough PL, Chang YF, Valentine BA. Gastric function in dogs with naturally acquired gastric *Helicobacter* spp. infection. Journal of Veterinary Internal Medicine. 1999; 13: 507–515.

Tucker S, Penninck DG, Keating JH, Webster CR. Clinicopathological and ultrasonographic features of cats with eosinophilic enteritis. Journal of Feline Medicine and Surgery. 2014; 16: 950–956.

Twedt DC. Vomiting. In: S Ettinger and EC Feldman, Eds. Textbook of Veterinary Internal Medicine. 7th edn. Saunders, Elsevier. 2010: 195–200.

Van der Gaag I. The histological appearance of peroral gastric biopsies in clinically healthy and vomiting dogs. Canadian Journal of Veterinary Research. 1988; 52: 67.

Van der Gaag I, Happe RP. Follow-up studies by peroral gastric biopsies and necropsy in vomiting dogs. Canadian Journal of Veterinary Research. 1989; 53: 468–472.

Walter MC, Matthiesen DT. Acquired antral pyloric hypertrophy in the dog. Veterinary Clinics of North America: Small Animal Practice, 1993; 23: 547–554.

Webb C, Twedt DC. Canine gastritis. Veterinary Clinics of North America: Small Animal Practice. 2003; 33: 969–985, v–vi.

17

Ulcerative Colitis

Liza S. Köster

Introduction

Granulomatous colitis (GC) is also known as histiocytic ulcerative colitis (HUC) in the veterinary literature and afflicts both Boxer dogs but also non-Boxer dogs. This condition was first described in dogs in 1965 and is characterized by diffuse inflammation of the colon, cecum, and rectum with infiltration of periodic acid-Schiff (PAS) positive macrophages of the lamina propria and stroma of the submucosa with accompanying epithelial and submucosal ulceration (German *et al.* 2000; Van Kruiningen 1967). In human Crohn's disease and ulcerative colitis there is mounting evidence supporting the role of enteric microflora (Simpson *et al.* 2006). These conditions have increased number of bacteria but reduced diversity, and many patients will demonstrate clinical response to antimicrobial therapy. Host factors will also play a role, with individual susceptibility found in individuals with genetic defects in pathogen recognition receptors like toll-like receptors (TLR). Simpson and others proposed that an uncharacterized infectious agent or an abnormal mucosal flora is involved in the etiopathogenesis of GC (Simpson *et al.* 2006). Enteroinvasive *E. coli* was determined to be the invasive bacteria found in the mucosal biopsies, although the role of infectious diseases had been speculated on in prior studies, including culture of

bacteria from regional lymph nodes and immunostaining for anti-*E coli* antibody, among other organisms in macrophages on formalin-fixed colon and colic lymph nodes (Van Kruiningen 1967; Van Kruiningen, Civco, and Cartun 2005). These strains of *E. coli*, adherent and invasive *E. coli* (AIEC), are similar to those found in Chrohn's disease (Craven *et al.* 2010). It is assumed that host mucosal immunity is compromised allowing opportunistic invasion by *E. coli* strains. This condition has been described to respond within 7 days and dogs remain in remission at a 21-month follow-up, after a prolonged course of antibiotics, either enrofloxacin on its own or in combination with metronidazole and amoxicillin (Hostutler *et al.* 2004).

Diagnosis

HUC is accountable for an estimated 14% of cases of colitis that present to an academic hospital over a 20 year period in Australia, but reports in the United States are more conservative, in the region of 2% and on the decline, yet there is an increasing number of reports in the United Kingdom (Churcher and Watson 1997). The disease has been described typically in Boxers younger than 4-years of age, more commonly female (German *et al.* 2000; Churcher and Watson 1997), but reports include French bulldog

Chronic Disease Management for Small Animals, First Edition. Edited by W. Dunbar Gram, Rowan J. Milner and Remo Lobetti.
© 2018 John Wiley & Sons, Inc. Published 2018 by John Wiley & Sons, Inc.

(Gaag *et al.* 1978; Manchester *et al.* 2013), Beagle (Carvallo *et al.* 2015), Mastiff, Alaskan Malamute, Doberman Pincher (Stokes *et al.* 2001), and Bulldog (Hostutler *et al.* 2004). There is one case report documenting this condition in a cat (Van Kruiningen and Dobbins 1979). This disease presents much like other causes of chronic colitis – diarrhea characterized by increased frequency of defecation, tenesmus, urgency, hematochezia, and excessive mucus – but in severe cases, weight loss and inappetence can occur (Churcher and Watson 1997).

HUC should be considered as an etiology of chronic colitis in a dog with a typical signalment, namely young, usually female, Boxer breed, although other breeds have been diagnosed with this condition. Failure to respond to supportive care, including dietary manipulation, specifically a low residue prescription diet, anthelminthic dosing, and sulfasalazine should prompt an investigation. A minimum database may detect systemic complications including hypoalbuminemia due to protein-losing enteropathy. Differentials diagnoses for the chronic colitis include hypoadrenocorticism, adverse food reaction, dietary allergy or intolerance, parasitic, infectious, neoplastic, motility disorders, strictures, and irritable bowel syndrome. Fecal investigation should include flotation techniques using zinc sulphate fecal flotation for *Giardia*, and *Trichuris* spp., PCR for *Giardia* spp., *Salmonella* spp., *Cryptosporidium* spp., and *Clostridium perfringes* enterotoxin A gene, which can all result in large bowel clinical signs. The necessity to perform these tests is dictated by the history of the dog's housing environment and diet fed, with high-density housing and a raw meat diet being the greatest risk factors. Rectal scrapes may be helpful in identifying *Histoplasma* spp. or Pythiosis, although the latter is incredibly challenging to diagnose, often requiring a combination of ultrasound, biopsy, and serology. Ultrasound of the colon wall, examining for layering may be helpful, with transmural thickening and loss of layering indicative of infiltrative neoplasia like lymphoma and *Pythium insidiosum*. Diagnosis requires endoscopic biopsy after fasting for 48-hours and preparation of the colon with laxatives and enemas.

Proctoscopy will reveal inflamed, hyperemic mucosa in all cases with scattered hemorrhagic foci (Churcher and Watson 1997). The mucosa is also described as being friable and bleeds easily. Confirmation of the diagnosis is made by demonstrating the characteristic histopathology of infiltration by PAS-positive staining macrophages. In addition, special stains to aid in infectious agent identification would include, Gomori methenamine stain, Gram, and modified Steiner. Fluorescent in situ hybridization (FISH) with a probe against eubacterial 16S rRNA is a sensitive method of detecting bacteria on formalin samples.

Therapy

There is staggering evidence to support the role of infectious agents in the pathogenesis of HUC in dogs. No immunosuppressive therapy should be instituted if this condition is suspected and efforts should be made to confirm AIEC, either with special stains or FISH techniques, which is considered the most sensitive of tests.

Empirical treatment with antimicrobials and immunosuppressive therapy has resulted in poor outcomes on dogs with GC (Hostutler *et al.* 2004). In contrast, dogs have a reported dramatic improvement of the colonic histologic pattern and a significant weight gain after treatment with enrofloxacin (Hostutler *et al.* 2004; Davies *et al.* 2004; Mansfield *et al.* 2009). Enrofloxacin, is currently the recommended treatment in dogs with GC at a dose of 5–10 mg/kg, orally, daily for 6–10 weeks. Enrofloxacin is a bactericidal antibiotic with a highly effective broad gram-negative spectrum, it is also specific effect against *Mycobacterium, Mycoplasma, Chlamydia,* and rickettsia, but another important characteristic that plays a role in its success of treating HUC is its ability to penetrate macrophages. Chloramphenicol has also been described as an effective antimicrobial agent in dogs with GC (Van Kruiningen *et al.* 1965).

Antimicrobial resistance is described as a fairly common occurrence in dogs treated for GC (Craven *et al.* 2010). Persistent intra-mucosal *E. coli* can be demonstrated in mucosa using FISH technique in dogs that become antimicrobial unresponsive (Mansfield *et al.* 2009). Various *E. coli* strains were isolated and cultured from dogs with GC (n = 14), which translates to approximately two to three strains per dog, which were incidentally similar to the *E. coli* strains found in healthy dogs (n = 17). It appears that the antimicrobial-resistant individuals are the same dogs carrying antimicrobial-resistant strains. However, almost half of the *E. coli* strains from dogs with GC were resistant to not only enrofloxacin (6/14) but also chloramphenicol, trimethroprim sulfas, and rifampicin (4/14), and these dogs had a poor outcome (Craven *et al.* 2010). It remains to be seen if perhaps multidrug combinations that include tetracyclines, trimethropim, and ciprofloxacin may have a synergistic effect in overcoming resistance of *E. coli* strains as is seen in the case of Crohn's disease (Craven *et al.* 2010).

Quality of Life

Prior to the elucidation of the role of adherent and invasive *E.coli*, and the response to antibiotic therapy, this condition had a very grave prognosis. Usually there was minimal response reported to dietary modification, sulfasalazine, and immunosuppressive therapy. As early as when the disease was described in dogs, the outcome improved in instances where multimodal therapy, including antibiotics like chloramphenicol and tylosin were included in the protocol (Van Kruiningen *et al.* 1965). Treatment with enrofloxacin will lead to a rapid resolution and durable remission in dogs (Hostutler *et al.* 2004). Appropriate use of medications, specifically adequate duration of treatment, and compliance of owner and patient will help overcome resistant strains of *E. coli*. The importance of adequate dose regimens should be emphasized to owners, as the clinical manifestation of antibiotic-resistant strains will lead to antibiotic refractory clinical signs.

References

Carvallo FR, Kerlin R, Fredette C, et al. Histiocytic typhlocolitis in two colony Beagle dogs. Experimental and Toxicologic Pathology, 2015; 67: 219–221.

Churcher RK, Watson AD. Canine histiocytic ulcerative colitis. Australian Veterinary Journal. 1997; 75: 710–743.

Craven M, Dogan B, Schukken A, et al. 2010. Antimicrobial resistance impacts clinical outcome of granulomatous colitis in boxer dogs. Journal of Veterinary Internal Medicine. 2010: 24: 819–824.

Davies DR, O'Hara AJ, Irwin PJ, Guilford WG. 2004. Successful management of histiocytic ulcerative colitis with enrofloxacin in two Boxer dogs. Australian Veterinary Journal. 2004; 82: 58–61.

Gaag I, Toorenburg JIK, Voorhout G, et al. Histiocytic ulcerative colitis in a French Bulldog. Journal of Small Animal Practice, 1978; 19: 283–290.

German AJ, Hall EJ, Kelly DF, Watson AD, Day MJ. An immunohistochemical study of histiocytic ulcerative colitis in boxer dogs. Journal of Comparative Pathology. 2000; 122: 163–175.

Hostutler RA, Luria BJ, Johnson SE, et al. Antibiotic-responsive histiocytic ulcerative colitis in 9 dogs. Journal of Veterinary Internal Medicine. 2004;18: 499–504.

Manchester A, Hill S, Sabatino B, et al. Association between granulomatous colitis in French Bulldogs and invasive Escherichia coli and response to fluoroquinolone antimicrobials. Journal of Veterinary Internal Medicine, 2013; 27: 56–61.

Mansfield CS, James FE, Craven M, et al. Remission of histiocytic ulcerative colitis in Boxer dogs correlates with eradication of invasive intramucosal *Escherichia coli*. Journal of Veterinary Internal Medicine. 2009; 23: 964–969.

Simpson KW, Dogan B, Rishniw M, et al. Adherent and invasive *Escherichia coli* is associated with granulomatous colitis in boxer dogs. Infection and immunity, 2006; 74: 4778–4792.

Stokes JE, Kruger JM, Mullaney T, Holan K, Schall W. Histiocytic ulcerative colitis in three non-boxer dogs. Journal of the American Hospital Association, 2001; 37: 461–465.

Van Kruiningen H. Granulomatous colitis of boxer dogs: comparative aspects. Gastroenterology. 1967; 53: 114.

Van Kruiningen HJ, Dobbins WO, 3rd. Feline histiocytic colitis. A case report with electron microscopy. Veterinary Pathology. 1979; 16: 215–222.

Van Kruiningen H, Civco I, Cartun R. The comparative importance of *E. coli* antigen in granulomatous colitis of Boxer dogs. Apmis, 2005; 113(6): 420–425.

Van Kruiningen H, Montali R, Strandberg J, Kirk R. A granulomatous colitis of dogs with histologic resemblance to Whipple's disease. Pathologia Veterinaria Online, 1965; 2: 521–544.

18

Mega-Colon

Liza S. Köster

Introduction

Mega-colon refers to a condition where the colon is hypomotile manifesting in obstipation, with dilation or hypertrophy of the colon leading to fecal impaction and is caused by either congenital or acquired diseases (Byers, Leasure, and Sanders 2006). Congenital forms include aganglionosis (reported in an 11-week old kitten), Manx deformity or a feature of *situs inversus* (White 2002; Roe, Syme, and Brooks 2010).

Acquired mega-colon is either, secondary to chronic mechanical or functional bowel obstruction, or primary, also known as idiopathic. Obstructive mega-colon manifests as hypertrophic mega-colon, whereas a primary dysmotility disorders such as idiopathic mega-colon cause the colon to become dilated in the end-stage of the disease (Byers *et al.* 2006). Of cases, 62% are idiopathic, with 23% due to pelvic canal stenosis due to malunion of a pelvic fracture, or deformity, 6% nerve injury related to Manx sacral spinal cord deformity (Washabau 2003). Other reasons cited include complications from colopexy, colonic neoplasia, neuromuscular dysfunction caused by dysautonomia, rectal stricture, and metabolic or endocrine disease. The vast majority of cats with mega-colon, that is, idiopathic mega-colon will not have primary neurological disease. The unknown pathology afflicts colonic smooth muscle leading to generalized dysfunction and absence of motility.

Idiopathic mega-colon is most commonly described in the domestic shorthair, Siamese, and domestic long-hair cats with the mean age of onset being 7 years and 11 months (range 9 months to 17 years) but mostly observed in middle aged male cats (Trevail *et al.* 2011; Washabau 2003). Cats will have a history of tenesmus, dyschezia, occasional systemic signs including anorexia, weight loss, and vomiting. Clinical findings include dehydration, abdominal pain, and mesenteric lymphadenopathy (Washabau 2003). A potential sequel to the anorexia from mega-colon in the cat is hepatic lipidosis (Salas 2003).

Mega-colon, both dilated and hypertrophic mega-colon in dogs, is rarely described. Reported breeds include, German Shepherd Dog, Rottweiler, Giant Schnauzer, Sharr Mountain dog, Hungarian Kuvasz, Caucasian Shepherd, Sarplaninanc, and the English Mastiff. The most common form is secondary, with only 25% of cases being idiopathic (Prokić *et al.* 2010). A case series described this condition as more common in male dogs, dogs that received low levels of exercise, and had a history of chronic constipation, in the preceding five to 26 weeks (Nemeth, Solymosi, and Balka 2008). The underlying causes include, pelvic canal stenosis, lumbar and sacral spinal injuries, hindlimb fractures.

Chronic Disease Management for Small Animals, First Edition. Edited by W. Dunbar Gram, Rowan J. Milner and Remo Lobetti.
© 2018 John Wiley & Sons, Inc. Published 2018 by John Wiley & Sons, Inc.

The highest risk factor in dogs include a bone diet and low levels of physical activity (Nemeth *et al.* 2008; Prokić *et al.* 2010). Common historical complaints documented were persistent tenesmus, dyschezia, and obstipation refractory to medical management. Clinical signs included distended colon filled with hard feces, and abdominal pain (Nemeth *et al.* 2008). The histopathology is characterized by severe hypertrophy of the smooth muscle.

Diagnosis

Cats are often classified as having mega-colon in studies if they have constipation that is refractory to medical therapy for more than 3 months, had three of more bouts of constipation, and subsequently required sub-total colectomy (Trevail *et al.* 2011). The most common clinical sign is tenesmus, but other signs include, lethargy, dehydration, anorexia, and occasionally vomiting. This includes cats with idiopathic mega-colon, and known etiologies including pelvic fractures with malunion causing hypertrophic mega-colon or dysautonomia. Clinical features of dysautonomia, include mydriasis with depressed direct and consensual pupillary light reflex, dysuria with distended urinary bladder, dry mucous membranes, prolapsed third eyelid, and dysphagia (Sharp, Nash, and Griffiths 1984). The predominant clinical signs of hypertrophic mega-colon in the dog are tenesmus, weight loss, anorexia, and vomiting (Nemeth *et al.* 2008). Some dogs had reported anemia, or elevated packed cell volume (Nemeth *et al.* 2008).

Investigation should include a thorough physical examination with careful attention of abdominal palpation, minimum database that includes hematology, biochemistry, fecal analysis, and urinalysis. A rectal examination, conscious in the dog or under anesthesia in the cat or painful dog, can be helpful in gauging the pelvic canal size in the case of a malunion, or if there are other rectal pathologies including stricture, masses,

rectal diverticula, foreign body, or inflammation (Washabau 2003). Although the role of hypothyroidism and obesity in the pathogenesis of mega-colon is tenuous, it has been described in several cases and should warrant consideration. A full neurological examination should be conducted. If neurological disease is found, this may warrant further diagnostics including advanced imaging studies, cerebrospinal fluid analysis, infectious disease screen, or electrophysiologic studies to characterize and confirm the pathology. Abdominal and pelvic radiography serves two purposes, first to confirm the dilated colon (Figure 18.1) and second to exclude pelvic or spinal malformations or injuries, but orthopedic diseases may require computed tomography.

Mega-colon in cats is confirmed radiographically after appropriate history and clinical findings support a suspicion.

Therapeutics

If the mega-colon is secondary and hypertrophic, the underlying cause should be addressed. In the case of pelvic canal stenosis of less than 6-months duration, a pelvic osteotomy is indicated (Washabau 2003; MacPhail 2002). The primary pathogenesis of idiopathic mega-colon is smooth muscle dysfunction rather than neurological disease leading to dysmotility, which infers that therapeutics should be aimed at stimulating colonic smooth muscle contraction (Washabau and Holt 1999). However, in end-stage mega-colon, fiber supplements and prokinetics are unlikely to have much benefit. Medical management comprises of short-term resolution of the fecal impaction, which requires manual evacuation of the bowels under anesthesia using lubrication and enemas, usually after 24-hours of rehydration, and long-term management by utilizing stool softeners, prokinetics, and dietary changes. Obstipation due to mega-colon exceeding 6-months should be managed with a subtotal colectomy (Washabau 2003). This technique,

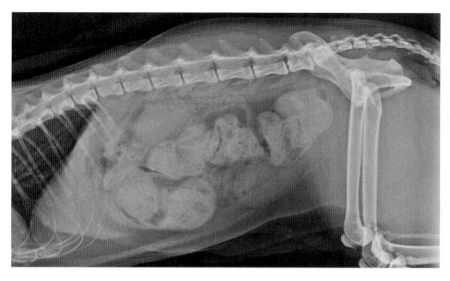

Figure 18.1 Right lateral abdominal radiograph in a skeletally mature domestic shorthair cat diagnosed with idiopathic mega-colon. The colon is severely dilated and filled with fecal material. (With permission, Dr Carla Chow, Nine Lives, The Cat Hospital, Hong Kong.)

as opposed to a colectomy, is preferred as long-term cats that had the ileocolic junction preserved had improved stool consistency, it is also thought to minimize bacterial ascension (Sweet, Hardie, and Stone 1994). In hypertrophic canine mega-colon, constipation that is refractory to medical therapy for more than 2-months then subtotal colectomy, preserving the ileocecal junction, is recommended with the best long-term outcome (Nemeth *et al.* 2008).

The first line of treatment should employ enemas and deobstipation. Hydration of the patient followed by a warm water or 0.9% saline (5–10 ml/kg body weight) enema, with or without a surgical lubricant, is performed in hospital over several days (MacPhail 2002). Dehydration contributes to colonic water absorption, which hardens fecal matter and should be addressed. Thereafter osmotic laxatives can be used, but emollient, lubricant, and stimulant laxatives are not indicated in mega-colon. Lactulose is a poorly absorbed carbohydrate that is hydrolyzed to a fatty acid by the colonic microflora. These metabolites exert osmotic pressure and draw fluid into the colon (Davenport, Remillard, and Carroll 2010). Cats with

longstanding mega-colon are unlikely to respond to lactulose laxatives.

Dietary intervention is helpful in feline constipation. Key components of the diet that need to be addressed include, water intake, fiber content, and digestibility (Davenport *et al.* 2010). Emphasis should be placed on providing access to fresh water in multiple locations in the pet's living environment. The inclusion of canned sweet potato and pumpkin, not only increase fiber content but also has over 90% water. Dietary fiber with low solubility, are bulk-forming laxatives, distend motility by distending the colon, and can form dry stool, an unattractive option for mega-colon. It is recommended that the diet not exceed 5% dry matter crude fiber. Soluble fiber including pectins, canned pumpkin, guar gum, and psyllium are options that are more appropriate. The intestinal bacteria, producing short-chain fatty acids, altering colonic microenvironment, will ferment some of these soluble fibers. Short-chain fatty acids are known to have a strong impact on the colonic microenvironment and serve as nutrients for the colonocytes. Psyllium enriched, and chicory pulp, fructo-and mano-oligosacharides containing, dry diets has been trialed in cats for the management of constipation (Freiche *et al.* 2011). Palatability was considered excellent and most cats were considered to have improved by 2 months with fecal consistency having improved considerably and the use of cisapride and lactulose decreased considerably (Freiche *et al.* 2011). It is generally recommended that highly digestible diet be fed to cats and dogs with mega-colon, and dividing meals will also limit the amount of ingesta reaching the large bowel (Davenport *et al.* 2010). In dogs, an additional intervention that can be helpful is post-prandial leash walking, as gastro-colic reflex and exercise will stimulate defecation (Davenport *et al.* 2010).

Various prokinetics can be considered in both cats and dogs (Table 18.1). Cisapride has shown to stimulate smooth muscle contraction along the entire length of the colon (Hasler and Washabau 1997; Washabau and Sammarco 1996). Certain H_2-receptor antagonists, ranitidine and nizatadine, but not cimetidine or famotidine, will also stimulate the colon along its entire length stimulating peristalsis (Hall and Washabau 1997). The mechanism of action is acetylcholinesterase inhibition, increasing the binding of acetylcholine that can bind to smooth muscle muscarinic receptors. Motilin-like drugs including erythromycin accelerate canine colonic transit, and has been shown to stimulate canine, but not feline colonic smooth muscle in vitro (Washabau 2003). Lastly sympathomimetics can be considered, bethanechol a cholinomimetic binds muscarinic cholinergic receptors stimulating gastrointestinal motility (Washabau 2003). Misoprostol, a prostaglandin E_1 analogue, has been shown in vitro to stimulate feline colonic smooth muscle but there are no in vivo studies (Mosenco, Meltzer, and Kennedy 2003). Medical management alone using cisapride, is estimated to be effective in 35% of cases of dogs with hypertrophic mega-colon (Prokić *et al.* 2010). Drugs with similar prokinetic effect include prucalopride and tegaserod (Table 18.1). Tegaserod can be administered intravenously, with equal benefit noted at the high and low end of the dose range, and it has no

Table 18.1 List of drugs used in megacolon in the canine and feline patient.

Medical therapy	Mechanism of action	Dosage
Lactulose	Hypersomolar laxative	
Cisapride	Prokinetic, a serotonergic 5-HT$_4$ agonist	0.1–0.5 mg/kg, orally, TID to QID in dogs and cats Up to 1 mg/kg in dogs
Prucalopride*	Prokinetic, a potent partial 5-HT$_4$ and other 5_HT receptors	0.02–1.25 mg/kg, oral or intravenous in dogs 0.64 mg/kg, cats
Tegaserod	Potent 5-HT$_4$ and weak 5-HT$_{1D}$ receptor agonist	0.05–0.1 mg/kg, intravenously, BID, in dogs
Erythromycin	Motilin-like drug	0.5–1 mg/kg, orally or intravenously, TID
Ranitidine	Acetylcholinesterase inhibitor	1–2 mg/kg, orally, BID to TID
Nizatadine	Acetylcholinesterase inhibitor	2.5–5 mg/kg, orally, SID
Bethanechol	Cholinomimetic	5–15 mg/dog, orally, TID

Abbreviations: BID, twice daily; QID, four times daily; SID, once daily; TID, three times daily.
* Not approved in the USA.
Source: Adapted from Washabau 2003. Reproduced with permission of Elsevier.

effect on QT interval prolongation. Prucalopride is not registered for use in the United States by the Food and Drug Administration, although approved for use in Europe and Canada.

Quality of Life

Congenital aganglionosis would be expected to have both short-term and long-term complications and a reasonably poor prognosis would be realistic. This disease would require intensive owner commitment to performing daily enema procedures. Surgery is indicated in infants with this condition overall having a good long-term outcome, 86% of patients had excellent anorectal function, and appeared well adjusted in a long-term follow-up study (Moore, Albertyn, and Cywes 1996). Subtotal colectomy could be considered in canine and feline pediatric patients with congenital mega-colon. Secondary mega-colon potentially would carry a fair prognosis if the underlying cause can be corrected within 6 months, for example, pelvic osteotomy. In cats, there are reported excellent long-term outcomes after subtotal colectomy although intestinal anastomosis dehiscence carries an 80% mortality rate (Wylie and Hosgood 1994). Postoperative constipation rates can be as high as 45%, requiring euthanasia or further surgery (Sweet *et al.* 1994). In dogs with acquired mega-colon, excellent short-term outcome, with complete recovery reported within 28 days in one study with a combination of both surgical and medical management (Prokić *et al.* 2010). Surgical management of eight large breed dogs with hypertrophic mega-colon allowed return of normal defecation within 5 to 10 weeks (Nemeth *et al.* 2008). Despite no intraoperative complications, one dog in this study suffered fatal septic peritonitis postoperatively.

Quality of life considers many facets such as physical and emotional suffering, and specifically pain. The distress experienced by the pet owner/carer should not be ignored and contributes significantly to outcome due to this effect on compliance. Concerns of pet owner/carer that is responsible for chronic medical management of a dog or cat include the impact of the medical management on work and social life, the constant need for veterinary visits, worry that the cat or dog may need hospitalization, the inability to leave the pet in a boarding facility, and the deep concern that the pet may be suffering. Ultimate success of managing a chronic disease requires addressing these quality-of-life concerns.

The diagnosis of congenital mega-colon has implications in terms of long-term outcome. In humans, 6.1% of children suffered a long-term complication of fecal soiling postoperatively (Moore *et al.* 1996). A similar complication in a dog or cat may not manifest in psychosocial maladjustment but certainly could be a cause for owner stress.

The underlying etiology of secondary mega-colon will impact on the quality of life of both the pet and the owner. Dysautonomia is an obvious example of a patient that is completely dependent on medical management and nursing by the owner. In a study that monitored the long-term response to treatment of 40 cats diagnosed with feline dysautonomia, only nine of the cats survived, and a full year was required for recovery, no doubt a testament to the perseverance of the owners (Sharp *et al.* 1984).

Cats or dogs that have persistent obstipation despite medical management are candidates for subtotal colectomy, which is considered a satisfactory option as opposed to euthanasia, which would be the probable outcome, assuming there are no financial limitations. Perioperative complications, including dehiscence and peritonitis, need to be discussed, although long-term complications are minimal.

References

Byers CG, Leasure CS, Sanders NA. Feline idiopathic megacolon. Compendium on Continuing Education for the Practising Veterinarian-North American Edition, 2006; 28: 658.

Davenport DJ, Remillard RL, Carroll M. Constipation/obstipation/megacolon. In: MS Hand, CD Thatcher, RL Remillard, P Roudebush, and BJ Novotny, Eds. Small Animal Clinical Nutrition. Mark Morris Institute. 2010: 1120–1123.

Freiche V, Houston D, Weese H, et al. Uncontrolled study assessing the impact of a psyllium-enriched extruded dry diet on faecal consistency in cats with constipation. Journal of Feline Medicine and Surgery. 2011; 13: 903–911.

Hall JA, Washabau RJ Gastrointestinal prokinetic therapy: Acetylcholinesterase inhibitors. The Compendium on Continuing Education for the Practicing Veterinarian. 1997; 19(5): 615–620.

Hasler AH, Washabau RJ. Cisapride stimulates contraction of idiopathic megacolonic smooth muscle in cats. Journal of Veterinary Internal Medicine. 1997; 11(6): 313–318.

MacPhail C. Gastrointestinal obstruction. Clinical Techniques in Small Animal Practice, 2002; 17: 178–183.

Moore S, Albertyn R, Cywes S. Clinical outcome and long-term quality of life after surgical correction of Hirschsprung's disease. Journal of Pediatric Surgery. 1996; 31: 1496–1502.

Mosenco A, Meltzer K, Kennedy D. Prostanoids stimulate duodenal and colonic smooth muscle contraction. Journal of Veterinary Internal Medicine. 2003; 17: 447.

Nemeth T, Solymosi N, Balka G. Long-term results of subtotal colectomy for acquired megacolon in eight dogs. Journal of Small Animal Practice. 2008; 49: 618–624.

Prokić B, Todorović V, Mitrović O, Vignjević S, Savić-Stevanović V. Ethiopathogenesis, diagnosis and therapy of acquired megacolon in dogs. Acta Veterinaria, 2010; 60: 273–284.

Roe KA, Syme HM, Brooks HW. Congenital large intestinal hypoganglionosis in a domestic shorthair kitten. Journal of Feline Medicine and Surgery. 2010; 12: 418–420.

Salas E. Hepatic lipidosis in a Maine coon cat secondary to megacolon. Senior seminar Cornell University. 2003.

Sharp NJH, Nash AS, Griffiths IR. Feline dysautonomia (the Key-Gaskell syndrome): a clinical and pathological study of forty cases. Journal of Small Animal Practice. 1984; 25: 599–615.

Sweet D, Hardie E, Stone E. Preservation versus excision of the ileocolic junction during colectomy for megacolon: A study of 22 cats. Journal of Small Animal Practice. 1994; 35: 358–363.

Trevail T, Gunn-Moore D, Carrera I, Courcier E, Sullivan, M. Radiographic diameter of the colon in normal and constipated cats and in cats with megacolon. Veterinary Radiology and Ultrasound. 2011; 52: 516–520.

Washabau RJ. Gastrointestinal motility disorders and gastrointestinal prokinetic therapy. Veterinary Clinics of North America: Small Animal Practice. 2003; 33: 1007–1028.

Washabau RJ, Holt D. Pathogenesis, diagnosis, and therapy of feline idiopathic megacolon. Veterinary Clinics of North America: Small Animal Practice. 1999; 29: 589–603.

Washabau RJ, Sammarco J. Effects of cisapride on feline colonic smooth muscle function. American Journal of Veterinary Research. 1996; 57: 541–546.

White RN. Surgical management of constipation. Journal of Feline Medicine and Surgery. 2002; 4: 129–138.

Wylie KB, Hosgood G. Mortality and morbidity of small and large intestinal surgery in dogs and cats: 74 cases (1980–1992). Journal of the American Animal Hospital Association. 1994; 30(5): 469–474.

19

Inflammatory Bowel Disease

Iwan A. Burgener

Introduction

Intestinal epithelial cells serve as a barrier between the body and viruses, bacteria, and parasites present in the intestinal lumen. Rather than being a passive barrier, the intestinal epithelium is an active participant in the mucosal immune response through antigen processing and presentation, secretion of cytokines, and recruitment of inflammatory cells in response to pathogens and their products. The gastrointestinal-associated lymphoid tissue (GALT) is the largest and most complex immunological organ of the body and must be capable of mounting a protective immune response to pathogens, while maintaining tolerance to harmless environmental antigens such as commensal bacteria and food. The breakdown of this tolerance is a key factor in the development of chronic intestinal inflammation.

In the dog and cat, inflammatory bowel disease (IBD) is the collective term for a group of chronic enteropathies characterized by persistent or recurrent gastrointestinal signs and inflammation of the gastrointestinal tract (Simpson and Jergens 2011). The specific steps that lead to IBD and the basis for phenotypic variation and unpredictable responses to treatment are not known. The breakdown of immunologic tolerance to luminal antigens (bacteria and dietary components) is thought to be critical, perhaps resulting from disruption of the mucosal barrier, dysregulation of the immune system, or disturbances in the intestinal microflora (Burgener *et al.* 2008; Dandrieux, Bornand, and, Burgener 2008; Xenoulis, Palculict, and Allenspach 2008). Until recently, histiocytic ulcerative colitis (HUC) was also considered a special form of IBD of unknown etiology, however, it has now been identified as being caused by an adherent and invasive phenotype of *E.coli* (Simpson *et al.* 2006). These findings elucidated the success of the antibiotic therapy for HUC, which included enrofloxacin (Hostutler *et al.* 2004).

Diagnosis

Chronic enteropathies are frequently encountered in dogs and cats, resulting in diarrhea and occasionally vomiting (Allenspach *et al.* 2007). The clinician faced with a case usually performs an extensive workup to exclude extra-gastrointestinal causes for diarrhea and vomitus (e.g., liver, kidney, hypoadrenocorticism (dogs), hyperthyroidism (cats)) as well as disorders such as pancreatic diseases, chronic parasitic or bacterial infections, and tumors. Diagnostics performed to rule out underlying disorders include a complete blood count (CBC), serum biochemical analysis (incl. bile acids/ammonium), urinalysis, hormonal testing

Chronic Disease Management for Small Animals, First Edition. Edited by W. Dunbar Gram, Rowan J. Milner and Remo Lobetti.
© 2018 John Wiley & Sons, Inc. Published 2018 by John Wiley & Sons, Inc.

(ACTH stimulation test in dogs, T4 in cats), parasitic and bacterial analysis of fecal samples, abdominal ultrasonography, and assessment of serum concentration of trypsin-like immunoreactivity (TLI), pancreatic specific lipase (PLI), serum cobalamin and folate concentrations. If there is no obvious underlying infectious, parasitic, pancreatic, neoplastic, endocrinologic or metabolic disease identified, these animals are mostly undergoing a trial therapy +/- endoscopy and are retrospectively diagnosed by the response to treatment as antibiotic-responsive diarrhea (ARD; Tylosin-responsive chronic diarrhea (Westermarck *et al.* 2005); nowadays better dysbiosis), food-responsive diarrhea (FRD) or inflammatory bowel disease (IBD; also called steroid-responsive diarrhea).

Investigation of the intestinal microflora in dogs with IBD is difficult. One attempt to non-invasively assess the impact of the intestinal microflora is the measurement of serum cobalamine and folate concentrations. Cobalamine is absorbed via a receptor-mediated mechanism in the terminal ileum, and folate is absorbed in the jejunum. Theoretically, the increased number of bacteria should increase the serum level of folate and decrease the levels of cobalamine, because bacteria synthesize folate and bind cobalamine. However, the sensitivity and specificity of these measurements are low (sensitivity 5–30%, specificity 30–100%; German *et al.* 2003). Molecular methods, such as molecular fingerprinting or pyrosequencing to detect bacteria in the duodenal juice or in biopsies will possibly be helpful to understand the impact of the microflora on disease mechanism in the future (Xenoulis *et al.* 2008).

The diagnosis of IBD therefore involves careful integration of signalment (for breed predispositions see Simpson and Jergens 2011), home environment, history, physical findings, clinicopathologic testing, diagnostic imaging, and histopathology of intestinal biopsies. Furthermore, IBD is associated with histopathology evidence of inflammation in the intestinal mucosa with the infiltration of the gastric, small and/or large intestinal wall with inflammatory cells. The nomenclature reflects the predominant cell types present, with lymphocytic-plasmacytic enteritis (LPE) being the most commonly reported form. Most lymphocytes and plasma cells are in the lamina propria and crypt dilatation and loss of surface epithelial cells are often associated with this form. Eosinophilic (gastro-) enteritis is less common. Patients may reveal a peripheral eosinophilia, which may be one component of the hypereosinophilic syndrome. This form occurs uncommonly, and the animals affected tend to be younger. Endoparasites, infectious agents, and food allergy have all been incriminated in this form, but none have been proven. Regardless, it is prudent to investigate and eliminate these potential etiologies first since treatment of eosinophilic enteritis tends to be more difficult than that of LPE. Granulomatous enteritis is rare and usually presents as a segmental, thickened, partially obstructed segment of bowel. The ileum and colon appear to be affected most commonly. It is important to eliminate inflammation secondary to fungal disease, intestinal parasites, feline infectious peritonitis, and foreign material. Treatment of this form remains controversial, although most advocate surgical resection if possible.

Therapeutics

Most clinicians start with a strict elimination diet for at least 6–8 weeks to exclude FRD. In regard to the diet used for the treatment trial, there are different possibilities to consider. The first one consists of feeding exclusively a nutritionally balanced, highly digestible novel protein diet, where the protein source must not have been fed to the animal before. The second possibility consists of feeding diets with hydrolyzed proteins with the idea that these proteins are too small to evoke an allergic reaction. Nevertheless, it is clinically impossible to differentiate between a true food allergy and just food intolerance. If not responding, these animals can subsequently be treated with a 4–6 week course of antibiotics such as metronidazole or tylosin (Westermarck *et al.* 2005). If they respond to this treatment, they are considered to suffer from ARD, nowadays referred to as intestinal dysbiosis.

Dogs with persistent signs of chronic enteropathy that are neither responding to elimination diet nor antibiotics are finally considered to be suffering from idiopathic IBD and are given glucocorticoids (mostly prednisolone) as the mainstay of therapy. Prolonged treatment with corticosteroids can be frustrating because of the numerous side-effects associated with it. Especially in large breed dogs, polyuria/polydipsia may become unbearable for the owners. When used in combination with other immuno-suppressive drugs like azathioprine, the required dosage of corticosteroids and the associated side effects can eventually be decreased or the dogs can be weaned off corticosteroids sooner. For cases showing severe side-effects with prednisolone, oral budesonide might be an option, but initial studies in dogs with IBD are not very convincing in regard to reduction of side-effects. A number of dogs treated with immunosuppressive doses of corticosteroids will show either no response at all to the drug or will experience a clinical relapse after weeks to months of treatment. Cyclosporine (Allenspach *et al.* 2007) and chlorambucil (Dandrieux *et al.* 2013) have been shown to be effective in steroid refractory IBD. Cobalamine supplementation for hypocobalaminemia, increased omega-3 fatty acids (Ontsouka *et al.* 2012) and probiotics may perhaps not help in all cases, but they share the potential to ameliorate the clinical problems. The most important treatment options are summarized in Table 19.1.

Table 19.1 The most important therapeutic options for IBD in dogs and cats.

	Active ingredient	Dosage
Nutritional management	Novel protein or hydrolyzed diet	For at least 6–8 weeks, mostly improvement within 2 weeks
	High fiber diet +/− psyllium	Sometimes helpful for large intestinal problems
Immunosuppressive	Prednisolone	1 mg/kg PO BID and taper after resolution of signs
	Budesonide	1–3 mg PO SID (per dog) 1 mg PO SID (per cat)
	Cyclosporine	5 mg/kg PO SID (dog)
	Chlorambucil	2 mg/kg PO every second day (cat) 2–6 mg/m^2 PO SID (cat) 4–6 mg/m^2 PO SID (dog) Treat for 7–21 days, then reduce
	Azathioprine	2 mg/kg PO SID (dog)
Antimicrobials	Metronidazole	10–20 mg/kg PO BID (dog, cat)
	Tylosin	10–40 mg/kg PO BID (dog, cat) 25 mg/kg PO SID (dog)
	Enrofloxacin	5–10 mg/kg PO SID (dog) (histiocytic ulcerative colitis)
Anti-inflammatory: 5-aminosalicylates (Sometimes used for colitis)	Sulfasalazine Olsalazine/mesalamine	10–30 mg/kg PO BID-TID (dog) 10–20 mg/kg PO SID (cat) 10–20 mg/kg PO TID (dog)
Cobalamine		SC q1week for at least 6 weeks. Cat/dog < 5 kg 250 µg Dog 5–15 kg 400 µg Dog 15–30 kg 800 µg Dog 30–45 kg 1200 µg Dog > 45 kg 1500 µg

Quality of Life for Patient and Caregiver

The clinical course of IBD in dogs is characterized by spontaneous exacerbations and remissions, which makes the assessment of disease burden difficult. Therefore, a scoring system for the evaluation of the canine IBD activity (CIBDAI) was developed (Jergens *et al.* 2003; see Table 19.2). This scoring system was compared to serum concentrations of C-reactive protein (CRP), haptoglobin (HAP), alpha-acid glycoprotein (AGP), and serum amyloid A (SAA), as well as histology scores derived from endoscopic biopsy specimens. Among IBD dogs, the CIBDAI showed good correlation to both histology and HAP scores, but CRP also was a strong co-correlate of disease activity. The IBD dogs showed significantly decreased CIBDAI and CRP values but significantly increased HAP concentrations after medical therapy compared to pretreatment values. Therefore, the CIBDAI is a reliable measure of inflammatory activity in canine IBD and the effect of therapy. Three other factors (albumin levels, ascites and peripheral edema, and pruritus) were added to the CIBDAI to get the CCECAI (canine chronic enteropathy clinical activity index; Allenspach *et al.* 2007), another activity index for the disease. Both indices are quite simple to determine and are very helpful tools to evaluate clinical severity of the disease, progression or treatment success, and therefore also the quality of life.

Table 19.2 Canine inflammatory bowel disease activity index (CIBDAI).

Clinical symptoms assessed	Score
Attitude/activity	0–3
Appetite	0–3
Vomiting	0–3
Stool consistency	0–3
Stool frequency	0–3
Weight loss	0–3

After summation of the scores, the total composite score is assessed as clinically insignificant disease (score 0–3), mild (score 4–5), moderate (score 6–8), or severe IBD (score 9 or greater).
Source: Jergens *et al.* 2003. Reproduced with permission of American College of Veterinary Internal Medicine.

References

Allenspach K, Wieland B, Gröne A, Gaschen F. Chronic enteropathies in dogs: evaluation of risk factors for negative outcome. Journal of Veterinary Internal Medicine. 2007; 21(4): 700–708.

Burgener IA, König A, Allenspach K, et al. Upregulation of toll-like receptors in chronic enteropathies in dogs. Journal of Veterinary Internal Medicine. 2008; 22: 553–560.

Dandrieux JR, Bornand VF, Burgener IA. Evaluation of lymphocyte apoptosis in dogs with inflammatory bowel disease. The American Journal of Veterinary Research. 2008; 69(10): 1279–1285.

Dandrieux JR, Noble PJM, Cripps PJ, German AJ, Scase TJ Comparison of a chlorambucil-prednisolone combination with an azathioprine-prednisolone combination for treatment of chronic enteropathy with concurrent protein-losing enteropathy in dogs: 27 cases (2007–2010). Journal of the American Veterinary Medical Association. 2013; 242(12): 1705–1714.

German AJ, Day MJ, Ruaux CG, Steiner JM, Williams DA, Hall EJ. Comparison of direct and indirect tests for small intestinal bacterial overgrowth and antibiotic-responsive diarrhea in dogs. Journal of Veterinary Internal Medicine. 2003; 17(1): 33–43.

Hostutler RA, Luria BJ, Johnson SE, et al. Antibiotic-responsive histiocytic ulcerative colitis in 9 dogs. Journal of Veterinary Internal Medicine. 2004; 18(4): 499–504.

Jergens AE, Schreiner CA, Frank DE, et al. A scoring index for disease activity in canine inflammatory bowel disease. Journal of Veterinary Internal Medicine. 2003; 17(3): 291–297.

Ontsouka EC, Burgener IA, Luckschander-Zeller N, Blum JW, Albrecht C. Fish-meal diet enriched in omega-3 PUFA and treatment of canine chronic enteropathies. European Journal of Lipid Science and Technology. 2012; 114(4): 412–422.

Simpson KW, Dogan B, Rishniw M, et al. Adherent and invasive *Escherichia coli* is associated with granulomatous colitis in boxer dogs. Infection and Immunity. 2006; 74(8): 4778–4792.

Simpson KW, Jergens AE. Pitfalls and progress in the diagnosis and management of canine inflammatory bowel disease. Veterinary Clinic of North America: Small Animal Practice. 2011; 41(2): 381–398.

Westermarck E, Skrzypczak T, Harmoinen J, et al. Tylosin-responsive chronic diarrhea in dogs. Journal of Veterinary Internal Medicine. 2005; 19(2): 177–186.

Xenoulis PG, Palculict B, Allenspach K, et al. (2008). Molecular-phylogenetic characterization of microbial communities imbalances the small intestine of dogs with inflammatory bowel disease. FEMS Microbiology Ecology. 2008; 66(3): 579–589.

20

Protein-Losing Enteropathy

Iwan A. Burgener

Introduction

Protein-losing enteropathy (PLE) is a syndrome in which there is excessive loss of proteins into the lumen of the gastrointestinal tract (Willard *et al.* 2000). PLE is identified when hypoalbuminemia occurs because the loss of albumin cannot be compensated by liver synthesis (Dossin and Lavoué 2011). In dogs, PLE has been described extensively, and certain breeds (Norwegian Lundehund, Basenji, Soft Coated Wheaten Terrier, German Shepherds, Rottweilers, and Yorkshire Terriers) appear to be at increased risk for PLE (Littman *et al.* 2000; Lecoindre, Chevallier, and Guerret 2010; Simpson and Jergens 2011; Equilino *et al.* 2015). Commonly reported causes of PLE include alimentary lymphoma, chronic intussusception, hookworm infestation, inflammatory bowel disease (IBD), or lymphangiectasia (Murphy *et al.* 2003). Food hypersensitivity reactions are also a documented cause of enteropathy and can be occult or associated with clinical signs of varying severity, including PLE. However, any disease causing gastrointestinal tract inflammation, infiltration, congestion, or bleeding can result in PLE (Hall and German 2010).

Identifying gastrointestinal tract disease in a dog with hypoproteinemia and ruling out cutaneous protein loss, renal protein loss, and hepatic insufficiency leads to a diagnosis of PLE (Willard *et al.* 2000). Enteric loss of

protein can occur by means of several mechanisms, including increased mucosal permeability to proteins, lymphatic obstruction, or mucosal erosion and has a greater effect on serum concentrations of proteins that typically have a low catabolic rate (Vaden *et al.* 2000).

Lymphangiectasia is a condition characterized by dilatation of the lymphatic vessels and leakage of lymph from the villi or from deeper portions of the intestinal wall into the intestinal lumen (Dossin and Lavoué 2011). The leakage of proteins, lipids, and lymphocyte-rich lymph into the intestinal lumen is responsible for the protein loss (i.e., PLE) and lymphopenia sometimes is observed. Lymphangiectasia may be primary (idiopathic or congenital) or secondary to other diseases that increase the hydrostatic pressure in the lymphatic vessels of the gastrointestinal tract due to infiltrates (e.g., IBD or alimentary lymphoma).

Diagnosis (see also Chapter 19 on IBD)

The first step when facing a dog or cat with a suspicion of PLE is to rule out other conditions associated with hypoalbuminemia such as renal loss (protein-losing nephropathy), lack of production (liver failure), third space loss (ascites or pleural effusion), or loss across the skin (burns). Therefore, the

Chronic Disease Management for Small Animals, First Edition. Edited by W. Dunbar Gram, Rowan J. Milner and Remo Lobetti.
© 2018 John Wiley & Sons, Inc. Published 2018 by John Wiley & Sons, Inc.

workup should include a urinalysis, protein-to-creatinine ratio, liver function test (bile acids or ammonia), and a search for inflammatory fluid accumulation within the thorax and abdomen.

Reported clinical signs include were diarrhea (91%), weight loss (74%), anorexia (56%) and lethargy (51%) (Lecoindre *et al.* 2010). In one study leukocytosis was detected in 20/29 dogs, whereof 14 had a high band count (Equilino *et al.* 2015). Serum biochemical analyses revealed that serum total protein, albumin, and total calcium concentrations were decreased in all 29 dogs (Equilino *et al.* 2015), whereas serum cobalamine concentrations were low in 75% of the dogs.

Serum concentration of C-reactive protein (CRP), an acute-phase reactant, can be useful as a prognostic marker in dogs with IBD (Jergens *et al.* 2003). However, in some studies in dogs (Allenspach *et al.* 2007; McCann *et al.* 2007), CRP concentration did not reflect the severity of IBD as assessed by use of the canine chronic enteropathy clinical activity index (CCECAI) or canine inflammatory bowel disease activity index (CIBDAI). A recent study (Equilino *et al.* 2015) showed that serum CRP concentration was high in most dogs with PLE and was significantly higher than in dogs with food-responsive diarrhea (FRD).

Alpha1-proteinase inhibitor (α1-PI) is present in plasma, interstitial fluid, and lymph, but is not usually found at high concentrations within the lumen of the gastrointestinal tract. Furthermore, α1-PI is resistant to proteolytic degradation and its molecular weight is similar to that of albumin. Therefore, it can be used as a marker for intestinal protein loss (Murphy *et al.* 2003). A study in Yorkshire Terriers revealed an association between serum α1-PI concentrations less than the lower limit of the reference interval and cobalamine deficiency (Grützner *et al.* 2013). This is suggestive of severe long-standing distal small intestinal disease, such as PLE, which has been reported frequently for this breed. In a recent study with PLE dogs secondary to IBD, serum α1-PI concentration

was significantly lower in PLE than FRD and 50% of the dogs yielded α1-PI values below the lower end of the reference range (Equilino *et al.* 2015).

The heterodimeric protein complex calprotectin binds calcium and zinc, is expressed and released from infiltrating myelomonocytic cells at sites of inflammation, and has the potential to differentiate between healthy dogs from those with inflammatory conditions, such as IBD (Heilmann, Suchodolski, and Steiner 2008). S100A12, a calcium-binding protein of the S100 superfamily that is mainly localized in granulocytes and mononuclear inflammatory cells appears to be a sensitive and specific biochemical marker of chronic gastrointestinal inflammation in humans. A test for S100A12 protein detection in serum and fecal samples from dogs has recently been developed and validated (Heilmann *et al.* 2011). Serum calprotectin and S100A12 concentrations were mostly elevated in dogs with PLE secondary to IBD (Equilino *et al.* 2015), but did not differ significantly between PLE and FRD.

Ultrasonographic findings in 29 dogs with PLE (Equilino *et al.* 2015) included stomach wall thickening in 5 dogs and abnormalities of the intestinal wall (stippling, striations, or loss of wall layering) in 26 dogs (segmental abnormalities in 14 dogs and generalized abnormalities in 12 dogs). The duodenum and jejunum were involved in almost all cases, whereas only 1 dog showed colonic changes on ultrasound. Abdominal effusion was present in 22 dogs (mild effusion in 16 dogs and moderate effusion in 6 dogs), and the mesentery was assessed as hyperechoic in 21 dogs. Abdominal lymph nodes were rarely enlarged.

Endoscopic and histopathology findings in 29 dogs with PLE (Equilino *et al.* 2015) showed evidence of gastric fibrosis (N = 17) and lymphocytic-plasmacytic gastritis (N = 16). Histopathology abnormalities in the duodenum were identified in all dogs: lymphocytic-plasmacytic inflammation (N = 29), lymphangiectasia (N = 21), eosinophilic inflammation (N = 9), and fibrosis (N = 9).

There was no correlation found between severity of intestinal inflammation in histopathology and findings in abdominal ultrasound. Lecoindre *et al.* (2010) also found that most PLE cases where associated with moderate to severe inflammatory infiltrates (86%), associated with dilatation of intestinal crypts (71%) and lymphangiectasia (62%).

Therapeutics (see also Chapter 19 on IBD)

The treatment of PLE is complicated by the variety of different underlying etiologies. Thus, the focus of treatment is to identify and correct or control (if possible) any underlying cause (e.g., IBD, lymphoma, gastric ulcers, giardiasis, histoplasmosis) and then to reduce the leakage of lymph and protein across the gut wall through non-specific but appropriate diet and/or drug therapy (Zoran 2014). Treatment of specific diseases that may cause PLE, such as IBD, alimentary lymphoma, or infectious diseases like histoplasmosis are beyond the scope of this chapter and can be found elsewhere. The non-specific therapy of PLE has four main goals, namely provide adequate nutritional support, increase oncotic pressure, reduce inflammation associated with leakage of lymph and crypt lesions; and address or prevent complications, especially thromboembolic events (Dossin and Lavoué 2011; Zoran 2014).

The two most important aspects in regard to nutritional support are the replenishment of the proteins lost to allow recovery of protein functions (e.g., albumin, clotting factors, anti-thrombin) and muscle mass and to provide enough energy in the diet while avoiding too much fat that the GI tract is unable to digest. A very detailed review of these aspects can be found elsewhere (Zoran 2014). The most efficient way to provide long-term oncotic support is to address and potentially cure the primary disease. In critical cases, hydroxyethyl starches are used at a maximal dosage rate of 20–30 ml/kg/day (Dossin and Lavoué 2011). However, they only provide short-term support and may, at higher dosages, impair coagulation. Fresh frozen plasma may be used to increase the albumin and provide coagulation factors, and anti-thrombin. However, a large volume of plasma is required to significantly increase the albumin concentration. Coagulation should be monitored in patients with severe PLE because hypercoagulability and thrombosis have been reported. In these cases, fresh frozen plasma can be used to increase anti-thrombin and coagulation factors.

Quality of Life

With PLE, the quality of life is often correlating with the albumin level. With severe hypoalbuminemia (<15 g/l), muscle atrophy/muscle wasting, ascites, and possibly pleural effusions can occur. Furthermore, the level of complications rises as well due to a severe decrease of anti-thrombin and coagulation factors.

The clinical course of IBD and PLE is characterized by spontaneous exacerbations and remissions, which makes assessing the disease burden difficult. The scoring system for the evaluation of the canine IBD activity (CIBDAI and CCECAI) (Allenspach *et al.* 2007; Jergens *et al.* 2003) can also be used for PLE and is a reliable measure of inflammatory activity in canine PLE and the effect of therapy. These indices are quite simple to determine and are very helpful tools to evaluate clinical severity of the disease, progression or treatment success, and therefore also the quality of life.

End of therapeutic intervention is dependent on the primary disease leading to PLE. Especially the cases with severe protein loss secondary to severe IBD might often use hydrolyzed diets and more than only prednisolone to stabilize. But even then, there remain certain cases that will not or only for a short time respond to any of the mentioned treatment options.

In a recent study with PLE secondary to IBD (Equilino *et al.* 2015), 6 of 29 dogs with PLE were still alive at the end-point of the study (survival time 730 to 2,347 days). The other 23 dogs were deceased, with a median survival time of 67 days (range, 2 to 2,551 days).

Owners of 17 dogs elected euthanasia because of lack of clinical improvement (survival time 2 to 874 days), whereas six dogs were euthanized or died because of other diseases.

References

Allenspach K, Wieland B, Gröne A, Gaschen F. Chronic enteropathies in dogs: evaluation of risk factors for negative outcome. Journal of Veterinary Internal Medicine. 2007; 21(4): 700–708.

Dossin O, Lavoué R. Protein-losing enteropathies in dogs. Veterinary Clinic of North America: Small Animal Practice. 2011; 41: 399–418.

Equilino M, Theodoloz V, Gorgas D, et al. Evaluation of serum biochemical marker concentrations and survival time in dogs with protein-losing enteropathy. Journal of the American Veterinary Medical Association, 2015; 246(1): 91–99.

Grützner N, Heilmann RM, Bridges CS, Suchodolski JS, Steiner JM. Serum concentrations of canine alpha1-proteinase inhibitor in cobalamin-deficient Yorkshire Terrier dogs. Journal of Veterinary Diagnostic Investigation. 2013; 25(3): 376–385.

Hall EJ, German AJ. Diseases of small intestine. In: SJ Ettinger and EC Feldmann, Eds. Textbook of Veterinary Internal Medicine, 7th edn. Saunders Elsevier, 2010: 1526–1572.

Heilmann RM, Lanerie DJ, Ruaux CG, Grützner N, Suchodolski JS, Steiner JM. Development and analytic validation of an immunoassay for the quantification of canine S100A12 in serum and fecal samples and its biological variability in serum from healthy dogs. Veterinary Immunology and Immunopathology. 2011; 144(3–4): 200–209.

Heilmann RM, Suchodolski JS, Steiner JM. Development and analytic validation of a radioimmunoassay for the quantification of canine calprotectin in serum and feces from

dogs. The American Journal of Veterinary Research. 2008; 69: 845–853.

Jergens AE, Schreiner CA, Frank DE, et al. A scoring index for disease activity in canine inflammatory bowel disease. Journal of Veterinary Internal Medicine. 2003; 17(3): 291–297.

Lecoindre P, Chevallier M, Guerret S. Les entéropathies exsudatives d'origine non néoplastique du chien: Étude rétrospective de 34 cas [Protein-losing enteropathy of non-neoplastic origin in the dog: a retrospective study of 34 cases] [in French]. Schweizer Archiv Fur Tierheilkunde. 2010; 152(3): 141–146.

Littman MP, Dambach DM, Vaden SL, Giger U. Familial protein-losing enteropathy and protein-losing nephropathy in Soft Coated Wheaten Terriers: 222 cases (1983–1997). Journal of Veterinary Internal Medicine. 2000; 14: 68–80.

McCann TM, Ridyard AE, Else RW, Simpson JW. Evaluation of disease activity markers in dogs with idiopathic inflammatory bowel disease. The Journal of Small Animal Practice. 2007; 48(11): 620–625.

Murphy KF, German AJ, Ruaux CG, Steiner JM, Williams DA, Hall EJ. Fecal α1-proteinase inhibitor concentration in dogs with chronic gastrointestinal disease. Veterinary Clinical Pathology. 2003; 32(2): 67–72.

Simpson KW, Jergens AE. Pitfalls and progress in the diagnosis and management of canine inflammatory bowel disease. Veterinary Clinic of North America: Small Animal Practice. 2011; 41(2): 381–398.

Vaden SL, Sellon RK, Melgarejo LT, et al. Evaluation of intestinal permeability and gluten sensitivity in Soft-Coated Wheaten terriers with familial protein-losing enteropathy, protein-losing nephropathy, or both. American Journal of Veterinary Research. 2000; 61(5): 518–524.

Willard MD, Helman G, Fradkin JM, et al. Intestinal crypt lesions associated with protein-losing enteropathy in the dog.

Journal of Veterinary Internal Medicine. 2000; 14(3): 298–307.

Zoran DL. Protein-losing enteropathies. In: JD Bonagura and DC Twedt, Eds. Kirk´s current veterinary therapy XV. Saunders Elsevier. 2014: 540–544.

21

Cholecystitis
Joanne L. McLean

Introduction

Cholecystitis is an apparently uncommon entity in small animals, with published information on the condition limited to small case series and clinical reports (Lawrence *et al.* 2015). Cholecystitis is a broad term describing inflammation of the gallbladder (GB) attributed to ascending infection from the intestinal tract or a hematogenous source of infection (bacterial or parasitic), blunt abdominal trauma, cystic duct occlusion (e.g., cholelithiasis), cystic artery thrombosis, or neoplasia. Choleliths are concurrently identified in some patients, but the causal role has yet been determined (Aguirre 2010). Cholecystitis can be categorized as non-necrotizing, necrotizing, or emphysematous (Richter and Pike 2014).

In non-necrotizing cholecystitis, inflammation of the GB may involve nonsuppurative or suppurative inflammation; may be associated with infectious agents, systemic disease, or neoplasia; or may reflect blunt abdominal trauma or GB obstruction by occlusion of the cystic duct (e.g., cholelithiasis, neoplasia, or choledochitis). Cystic duct occlusion incites GB inflammation secondary to bile stasis; this process is augmented by mechanical irritation by a cholelith (Center 2009).

Necrotizing cholecystitis is a more severe syndrome that may develop secondary to thromboembolism, blunt abdominal trauma, bacterial infection, extra-hepatic biliary obstruction (EHBO) (cystic duct obstruction or distal duct obstruction by choleliths, stricture, or neoplasia), or a mature gallbladder mucocele (causing tense GB distention). Extension of an inflammatory or neoplastic process from adjacent hepatic tissue also may be an underlying cause. Necrotizing cholecystitis can present with or without GB rupture (type 1 and II), or as a chronic syndrome associated with adhesions between the GB, omentum, and adjacent viscera (type 3). Bacteria are commonly cultured from the gallbladder wall (Center 2009).

Emphysematous cholecystitis/choledochitis is a rare manifestation of acute cholecystitis complicated by gas producing organisms (*E. coli, Clostridium* bacteria) and associated with gas within the wall or lumen of the GB or segments of the biliary tree. It is a rare disease entity in the dog and extremely rare in cats (Aguirre 2010). In dogs, it has been associated with diabetes mellitus, acute cholecystitis with or without cholecystolithiasis, traumatic ischemia, mature GB mucocele formation, and neoplasia.

Chronic Disease Management for Small Animals, First Edition. Edited by W. Dunbar Gram, Rowan J. Milner and Remo Lobetti.

Clinical and Diagnostic Findings

Cholecystitis is seen most commonly in older animals (median age 9½ years) with no apparent breed or sex predilection (Church and Mathiessen 1988), although one study showed an overrepresentation of Dachshunds (Lawrence *et al.* 2015).

Cholecystitis may be acute or chronic in nature. Signs of acute cholecystitis include abdominal pain (may only be postprandial), anorexia, vomiting, pyrexia, and icterus. Some animals may present with signs of hypodynamic shock especially when GB rupture or bile peritonitis is present. Signs of chronic cholecystitis are more vague, with a waxing and waning nature, making a diagnosis of chronic cholecystitis more challenging. Clinical signs may include intermittent anorexia, vomiting, and progressive weight loss.

Diagnosis is based on clinical signs, clinicopathologic features, and ultrasonographic imaging findings. Laboratory abnormalities present in cases of cholecystitis are very nonspecific and indistinguishable from other hepatobiliary diseases. Abnormalities seen may include variable leukocytosis, with or without toxic neutrophils or a left shift, hyperbilirubinemia and moderate to marked increases in liver enzyme activity, especially ALP and GGT. Abdominal radiography may reveal indistinct detail in the cranial abdomen consistent with focal peritonitis or rarely; the GB wall may become radio-dense due to dystrophic mineralization secondary to chronic inflammation. Choleliths may also be seen and in cases of emphysematous cholecystitis, a spherical to ovoid gas opacity superimposed over the hepatic silhouette may be present.

Ultrasonography is the current gold standard for diagnosis of cholecystitis in small animals. Common ultrasonographic abnormalities include a thickened GB wall (Figure 21.1), intraluminal echogenic debris, presence of choleliths, signs of EHBO, or emphysema of the GB wall (Richter and Pike 2014). Pericholecystic fluid and omental

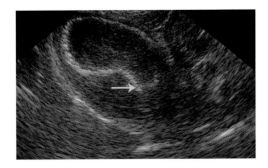

Figure 21.1 Ultrasound image of a dog with cholecystitis. There is a markedly echogenic and thickened gall bladder wall. The gall bladder is filled with echogenic fluid and sediment, and dilation of the proximal cystic duct also appears to be present (arrow).

adhesions may also be detected. Ultrasound is highly sensitive for the identification of GB rupture (86% sensitivity). Loss of GB wall continuity, hyperechoic fat in the cranial peritoneal cavity and presence of pericholecystic fluid or free abdominal fluid are all supportive of GB rupture (Richter and Pike 2014).

Percutaneous ultrasound-guided cholecystocentesis is also a relatively safe, minimally non-invasive diagnostic procedure that can prove useful in making both a diagnosis and in aiding in medical management of cases with cholecystitis. Bile samples should be sent for both cytological and aerobic/anaerobic culture with antimicrobial sensitivity testing. Complications of this procedure include intraperitoneal bile leakage, hemorrhage, hemobilia, bacteremia, and vasovagal reactions that may result in ventilator arrest, severe bradycardia, and death (Center 2009). To avoid bile leakage, it is recommended that the GB be drained completely during cholecystocentesis (Aguirre 2010).

Therapeutic Management

Both medical and surgical management is available for patients with cholecystitis. Medical management is indicated in cases of non-necrotizing cholecystitis where the GB wall integrity does not appear compromised on abdominal ultrasound. When embarking on medical treatment it is important that the pet owner be warned of the possible need for surgical intervention in the future either if medical management is unsuccessful in resolving the infection or if biliary rupture/EHBO subsequently occurs. Medical management typically consists of intravenous fluid therapy, antibiotic and analgesic therapy, anti-emetic and gastro-protectant therapy, if indicated, and the use of choleretics such as ursodiol. The choice of antibiotic therapy should ideally be guided by bacterial cultures of bile samples retrieved via cholecystocentesis. In one study 62% of patients with cholecystitis had positive cultures, with *E. coli, Enteroccoccus spp, Bacteroides spp, Streptococcus spp* and *Clostridium spp* being the most commonly isolated bacteria (Wagner, Hartmann, and Trepanier 2007). Thus without bile samples for culture, empiric antibiotic therapy effective against gram negative bacteria and anaerobic bacteria is advised. Such antibiotics would include cefoxitin, metronidazole, and/or enrofloxacin. Antibiotics should be continued for a minimum of 4 weeks and potentially longer to ensure complete resolution of the infection.

Regular monitoring of patients during medical therapy (at least 3 weekly) is imperative and should include serial ultrasonographic examination of the GB and serum liver enzyme activity analyses. Frequent communication with pet owners on their perception of the status of their dog's clinical condition is also important. Progression of the disease in any fashion on serial examinations should warrant immediate surgical intervention. Euthanasia may unfortunately need to be considered in cases where medical management is unsuccessful in resolving the infection and controlling clinical signs and cost constraints prohibit surgery.

In patients with necrotizing or emphysematous cholecystitis where there is ultrasonographic evidence of severe GB wall compromise or GB rupture, surgical intervention in the form of cholecystectomy is advised. In some cases, placement of a temporary biliary stent or a cholecystoenterostomy may also be required to circumvent a permanently occluded distal common bile duct, but should be carefully considered because of the high rate of complications, especially in cats. During surgery samples of bile, gallbladder wall, choleliths, and liver tissue should also always be submitted for histopathology and aerobic and anaerobic culture.

Preoperative management of cholecystitis should focus on restoration of fluid and electrolyte status (these patients often have severe cardiovascular compromise or sepsis), appropriate analgesia, and treatment with broad-spectrum antibiotics effective against enteric opportunists. Patients with chronic EHBO may also have a coagulopathy due to a relative deficiency of vitamin K from altered hepatobiliary excretion of bile acids required for vitamin K absorption (Richter and Pike 2014). It is, therefore, recommended that coagulation profiles be performed pre-operatively and failing that, prophylactic vitamin K (0.5–1.5 mg/kg IM or SC) or a fresh frozen plasma transfusion be administered.

If only the gallbladder is involved, and in the absence of neoplasia, simple cholecystectomy may be curative with a long-term survival and good quality of life expected. If the common bile, cystic, or hepatic ducts are involved, a more guarded prognosis is warranted, and long-term antibiotic therapy recommended. Patients having undergone biliary tree decompression by placement of a biliary stent or by biliary enteric-anastomoses are also more susceptible to future retrograde septic cholangitis and choledochitis. Owners should be instructed to monitor such patients for pyrexia, inappetance, vomiting, and signs of cyclic illness. A complete blood count and liver enzyme activity levels should be assessed every 3–4 months. Chronic or intermittent antimicrobial administration may be needed to control ascending cholangitis in these patients. Fortunately, illness is usually transient and responsive to antibiotics.

References

Aguirre A. Diseases of the gallbladder and extrahepatic biliary system. In: SJ Ettinger and EC Feldman, Eds. Textbook of veterinary internal medicine, 7th edn. Elsevier Saunders. 2010: 1689–1695,

Center SA. Disease of the gallbladder and biliary tree. Veterinary Clinics of North America Small Animal Practice. 2009; 39: 543–598.

Church EM, Matthiesen DT. Surgical treatment of 23 dogs with necrotizing cholecystitis. Journal of the American Animal Hospital Association. 1988; 24: 305–310.

Lawrence YA, Ruaux CG, Nemanic S, Milovancev M. Characterization, treatment and outcome of bacterial cholecystitis and bactibilia in dogs. Journal of the American Veterinary Medical Association. 2015; 246: 982–989.

Richter KP and Pike FS. Extrahepatic biliary tract disease. In: JD Bonagura and DC Twedt, Eds. Kirk's current veterinary therapy XV. Elsevier Saunders. 2014: 602–605,

Wagner KA, Hartmann FA, Trepanier LA. Bacterial culture results from liver, gallbladder, or bile in 248 dogs and cats evaluated for hepatobiliary disease: 1998–2003. Journal of Veterinary Internal Medicine. 2007; 21: 417–424.

Further Reading

Neer TM. A review of disorders of the gallbladder and extrahepatic biliary tract in the dog and cat. Journal of Veterinary Internal Medicine. 1992; 6: 186–192.

22

Biliary Mucocele

Joanne L. McLean

Introduction

Although the disease has been recognized for several decades, the incidence of gallbladder (GB) mucoceles (MCs) in dogs appears to have rapidly increased over the last 20 years (Malek *et al.* 2013). GB MCs are now considered the most common causes of extrahepatic biliary disease in the canine patient and the most common reason for performing biliary surgery in this species (Hottinger 2014). Whether this apparent increase is as a result of increased awareness of the disease together with early detection by improved abdominal ultrasonography, or a true increase in incidence of the disease, is still unknown (Malek *et al.* 2013).

A GB MC is defined as accumulation of mucous and inspissated bile salts within the fundus of the GB causing GB distention. The MC develops because of the progressive accumulation of tenacious, mucin-laden bile in the GB, which may extend into the cystic duct, common bile-duct, and hepatic ducts. This accumulation leads to pressure ischemic necrosis of the GB or cystic duct wall, opportunistic bacterial infections and potentially GB or cystic duct/common bile duct rupture with subsequent bile peritonitis (Hottinger 2014). On histopathology, it is characterized by cystic mucinous epithelial hyperplasia of the GB wall with inflammatory infiltrates but rarely with an infectious etiology being recognized. Grossly a MC appears as an accumulation of shiny green-black gelatinous material with lamellar striations within the GB lumen.

Pathogenesis

In humans, functional or structural obstruction of the cystic or common bile duct is the most common cause for GB MCs, this, however, has not been shown to be the case in dogs. In dogs, impaired GB motility and abnormalities in cholesterol and lipid metabolism appear to be the primary factors in disease development. Delayed GB emptying allows for accumulation of concentrated bile salts, which stimulates mucous production by the epithelial lining of the GB (Tsukagoshi *et al.* 2012).

Conditions shown to be associated with poor GB motility and abnormal cholesterol and lipid metabolism include some endocrinopathies (diabetes mellitus (DM), hypothyroidism, and Cushing's disease), exogenous administration of corticosteroids as well as some dyslipidemias (hypertriglyceridemia, hypercholesterolemia). Dogs with Cushing's disease are 29 times more likely to have an MC than those without the disease and there is significant association between GB MC and hypothyroidism (Mesich *et al.* 2009). Complete resolution of spontaneous

Chronic Disease Management for Small Animals, First Edition. Edited by W. Dunbar Gram, Rowan J. Milner and Remo Lobetti.
© 2018 John Wiley & Sons, Inc. Published 2018 by John Wiley & Sons, Inc.

GB MCs has been shown in two dogs when treatment of concurrent hypothyroidism was initiated (Walter *et al.* 2008).

Another study looking at the effect administration of hydrocortisone has on bile acid composition demonstrated a reversible change in the bile acid composition in treated dogs compared to controls, with increased concentrations of the more hydrophobic unconjugated bile acids seen. The shift to less water soluble, more hydrophobic caustic bile acids may be responsible for mucosal irritation and hence trigger mucinous hyperplasia (Kook *et al.* 2011).

There is a potential genetic component to the disease as it has been shown that there is significant association of a mutation in the ABCB4 gene in Shetland sheepdogs and other dogs with biliary MCs (Mealey *et al.* 2010). This gene is responsible for encoding for the secretion of phosphatidyl choline (PC) across the bile canaliculi. PC is responsible for reducing bile salt cytotoxicity and protecting the biliary mucous from damage. The toxic bile acids are thought to be responsible for the cystic epithelial pathology that manifests.

Diagnostics

As with any disease process, diagnosis of a GB MC requires assimilating data from the signalment of the patient, owner history, clinical signs, clinical examination findings, laboratory data, and diagnostic imaging findings.

GB MCs commonly present in middle-aged to old dogs, with no definitive breed predisposition although they are overrepresented in Shetland Sheepdogs, Cocker Spaniels, Miniature Schnauzers and Dachshunds. There is no apparent sex predilection. Because MCs are thought to develop slowly; presenting clinical signs are variable with a waxing and waning nature. In fact, MCs are often detected as incidental findings on routine abdominal ultrasonography when the animal is showing no clinical signs of systemic disease. In the majority of cases subacute to chronic non-specific, vague clinical signs are seen including vomiting, anorexia, lethargy, diarrhea, polyuria-polydipsia, icterus, dehydration, tachycardia, tachypnea, and abdominal discomfort. Alternatively, patients may present with signs of acute abdomen associated with extrahepatic bile duct obstruction, pancreatitis or bile peritonitis. Pyrexia, if present, is often associated with bacterial cholecystitis or bile peritonitis.

Routine clinico-pathological abnormalities seen are indistinguishable from other hepatobiliary diseases and certain endocrinopathies and are not particularly useful in making a diagnosis. These include increases in serum liver enzyme activity (ALP, ALT, and GGT), hyperbilirubinemia, hypertriglyceridemia, and hypercholesterolemia. Neutrophilic leucocytosis, often with a left shift, can occur with bile peritonitis and bacterial cholecystitis.

Abdominal radiographs are not adequate for making a definitive diagnosis but are useful for excluding other causes of acute abdomen or vomiting such as gastrointestinal obstruction, or abdominal masses and other hepatobiliary diseases including acute liver injury, neoplasia, and choleliths.

Abdominal ultrasound is the preferred and most sensitive diagnostic test for GB MCs, which have distinct ultrasonographic characteristics. The tenacious mucin along the GB wall is visualized as a hypoechoic rim. The central contents are hyperechoic and non-gravity dependent with ballottement or re-positioning of the patient. Radiating striations extend from the GB wall centrally as the MC matures, creating the described "kiwi-fruit" appearance (Figure 22.1) (Besso *et al.* 2000, Hottinger 2014). Ultrasonography may also detect signs of extrahepatic biliary obstruction as the mucinous bile extends into the cystic, common, and hepatic ducts. Ultrasonographic features of GB wall necrosis

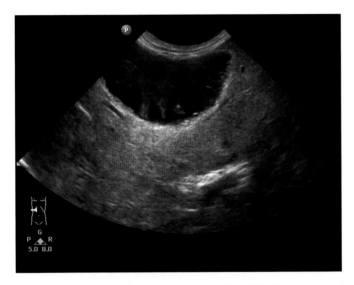

Figure 22.1 Longitudinal ultrasound image of a gallbladder mucocele demonstrating the characteristic "kiwi-fruit" or stellate appearance. The mucin layer is hypoechoic while the hyperechoic bile is centrally located. (Courtesy Dr R. Friedlein, Fourways Veterinary Hospital, South Africa.)

or early rupture of the GB include an irregular outline or defect to the GB wall, hyperechoic surrounding mesenteric fat or a hypoechoic halo of fluid surrounding the GB itself (Besso *et al.* 2000). One disadvantage of ultrasonography in these cases however, is that it lacks the sensitivity to accurately assess the presence of pressure necrosis of the GB wall or cystic duct which can lead to eventual rupture and subsequent bile peritonitis in some cases.

Because historical and presenting signs are often so vague and laboratory abnormalities seen so non-specific, often many animals are presumed to be suffering from other medical conditions such as pancreatitis or chronic gastrointestinal diseases such as IBD, especially when diagnostic imaging tools such as abdominal ultrasonography are not readily available to the clinician. It is, therefore, imperative that the clinician carefully reviews all available information and refers cases to institutes where ultrasonography is available to achieve an accurate and timely diagnosis. Often however, a diagnostic conundrum can occur when other concomitant disease processes such as pancreatitis or cholangiohepatitis are present. In these cases, it becomes a diagnostic challenge to decide whether the GB MC present is an incidental finding or contributing to the clinical signs seen.

Therapeutic Management

Both medical and surgical treatments have been reported for the management of GB MC, with surgery (cholecystectomy with retrograde lavage of the common bile duct), considered the treatment of choice in all cases of GB MC. Cholecystotomy or cholecystoenterostomy are not recommended as recurrence can be a problem and necrosis of the GB wall may not be visually evident during surgery but can lead to postoperative GB rupture and bile peritonitis. Discretion can be used in determining the timing of surgery in dogs with an intact GB. Dogs without clinical signs and that do not have signs of GB leakage on abdominal ultrasound can have surgery on an elective basis. In dogs with clinical signs, however surgery should be considered more urgent and in cases of GB rupture with or without bile peritonitis, surgery should be considered an emergency procedure.

Long-term prognosis is excellent for patients that survive the perioperative period. Unfortunately, the perioperative prognosis for dogs having undergone surgery is guarded with the mortality rates ranging from 21% to 32% (Pike *et al.* 2004; Worley, Hottinger, and Lawrence 2004; Aguirre *et al.* 2007). No concrete preoperative survival prognosticators have been demonstrated and even dogs with biliary tract rupture and bile peritonitis have been shown not to fare worse than those with an intact GB. Postoperatively, hypotension and a high serum lactate have been shown to be very highly associated with mortality (Malek *et al.* 2013). Common postoperative complications include pneumonia, pancreatitis, pulmonary thromboembolism, and bile peritonitis. Preoperative and postoperative pancreatitis as a reported complication in fact has a high enough incidence to warrant recommendation of preventative measures such as withholding food 24–48 hours postsurgery and close monitoring of pain and comfort levels in the perioperative period. Samples of the liver, GB wall, and bile should be routinely collected during surgery for histopathology and bacterial culture. Copious abdominal lavage is indicated if bile spillage has occurred during surgery or if biliary tract rupture is present.

Postoperative management should include a broad-spectrum antibiotic until bacterial culture results are available, intravenous fluid therapy, antiemetic and gastro-protective agents in symptomatic patients, adequate analgesia, and close monitoring of blood pressure, serum lactate, heart rate, and respiratory rate. Long-term management should also include a low-fat diet and ursodiol. Often antibiotic therapy is continued for at least 2 weeks postoperatively. Many patients with GB MCs also have a degree of histopathological liver abnormalities evident on biopsy including bile duct hyperplasia, portal fibrosis, cholangiohepatitis, nodular regeneration, and hepatocellular vacuolar changes. Despite these changes, in most patients liver enzyme activities return to normal after surgery. Concurrent liver disease does however remain in some patients, which may require ongoing long-term medical management. In addition, in all patients, concurrent endocrinopathies and dyslipidemias should be addressed.

Medical therapy in the majority of cases is unable to transform a semisolid MC into liquid bile and should only ever be considered in patients that are asymptomatic and have normal liver enzyme activities. One report however does claim successful management of two symptomatic dogs with clinical signs attributable to GB MC's and underlying hypothyroidism, but in this report the authors do caution that surgery is still the preferred method of management (Walter *et al.* 2008). Medical management may also unfortunately have to be considered in symptomatic patients when the pet owner has severe cost constraints that preclude surgery or when the pet owner considers the perioperative mortality rates unacceptable. Medical management however can never be considered in patients with confirmed biliary rupture with or without bile peritonitis or where ultrasonographic signs of extrahepatic biliary obstruction are present. When embarking on medical treatment in symptomatic patients it is also imperative that the pet owner be warned of the possible need for surgery in the future either if medical management is unsuccessful in alleviating or controlling clinical signs to acceptable levels or if biliary rupture/extrahepatic bile duct obstruction subsequently occurs.

Medical management consists of feeding a low-fat diet and the use of ursodiol (10–15 mg/kg SID) as well as broad-spectrum antibiotics and analgesic agents if required (buprenorphine, tramadol). Some patients may also benefit from the use of antiemetic agents (metoclopramide, maropitant) and gastroprotectants (omeprazole, ranitidine, sucrulphate) if vomiting and anorexia are unrelenting. Ursodiol is administered to improve the bile acid profile, to protect hepatocytes and biliary epithelium against the injurious effects of bile stasis and to promote choleresis. Some evidence also exists that ursodiol upregulates canalicular transporters and thus may be beneficial in dogs with transporter gene defects (Hottinger 2014). Other agents with antioxidant properties such as SAMe have also been postulated to have some benefit in medical management of GB MCs. Investigation into the presence of underlying endocrinopathies (DM, Cushing's, hypothyroidism) and treatment of those conditions as well as cessation of exogenous steroid therapy is also important in these cases. Medical management is often life-long and requires good pet owner compliance and dedication. Regular examinations (at least 6 weekly), which should include serial ultrasonographic examination of the GB and serum liver enzyme activity analyses, are imperative. Frequent communication with pet owners on their perception of the status of their dog's clinical condition is also important. Progression of the disease in any fashion on serial examinations should warrant immediate surgical intervention. Euthanasia may unfortunately need to be considered in cases where medical management is unsuccessful in controlling the animal's clinical signs to an acceptable level and cost constraints prohibit surgery.

References

Aguirre AL, Center SA, Randolph JF, et al. Gallbladder disease in Shetland Sheepdogs: 38 cases (1995–2005). Journal of the American Veterinary Medical Association. 2007; 231: 79–88.

Besso JD, Wrigley RH, Gliato JM, Webster CRL. Ultrasonographic appearance and clinical findings in dogs with gallbladder mucocele. Veterinary Radiology and Ultrasound. 2000; 41: 261–271.

Hottinger HA. Canine biliary mucocele. In: JD Bonagura and DC Twedt, Eds. Kirk's current veterinary therapy XV. Elsevier Saunders. 2014: e221–224,

Kook PH, Schellenberg S, Rentsch KM, Reusch CE, Glaus TM. Effect of twice-daily oral administration of hydrocortisone on the bile acids composition of gallbladder bile in dogs. American Journal of Veterinary Research. 2011; 72: 1607–1612.

Malek S, Sinclair E, Hosgood G, Moens NMM, Baily T, Boston SE. Clinical findings and prognostic factors for dogs undergoing cholecystectomy for gallbladder mucocele. Veterinary Surgery, 2013; 42: 418–426.

Mealey KL, Minch JD, White SN, Snekvik KR, Mattoon JS. An insertion mutation in ABCB4 is associated with gallbladder mucocele formation in dogs. Comparative Hepatology. 2010; 9: 6.

Mesich MLL, Mayhew PD, Paek M, Holt DE, Brown DC. Gallbladder mucoceles and their association with endocrinopathies in dogs: a retrospective case-controlled study. Journal of Small Animal Practice. 2009; 50: 630–635.

Pike FS, Berg J, King NW, Penninck DG, Webster CRL. Gallbladder mucocele in dogs: 30 cases (2000–2002). Journal of American Veterinary Medical Association. 2004; 224: 1615–1622.

Tsukagoshi T, Ohno K, Tsukamoto A, et al. Decreased gallbladder emptying in dogs with biliary sludge or gallbladder mucocele. Veterinary Radiology and Ultrasound. 2012; 53: 84–91.

Walter R, Dunn ME, d'Anjou M, Lecuyer M. Nonsurgical resolution of gallbladder mucocele in two dogs. Journal of the American Veterinary Medical Association. 2008; 232: 1688–1693.

Worley DR, Hottinger HE, Lawrence HJ. Surgical management of gallbladder mucocele in dogs: 22 cases (1999–2003). Journal of American Veterinary Medical Association. 2004; 225: 1418–1422.

Further Reading

Aguirre A. Diseases of the gallbladder and extrahepatic biliary system. In: SJ Ettinger and EC Feldman, Eds. Textbook of veterinary internal medicine, 7th edn. Elsevier Saunders. 2010: 1689–1695.

Crews LJ, Feeney DA, Jessen CR, Rose ND, Matise I. Clinical, ultrasonographic, and laboratory findings associated with gallbladder disease and rupture in dogs: 45 cases (1997–2007). Journal of the American Veterinary Medical Association. 2009; 234: 359–366.

23

Chronic Hepatitis

Ninette Keller

Introduction

Chronic hepatitis is one of the most common chronic hepatic conditions in dogs and cats and is characterized by ongoing inflammation with hepatocellular necrosis, regeneration, and fibrosis. Evidence of fibrosis usually indicates severe disease. Advanced fibrosis will progress to cirrhosis, which in turn leads to portal hypertension, ascites, and acquired portosystemic shunts. In cats the inflammation is more directed at the bile ducts causing cholangitis or cholangio-hepatitis.

Although there are many known causes of chronic hepatitis, in most cases the cause is never identified. Causes include drugs (anticonvulsants, non-steroidal anti-inflammatories, antibiotics acetaminophen, methimazole/carbimazole, anthelmintics, amiodarone), infectious diseases (leptospirosis, herpes virus, canine adenovirus-1, *Ehrlichia*, *Bartonella*), and toxins (xylitol, copper, aflatoxins, cycads).

Certain breeds are more prone to develop chronic hepatitis: West Highland White Terriers, Labrador Retrievers, Scottish Terriers, Skye Terriers, American and English Cocker Spaniels, Doberman Pinchers, Dalmatians, Bedlington Terriers, and Standard Poodles.

Diagnosis

Chronic hepatitis should be considered in cases with persistent elevated liver enzymes with a definitive diagnosis made on histopathology. The history and physical examination will vary from no visible clinical signs to marked clinical signs dependent on the amount of liver damage present.

Laboratory results include persistent elevated high liver enzymes and total bilirubin; the latter indicative of a poorer prognosis (Gomez *et al.* 2014). Important differential diagnoses such as neoplasia must be excluded, as both prognosis and management of the patient will change. Patients with persistent elevated liver enzymes with or without ultrasonographic changes should undergo a liver biopsy. Biopsies can be obtained via exploratory laparotomy, ultrasound-guided, and laparoscopy. Ensure to check clotting factors prior to any liver biopsy. Fine-needle aspirate cytology of the liver is often unrewarding (Bahr *et al.* 2013; Cole *et al.* 2002; Wang *et al.* 2004).

Common comorbidities seen with chronic hepatitis includes cirrhosis and end-stage liver failure with acquired portosystemic shunts forming. Clinical signs can include hypoglycemia, coagulopathies, ascites, and hepatic encephalopathy.

Chronic Disease Management for Small Animals, First Edition. Edited by W. Dunbar Gram, Rowan J. Milner and Remo Lobetti.
© 2018 John Wiley & Sons, Inc. Published 2018 by John Wiley & Sons, Inc.

Therapeutics

A combination of drugs are used and needed for the management of chronic hepatitis. Response to therapy is ideally measured by re-biopsing the liver a few months later, however, in many cases, this is not feasible and repeating the liver enzymes 4–6 weeks after initiating therapy may help to monitor response. Therapy is often a combination of therapies and focused on the following:

- Treat underlying cause if known, for example, copper toxicity
- Control inflammation and immune modulation
- Antioxidant therapy
- Anti-fibrotic therapy
- Manage hepatic encephalopathy
- Symptomatic therapy.

Copper Chelation

- Penicillamine 10–15 mg/kg BID on an empty stomach. May lead to anorexia and vomiting. Use with caution in cats.
- Trientine can be used as an alternative in patients that do not tolerate penicillamine. Dose 15 mg/kg BID. The drug is not readily available.
- Zinc can be added to help reduce copper levels and avoid accumulation of copper again. Dose is 100 mg q12hrs of elemental zinc. After 2–3 months, the dose can be halved. Zinc should also be administrated on an empty stomach.

Antibiotics

Paramount for infectious hepatitis, but may also help to decrease bacterial colonization in severe chronic hepatitis patients. Amoxicillin, metronidazole, and cephalosporins are most commonly used for 2–4 weeks. If using metronidazole lower the dose to 7.5–10 mg/kg BID due to hepatic metabolism.

Choleretic Drugs

Decreasing cholestasis has been shown to improve clinical signs. Increasing levels of bilirubin can cause increase cell permeability and fibrogenesis.

Ursodeoxycholic acid (UDCA) at a dose of 15 mg/kg per day helps to decrease cholestasis inflammation and fibrosis. There has been some concern that the use of UDCA in bile duct obstruction may cause rupture but this has been shown not to be the case. UDCA has been shown to decrease the secondary toxic changes in the liver in experimental cases with obstructive biliary disease.

Anti-inflammatories/Immune Modulating Drugs

Prednisolone/Prednisone at 1–2 mg/kg/day for 2–4 weeks then gradually tapering to a dose of 0.5 mg/kg every second day. Glucocorticoid treatment is continued for 4–6 months. Ideally, the liver should be re-biopsy 4 months after start of treatment to evaluate if long-term anti-inflammatories are needed. Dexamethasone at 0.2–0.4 mg/kg SID is preferred in patients with portal hypertension and/or ascites as it has less mineralocorticoid effects (Favier et al. 2013).

Other drugs used in this category with varying success include azathioprine (1–2 mg/kg SID then taper to every second day) or cyclosporine 5 mg/kg SID-BID. Azathioprine has been used with good success in human chronic hepatitis and has shown promise in Labradors with chronic hepatitis. Mycophenolate can also be considered in severe cases at a dose of 10–20 mg/kg BID. When using long-term drop dose by 25–50%. In cats, chlorambucil at 0.25 mg/kg every third day is used as an add-on after prednisolone if more immunosuppression is required.

Antioxidants

- S-Adenosylmethionine (SAMe) helps with cell replication and has a modulating influence on inflammation. SAMe is a natural metabolite of hepatocytes. Dose of 20 mg/kg SID on an empty stomach.

- Silymarin (Milk thistle) is a potent free-radical scavenger and has been used for centuries in human medicine as a hepatic antioxidant. Dose: 50–250 mg per day.
- SAMe and silymarin has been shown to have a synergistic effect when used together.
- Vitamin E and C also functions as antioxidants. Vitamin E by protecting membrane phospholipids from peri-oxidative damage and vitamin C is a soluble intracellular antioxidant. As dogs and cats normally synthesize them, it is uncertain whether or not supplementation is required.
- Vitamin E: 400–500 units per day. Vitamin C: 30 mg/kg every QID.
- N-acetylcysteine at 70 mg/kg TID are used mostly in drug toxicities.

Antifibrotics

- Corticosteroids, zinc, penicillamine, and colchicine are all used as antifibrotics.
- Corticosteroids are the most commonly used as it also helps with inflammation.
- Colchicine is the only specific anti-fibrotic drug. It stimulates the collagenase activity and has been used to arrest and resolve hepatic fibrosis. It can cause GI signs and should always be started at the lower end of the dose. Dose: 0.03 mg/kg/day. It should be avoided in patients with renal failure and has not been used in cats.
- Zinc dose – 100 mg daily for 4 months then decrease to 50 mg SID. It works best on an empty stomach.
- Losartan (angiotensin II inhibitor) has recently been shown in human medicine to prevent fibrosis. Dose: 0.25–0.5 mg/kg/day.

Diet

Palatability is paramount and a special diet should not be used at the cost of loss of appetite. There is a misconception that all liver patients should be on a low-protein diet; however, a low-protein diet is only advised in patients with hepatic encephalopathy. Adequate protein is important for hepatocyte regeneration. The protein should be of high quality and digestibility. Dairy and plant protein are better tolerated than animal protein in patients with hepatic encephalopathy. A high carbohydrate and moderate fat content diet can be considered, especially if the patient is prone to hypoglycemia or hyperammonemia.

Feeding smaller meals frequently helps to reduce fasting hypoglycemia and serves to increase protein tolerance.

Including moderate amount of dietary fiber has been shown to be advantageous as soluble fiber reduces availability and production of nitrogenous waste products by the gut. Insoluble fiber on the other hand helps bind toxic substances.

Commercial liver diets are low in copper and recommended for patients with copper toxicity. Avoid liver, shellfish, organs, and cereal in home-cooked meals, as all of these are high in copper.

Symptomatic Therapy

Clinical signs of nausea, vomiting, diarrhea, and gastrointestinal bleeding are relatively common in patients with chronic hepatitis. As the disease progress and in severe cases hepatic encephalopathy manifests and ascites (due to low protein levels and portal hypertension) may occur.

Anti-nausea Drugs

- Metoclopramide 0.5–1 mg/kg TID, if in hospital then a continuous rate infusion (CRI) works best at a dose of 1–2 mg/kg/day.
- Ondansetron 0.1–1 mg/kg SID-TID.
- Maropitant – NOT recommended in cases with liver disease.

Appetite Stimulants

Appetite stimulants that can be considered include cyproheptadine (0.2 mg/kg BID or 1–2 mg total dose for cats BID) and mirtazapine (0.5 mg/kg per day).

Gastro-Intestinal Bleeding

- Protein-pump inhibitors such as omeprazole at 1 mg/kg BID other dosages shown not to work.
- H2-blockers such as famotidine at 0.5–1 mg/kg per os or 0.5 mg/kg slow IV or sc SID-BID can also be used. Avoid the use of cimetidine in these patients due to its powerful P450 microsomal enzyme inhibition.
- Sucralfate at 0.25–1 gram BID-TID. Stagger medication, as sucralfate is more active in an acid environment and can bind other medications.

Ascites

Ascites can be managed with diuretics. The most commonly used diuretics include furosemide (2–4 mg/kg/day) and/or spironolactone (1–4 mg/kg/day). If the ascites is severe then abdominocentesis can be performed to make the patient more comfortable.

Hepatic Encephalopathy

- Enemas play a big role in managing cases with hepatic encephalopathy (HE). Enemas help to rid the patient of ammonia producing substrates (bacteria and protein). Slightly acidic enemas works best as they ionize the ammonia and prevents further absorption, for example, povidone iodine as a 10% solution.
- Antibiotics (metronidazole/amoxicillin) will help to decrease ammonia-producing bacteria.
- Lactulose helps to decrease the pH in the colon and converts ammonia to ammonium, which is poorly absorbed. Dose is 0.2–0.5 ml/kg TID. Aim is to produce soft stools and not diarrhea. Decrease dose if diarrhea occurs.

Management of Coagulopathies

Patients with advanced chronic hepatitis may suffer from coagulopathies due to vitamin K deficiency. Vitamin K1 can be supplemented at 0.5–2 mg/kg sc or per os SID. If actively bleeding then a plasma transfusion or whole blood transfusion should be considered. Fresh whole blood is preferred above stored blood as ammonia accumulates in stored blood.

Which Therapy is Best for the Patient?

Histopathology results can help choose the combination of treatment that may be needed. The severity of inflammation as well as presence of fibrosis would indicate that anti-inflammatories and antifibrotics are needed as well as other supportive care.

As maintenance therapy, most clinicians will use UDCA and an antioxidant (Vitamin E, SAMe or silymarin) in chronic hepatitis cases. If inflammation persists then low-dose prednisolone may be needed.

If severe clinical signs return or liver enzymes continue to increase then restart a course of antibiotics. Use a combination of anti-oxidants (they have a synergistic effect) and start anti-inflammatories if patient is not on any at time of relapse. If patient is already on prednisolone or other anti-inflammatories consider adding another immunosuppressive drug.

Expected Outcome/Adverse Reactions

Improvement is usually seen within 24–48 hours after start/change of treatment. Possible side effects may include vomiting and diarrhea with certain drugs (colchicine). Alkaline phosphatase levels will potentially increase if prednisolone is used and thus may make interpretation of response to therapy difficult.

Quality of Life for Patient and Caregiver

Prognosis is variable but for patients with fibrosis and for cirrhosis or signs of hepatic encephalopathy it is guarded. Patients with cirrhosis, coagulopathies, hypoglycemia, and hypoalbuminemia usually die within a month of diagnosis. For patients with mild to moderate chronic hepatitis the mean survival time is around 20–30 months (Raffan *et al.* 2009).

Quality of life includes free of pain, not vomiting, reasonable appetite, and reasona- ble amount of energy. If the patient continues to vomit, remains anorexic, or shows signs of end-stage liver failure (severe ascites, hepatic encephalopathy) then the decision for eutha- nasia should be considered especially if there is no or a poor response to medication.

References

Bahr K, Sharkey L, Murakami T, Feeney D. Accuracy of US-guided FNA of focal liver lesions in dogs: 140 cases (2005–2008). Journal of the American Animal Hospital Association. 2013; 49(3): 190–196.

Cole T, Center S, Flood S, et al. Diagnostic comparison of needle and wedge biopsy specimens of the liver in dogs and cats. Journal of the American Veterinary Medical Association. (2002). 220(10), 1483–1490.

Favier R, Poldervaart J, Van den Ingh T, Penning LRJ. A retrospective study of oral prednisolone treatment in canine chronic hepatitis. Veterinary Quarterly. 2013; 33(3): 113–120.

Gomez S, Bexfield N, Scase T, Holmes M, Watson P. Total serum bilirubin as a negative prognostic factor in idiopathic canine chronic hepatitis. Journal of Veterinary Diagnostic Investigation. 2014; 26(2): 246–251.

Raffan E, McCallum A, Scase T, Watson P. Ascites is a negative prognostic indicator in chronic hepatitis in dogs. Journal of Veterinary Internal Medicine. 2009; 23(1): 63–66.

Wang K, Panciera D, Al-Rukibat R, Radi Z. Accuracy of ultrasound-guided fine-needle aspiration of the liver and cytologic findings in dogs and cats: 97 cases (1990–2000). Journal of the American Veterinary Medical Association. 2004; 224(1): 75–78.

Watson JP. Chronic hepatitis in dogs: a review of current understanding of the aetiology, progression, and treatment. The Veterinary Journal. 2004; 167(3): 228–241.

Further Reading

Center SA. Metabolic, antioxidant, nutraceutical, probiotic, and herbal therapies relating to the management of hepatobiliary disorders. The Veterinary Clinics of North America: Small Animal Practice. 2004; 34: 67–172.

Favier RP. Idiopathic hepatitis and cirrhosis in dogs. The Veterinary Clinics of North America: Small Animal Practice. 2009; 39(3): 481–488.

24

Portosystemic Liver Shunts

Ninette Keller

Introduction

Portosystemic shunts (PSS) are a direct venous connection between the portal vein and the systemic circulation bypassing the liver parenchyma. Usually the venous return from the intestines, stomach, spleen, and pancreas flows into the portal vein and then through the sinusoidal network within the liver before draining into the hepatic veins and then into the caudal vena cava. PSS can be congenital or acquired. In acquired shunting the abnormal venous connections form due to chronic portal hypertension. Primary portal vein hypoplasia is another variation without portal hypertension leading to microscopic malformation of the hepatic vasculature (Christiansen *et al.* 2000).

Other conditions that can mimic clinical signs of liver failure include protein losing enteropathy and primary liver disease (cirrhosis and fibrosis). Micro-intrahepatic portosystemic shunts can be a challenging diagnosis and needs to be differentiated from liver cirrhosis and fibrosis, which can only be made with histopathology.

When blood bypasses the liver, it leads to atrophy of the liver and eventually to liver failure. A loss of liver function leads to toxin build-up and loss of products normally produced by the liver (albumin, urea, glucose and clotting factors).

Diagnosis

Patients with PSS may present with clinical signs associated with neurological, gastrointestinal, or urinary tracts with the most common finding being abnormal behavior (40–90% of cases). Up to 75% of cats will present with severe ptyalism. Affected animals are often much smaller than their littermates. The most severe clinical signs are usually seen within a few hours after feeding. Ammonium urate calculi occur in up to 30% of cases and may be the main clinical reason patients are presented. Patients with PSS may also have other congenital abnormalities such as cryptorchidism and heart murmurs.

Diagnostic Options

Various diagnostic tools are available for diagnosing portosystemic shunts, and the method chosen will depend on availability and technical skills. Computed tomography and magnetic resonance angiography are more readily available compared to scintigraphy and have a high sensitivity and specificity. Abdominal ultrasound can be a cost-effective way of diagnosing shunts but require a high skill level of the operator. Portography via laparotomy is also an option (Figure 24.1). Protein C levels have also been documented as an aid in differentiating

Chronic Disease Management for Small Animals, First Edition. Edited by W. Dunbar Gram, Rowan J. Milner and Remo Lobetti.
© 2018 John Wiley & Sons, Inc. Published 2018 by John Wiley & Sons, Inc.

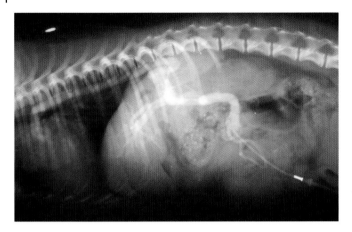

Figure 24.1 Contrast portogram showing extra-hepatic porto-caval shunt entering the caudal vena cava but with partial arborization of the liver.

primary portal vein hypoplasia from porto-systemic shunts. Protein C levels were over 70% increased in 88% of cases with primary portal vein hypoplasia and low in dogs with PSS (Gow *et al.* 2012; Kim *et al.* 2013).

Therapeutics

Hepatic encephalopathy requires quick intervention and can be managed with nil per os, intravenous fluids, lactulose (oral or per rectum), and anticonvulsants as needed to control seizure activity.

The biggest decision in patients with PSS is whether or not to have surgical correction. Surgery, however, is not an option for all patients or if there are cost constraints. Patients with primary portal vein hypoplasia or acquired shunts cannot be managed surgically and the correction of intrahepatic shunts is more technically difficult and requires advanced imaging equipment and skills for surgical correction.

A few long-term studies have been performed on patients with medical management alone. On average 50% of patients were euthanized within a year of diagnosis, but this does depend on the type of shunt. Surgery can have up to a 90% success rate in patients especially patients with extra-hepatic shunts (Greenhalgh *et al.* 2014).

Medical Management

Diet
Dietary protein should be restricted to the point where the patient's metabolic requirements are met without aggravating hepatic encephalopathy. The protein should be of high quality and readily digestible with dairy and plant protein better tolerated than animal protein. A high carbohydrate and moderate fat content diet can be considered especially if the patient is prone to hypoglycemia or hyperammonemia. Feeding smaller meals frequently helps to reduce fasting hypoglycemia and serves to increase protein tolerance. Including a moderate amount of dietary fiber has been shown to be advantageous as soluble fiber reduces availability and production of nitrogenous waste products by the gut. Insoluble fiber on the other hand helps bind toxic substances.

Oral Lactulose
Oral lactulose helps to decrease the pH in the colon and converts ammonia to ammonium, which is poorly absorbed. Dose is 0.2–0.5 ml/kg TID. Aim is to produce soft stools and not diarrhea. Decrease dose if diarrhea occurs.

Antibiotics
Antibiotics can assist in decreasing bacterial colonization. Amoxicillin, metronidazole, and cephalosporin are most commonly used for 2–4 weeks. If using metronidazole lower the dose to 7.5–10 mg/kg BID due to hepatic metabolism.

Expected Outcome

Long-term prognosis for patients on medical therapy alone is guarded to poor. The long-term prognosis in patients with extra-hepatic shunts post-surgery is good if there are no complications associated with surgery. In cases with intra-hepatic shunts, the prognosis depends on the surgical success rate with a complication rate as high as 75% reported. Cases with primary portal vein hypoplasia can do very well with medical management. In cats as discussed the prognosis remains poor even post-surgery especially if neurological signs occur.

Quality of Life

Prognosis is variable, but in patients with persistent seizures or hepatic encephalopathy, the prognosis is guarded. If the clinical signs of liver failure and/or hepatic encephalopathy cannot be managed then euthanasia should be considered. Quality of life for patients includes being free of pain, not vomiting, reasonable appetite and a reasonable amount of energy.

References

Christiansen J, Hottinger H, Allen L, Phillips L, Aronson L. Hepatic microvascular dysplasia in dogs: a retrospective study of 24 cases (1987–1995). Journal of the American Animal Hospital Association. 2000; 36(5): 385–390.

Gow A, Marques A, Yool D, et al. Dogs with congenital porto-systemic shunting (cPSS) and hepatic encephalopathy have higher serum concentrations of C-reactive protein than asymptomatic dogs with cPSS. Metabolic Brain Disease. 2012; 27(2): 227–229.

Greenhalgh S, Reeve J, Johnstone T, et al. Long-term survival and quality of life in dogs with clinical signs associated with a congenital portosystemic shunt after surgical or medical treatment. Journal of the American Veterinary Medical Association. 2014; 245(5): 527–533.

Kim S, Giglio R, Reese D, Reese S, Bacon N, Ellison G. Comparison of computed tomographic angiography and ultrasonography for the detection and characterization of portosystemic shunts in dogs. Veterinary Radiology and Ultrasound. 2013; 54(6): 569–574.

Further Reading

Cabassu J, Seim H, MacPhail C, Monnet E. Outcomes of cats undergoing surgical attenuation of congenital extrahepatic portosystemic shunts through cellophane banding: 9 cases (2000–2007). Journal of the American Veterinary Medical Association. 2011; 238(1): 89–93.

Caporali EH, Phillips H, Underwood L, Selmic, LE. Risk factors for urolithiasis in dogs with congenital extrahepatic portosystemic shunts: 95 cases (1999–2013). Journal of the American Veterinary Medical Association. 2015; 246(5): 530–536.

Fryer K, Levine J, Peycke L, Thompson J, Cohen N. Incidence of postoperative seizures with and without levetiracetam pretreatment in dogs undergoing portosystemic shunt attenuation. Journal of Veterinary Internal Medicine. 2011; 25(60): 1379–1384.

Mankin KM. Current concepts in congenital portosystemic shunts. The Veterinary Clinics of North America: Small Animal Practice. 2015; 45(3): 477–487.

Shawcross D, Jalan R. Dispelling myths in the treatment of hepatitic encephalopathy. Lancet, 2005; 365(9457): 431–433.

Weisse C, Berent A, Todd K, Solomon J, Cope C. Endovascular evaluation and treatment of intrahepatic portosystemic shunts in dogs: 100 cases (2001–2011). Journal of the American Veterinary Medical Association. 2014; 244(1): 78–94.

25

Hepatic Lipidosis

Tanya Schoeman

Introduction

Feline hepatic lipidosis (FHL) is a common and potentially fatal hepatopathy of cats characterized by excessive accumulation of triglycerides in the liver, with associated severe intrahepatic cholestasis and hepatic dysfunction (Zoran 2012). The primary form of the disease is idiopathic hepatic lipidosis (IHL) where over-conditioned cats that become anorexic are at increased risk, but the syndrome can also be seen secondary to other underlying disease conditions directly causing a catabolic state and prolonged anorexia. These diseases may include other liver diseases such as cholangio-hepatitis and extra-hepatic bile duct obstruction, but may also include diseases of other organ systems such as diabetes mellitus, neoplasia, hyperthyroidism, renal disease, pancreatitis, and small intestinal disease (Center 2005). The pathogenesis remains incompletely understood, but involves an imbalance between peripheral fat stores mobilized to the liver, hepatic use of fatty acids for energy, and hepatic dispersal of triglycerides (Armstrong and Blanchard 2009).

Anorexia, ranging from a few days to several weeks, often precedes development of FHL and is the most common presenting complaint. Anorexia in otherwise healthy cats may occur due to forced overly rapid weight loss, unintentional food deprivation, change to a diet unacceptable to the cat, a sudden change in lifestyle or stress such as boarding or surgery, but may also be associated with other systemic diseases (Armstrong and Blanchard 2009). Rapid weight loss is common and can be profound (often >25% of body weight), with concurrent sarcopenia. Other clinical signs include lethargy, depression, vomiting, diarrhea or constipation, and an unkempt, poor quality hair coat (Armstrong and Blanchard 2009). As the disease progresses and hepatic function deteriorates, icterus (about 70% of cases) and signs of hepatic encephalopathy such as severe depression, ptyalism, and seizures (<5% of cases) may develop (Dimski and Taboada 1995; Hill and Armstrong 2014). Ptyalism may also reflect nausea. Head or neck ventroflexion may occur with severe electrolyte imbalances (hypokalemia and/or hypophosphatemia) or thiamine deficiency (Center 2005).

Diagnosis

FHL is often suspected from typical history and physical examination findings. A complete blood count may be normal or reflect normocytic, normochromic non-regenerative anemia, poikilocytosis, large numbers of Heinz bodies and stress leukocytosis; an inflammatory leukogram may indicate concurrent disease (Hill and Armstrong 2014).

Chronic Disease Management for Small Animals, First Edition. Edited by W. Dunbar Gram, Rowan J. Milner and Remo Lobetti.
© 2018 John Wiley & Sons, Inc. Published 2018 by John Wiley & Sons, Inc.

Serum biochemistry usually shows evidence of intrahepatic cholestatic disease; indicated by moderate to marked elevations in alkaline phosphatase (ALP) enzyme activities, and hyperbilirubinemia. Alanine aminotransferase (ALT) and aspartate aminotransferase (AST) enzyme activities are often elevated as well, but not to the magnitude of ALP. γ-Glutamyltransferase (GGT) enzyme activities are normal to mildly increased (as opposed to increased GGT seen with other cholestatic disorders in cats) (Sherding 2000). Hypokalemia, hypophosphatemia, and/or hypomagnesemia are seen in some cats at presentation or may develop during treatment (Center 2005).

Urinalysis may show lipiduria and bilirubinuria (Armstrong and Blanchard 2009). Abnormalities in coagulation tests are commonly seen, most notably as a prolongation of the prothrombin time (PT). The coagulopathy in FHL is the result of vitamin K deficiency rather than decreased coagulation factor production due to liver failure. The PIVKA test may be a more sensitive indicator of prolonged clotting times, but this test is not always readily available (Hill and Armstrong 2014). Specific liver function testing is not necessary in most cases of FHL; bile acid testing is not indicated if the cat is bilirubinuric or hyperbilirubinemic (Center 2005).

Diagnostic imaging of the liver may be helpful in diagnosing IHL or ruling out other causes of illness. Abdominal radiography may show hepatomegaly. Abdominal ultrasound examination may show diffuse hyperechogenic appearance of the liver (Dimski and Taboada 1995).

A specific diagnosis is made by cytological identification of severe cytosolic vacuolization of the majority (80% or more) of hepatocytes without inflammation (Hill and Armstrong 2014). This can be obtained through ultrasound-guided fine-needle aspiration of the liver or a liver biopsy. Biopsies performed at the time of initial diagnosis are not advised, because these cats have a high risk of death. Fine needle aspiration is therefore preferred over biopsy for diagnosis of FHL as it is less invasive and generally provides samples that are adequate for establishing a presumptive diagnosis (Center 2005). However, cytological evaluation of a fine-needle aspirate from the liver is not accurate in diagnosing other hepatopathies, therefore an accompanying disease could potentially be missed. Liver biopsies are, therefore, indicated in cases where there is a failure to respond to treatment for FHL or if a high level of suspicion of other primary hepatic disorder(s) exists. Correction of any coagulopathy with Vitamin K_1 prior to performing liver aspirates or biopsies is essential (Center 2005).

Treatment

Treatment for FHL is aimed at correction of fluid and electrolyte abnormalities, nutritional support to meet protein and caloric needs, controlling complications of liver failure, and if present, treating concurrent systemic disorders.

Acute Therapy

- Intravenous fluids using a balanced polyionic crystalloid fluid is recommended (Armstrong and Blanchard 2009)
  - Cats with severe FHL are suspected to have impaired lactate metabolism, thus the use of lactated Ringer's solution should theoretically be avoided (Center 2005); however, the solution is commonly used with success by many clinicians (Hill and Armstrong 2014)
  - Avoid dextrose supplementation unless hypoglycemia is present, as dextrose supplementation promotes hepatic lipid deposition, inhibits fatty acid oxidation, and worsens electrolyte depletion (Hill and Armstrong 2014)
  - Correct all fluid and electrolyte imbalances before anesthesia is attempted for feeding tube placement (Armstrong and Blanchard 2009)

- Vitamin K$_1$: 0.5–1.5 mg/kg SC BID for three injections to treat coagulopathy
  - Allow adequate response interval after initiation of Vitamin K therapy before fine needle aspirates or biopsies of the liver are obtained (Center 2005)
- Supplement water-soluble vitamins
  - B-complex vitamins: Add to IV fluids (1–2 ml/L)
  - Cobalamin (Vitamin B$_{12}$): 250 µg SC once weekly for six weeks if decreased serum cobalamin is documented; this happens primarily where there is underlying gastrointestinal disease (Hill and Armstrong 2014)
  - Thiamine: 50–100 mg PO/cat/day for one week if severe ventroflexion of the neck is present (Center 2005)
- Enteral feeding
  - Enteral feeding must be initiated as early as possible. Oral forced feeding is not advised, as it is generally inadequate to provide enough calories to reverse FHL. Force-feeding can also be stressful and may exacerbate nausea and vomiting. It can also result in aversion to food, which may delay the return to voluntary food intake (Zoran 2012)
  - Provision of adequate calories to reverse the progression of FHL usually requires placement of a feeding tube. In critically ill cats with FHL, the stress of general anesthesia may be fatal thus the initial feeding should be given via a naso-esophageal tube (Hill and Armstrong 2014)
  - Once the cat is more stable, general anesthesia for long-term feeding tube placement can be safely accomplished (Zoran 2012)
- Appetite stimulants
  - Oral appetite stimulants such as mirtazapine or cyproheptadine are not recommended, as they are unreliable for ensuring the adequate caloric intake that is required for successful therapy for FHL (Hill and Armstrong 2014)
  - Oral diazepam should be avoided, as it can also cause idiosyncratic hepatic necrosis in cats (Zoran 2012)

- Blood transfusions are sometimes required for treatment of severe anemia (Center 2005)

Chronic Therapy

- Place an esophagostomy (or gastrostomy) tube for chronic long-term feeding
  - An esophagostomy (or gastrostomy) tube allows feeding of a blended solid canned food diet in the home environment until the FHL is resolved and adequate voluntary food intake resumes (Zoran 2012)
  - Diets selected for cats with FHL should ideally be high in protein and have lower amounts of carbohydrates, with the remaining calories coming from fat (Zoran 2012). Many commercially available diets meet these requirements including Maximum Calorie (IAMS Veterinary Formula) and Prescription Diets a/d or m/d (Hill's Pet Nutrition). Maximum Calorie is often preferred for tube feeding because of its high caloric density – it provides 2.1 kcal/ml, while most other commercial recovery-formula foods typically provide about 1 kcal/ml. A higher caloric density food allows daily energy requirements to be met with a lower total food volume (Hill and Armstrong 2014)
  - Do not restrict dietary protein unless overt signs of hepatic encephalopathy are present (Hill and Armstrong 2014)
  - Provide 40–60 kcal/kg/day. Start with tube feeding of ¼ to ½ of daily requirements, divided into four to six feedings. Gradually increase to daily requirements over three to four days (Zoran 2012)
  - Tube feeding is usually required for 3–6 weeks, pending clinical and biochemical improvement – total bilirubin concentration is expected to decrease by at least 50% within 7–10 days, although serum liver enzyme activities often require longer to decrease (Armstrong and Blanchard 2009)

- o Remove feeding tube only when the cat is eating on its own for at least a week (Zoran 2012).
- Control vomiting
  - o Vomiting is a common problem in cats with FHL and often persists during the first week of re-feeding despite gradual introduction of increasing meal volumes
  - o Maropitant 1 mg/kg SID IV, SC or PO is the drug of choice (Zoran 2012); however as the liver metabolizes maropitant, a dosage of 0.5 mg/kg is sometimes used. Maropitant may also provide visceral analgesia, which would be useful in cases with concurrent pancreatitis (Hill and Armstrong 2014)
  - o Metoclopramide 0.2–0.5 mg/kg TID SC/PO or CRI 1–2 mg/kg/day. Metoclopramide is a weak antiemetic in cats, but is commonly used for its prokinetic effects (Hill and Armstrong 2014)
  - o Ondansetron 0.1–1 mg/kg SID-BID IV/PO or dolasetron 0.5–1 mg/kg q SID-BId IV/PO is advised if vomiting persists (Zoran 2012)
  - o Famotidine 0.5–1 mg/kg q SID-BID IV/PO, a H$_2$ receptor antagonist, can be added in persistently vomiting cats to protect the lower esophagus from acid damage (Armstrong and Blanchard 2009)
- Dietary supplements (used empirically): Supplementation with specific micronutrients has been suggested by some authors (Center 2005). Until more evidence becomes available, the use of these supplements is based purely on clinician preference and experience. Clinicians should also consider that prescribing multiple supplements and medications might risk decreasing client compliance with feeding instructions.
  - o S-Adenosylmethionine (SAMe): 20 mg/kg PO OID (Zoran 2012)
  - o SAMe is an important hepatocellular metabolite and glutathione donor with hepatic and systemic antioxidant effects (Center 2005)

- o L-carnitine: 250–500 mg PO SID. L-carnitine is an essential cofactor for fatty acid oxidation; a relative carnitine deficiency is believed to exist in FHL (Center 2005)
- o Taurine: 250–500 mg PO SID for the initial 7–10 days of treatment. Taurine is an essential amino acid for cats and is required for bile acid conjugation; plasma taurine levels have been found to be decreased in many cats with FHL (Center 2005) Some recovery formula diets (for example Hill's a/d) are already high in taurine (Hill and Armstrong 2014)
- o Vitamin E (water soluble form): 50–100 units/cat PO SID, which is an important antioxidant (Center 2005).

Quality of Life

The two most important factors affecting the outcome in FHL are believed to be the presence of a serious or irreversible concurrent disease (which is more likely in an older cat) and how early enteral nutritional support is begun. A poorer prognosis is seen when concurrent pancreatitis is present, with hypokalemia and anemia also negative prognostic indicators (Hill and Armstrong 2014). In the absence of a fatal concurrent disease, recovery can be expected in approximately 80% or more of cases if enteral feeding is initiated early in the course of the disease and is sustained until voluntary food intake resumes. Owners should understand that tube feeding for 3–6 weeks or longer at home would be required for recovery. If owners are not prepared to commit for such a period to be active participants in their cats' recovery, then the decision to treat the cat should be reevaluated.

Careful consideration of the owner's financial situation should also form part of the decision whether to treat the cat or not. Establishing the diagnosis, identifying any underlying causes and initial management often requires several days of hospitalization, including anesthesia and feeding tube placement – this can be costly and time-consuming. However, if owners are prepared to commit financially, treating this disease can be ultimately rewarding. Once the cat has fully recovered, recurrence is unlikely unless an underlying, chronic cause is present.

References

Armstrong P, Blanchard G. Hepatic lipidosis in cats. The Veterinary Clinics of North America: Small Animal Practice. 2009; 39: 599–616.

Center S. Feline hepatic lipidosis. The Veterinary Clinics of North America: Small Animal Practice. 2005; 35: 225–269.

Dimski D, Taboada J. Feline idiopathic hepatic lipidosis. The Veterinary Clinics of North America: Small Animal Practice. 1995; 25: 357–373.

Hill S, Armstrong P. Feline hepatic lipidosis. In: JD Bonagura and DC Twedt, Eds. Kirk's Current Veterinary Therapy XV. Elsevier Saunders. 2014: 608–613.

Sherding RG. Feline jaundice. Journal of Feline Medicine and Surgery. 2000; 2: 165–169.

Zoran D. Diseases of the liver. In: SE Little, Ed. The cat: clinical medicine and management. Elsevier Saunders, St. Louis. 2012: 530–533.

Further Reading

Brown B, Maudlin GE, Armstrong J, Moroff SC, Maudin SG. Metabolic and hormonal alterations in cats with hepatic lipidosis. Journal of Veterinary Internal Medicine. 2000; 14: 20–26.

26

Feline Cholangitis

Tanya Schoeman

Introduction

Feline cholangitis (CCH) is the second most common form of liver disease in cats (Sherding 2000). The WSAVA Liver Standardization Group describes three different forms of cholangitis: neutrophilic, subdivided into acute and chronic forms; lymphocytic; and cholangitis associated with liver flukes (Twedt, Armstrong, and Simpson 2014). Because the primary starting point of the inflammatory disease in cats is the bile ducts (cholangitis), with inflammation extending to the hepatic parenchyma (cholangio-hepatitis) only with time and severity, the term cholangitis syndrome has become the preferred terminology (Twedt *et al.* 2014).

Neutrophilic (suppurative/exudative) CCH can be subdivided pathologically into an acute neutrophilic form (predominantly neutrophilic infiltration) and a chronic neutrophilic form (mixed cellular infiltrate of neutrophils, lymphocytes, and plasma cells). The cause of the acute form is thought to be bacterial from gastrointestinal origin, whereas the chronic form may represent a later stage of the same disease process, possibly triggered by persistent infection or inflammation. Bacterial entry by either the biliary system or hematogenous spread is possible. In lymphocytic (non-suppurative/lymphoplasmacytic) CCH, the cellular infiltrate consists mainly of lymphocytes and plasma cells. It tends to be more chronic and slowly progressive than neutrophilic CCH. Preliminary immunologic studies suggest that lymphocytic CCH could have an immune-mediated cause (Zoran 2012).

CCH has been described in a wide age range of cats, but cats with neutrophilic CCH tend to be younger (median age of 9 years) than those with lymphocytic CCH (median age 11.5 years) at the time of diagnosis (Sherding 2000). In some reports on lymphocytic CCH, a male predisposition was found, with Norwegian Forest cats overrepresented (Otte *et al.* 2012).

Affected cats with either type of CCH show clinical signs of anorexia, weight loss, lethargy, and vomiting. Cats are usually icteric, and a few may have ascites. Patients with neutrophilic CCH usually present for an acute onset of illness and pyrexia is often seen. In lymphocytic CCH, the signs are often intermittent and tend to wax and wane over months (Gagne *et al.* 1999). Polyphagia is sometimes seen in these cases. With neutrophilic CCH cats are usually febrile, dehydrated, and icteric and may have abdominal discomfort with palpation, while cats with lymphocytic CCH may have minimal physical examination abnormalities or may present icteric with hepatomegaly on abdominal palpation (Gagne *et al.* 1999).

Chronic Disease Management for Small Animals, First Edition. Edited by W. Dunbar Gram, Rowan J. Milner and Remo Lobetti.
© 2018 John Wiley & Sons, Inc. Published 2018 by John Wiley & Sons, Inc.

Frequent concurrent disorders in CCH cats include extra-hepatic bile duct obstruction, cholelithiasis, gall bladder abnormalities (sludge, cholecystitis), chronic subclinical pancreatitis, and inflammatory bowel disease. Because of the feline pancreatic and bile duct anatomy, it is common for cats to have CCH and pancreatitis simultaneously and in some cases; cats will also have concurrent IBD. The constellation of the three conditions occurring together is called triaditis. This combination is increasingly recognized in cats, and recent reports suggest 50–85 % of cats with one syndrome have all three diseases (Zoran 2012). Anorexia induced by CCH may also lead to secondary hepatic lipidosis (Twedt *et al.* 2014).

Diagnosis

A complete blood count may reveal mild non-regenerative anemia and variable leukocytosis. In one study, 33 % of the cats with lymphocytic CCH had leukocytosis, a lower percentage than for cats with neutrophilic CCH (Marolf *et al.* 2012). Cats with neutrophilic CCH tend to show neutrophilia with a left shift and/or toxic neutrophils, while cats with lymphocytic CHH may have lymphocytosis (Weiss, Armstrong, and Gagne 1997). Other laboratory findings seen in all types of CCH include elevated serum alanine aminotransferase (ALT), aspartate aminotransferase (AST), γ-glutamyltransferase (GGT), alkaline phosphatase (ALP) and hyperbilirubinemia. Many cats may show liver enzyme activities within reference range (Twedt *et al.* 2014). Hyperglobulinemia is sometimes seen in cases with lymphocytic CCH (Center 2009). Fasting and postprandial bile acids are often increased (Weiss *et al.* 1997). Coagulation tests may also be abnormal (Zoran 2012).

Most cats with CCH often have a normal ultrasound examination, including liver size, echogenicity and biliary systems (Marolf *et al.* 2012). When abnormalities were present, they included hepatomegaly, hyperechogenic appearance of the liver, dilated common bile duct, and echogenic gall bladder contents. Ultrasound changes in the liver and biliary system are similar for both neutrophilic CCH and lymphocytic CCH, but lymphocytic CCH cats are less likely to have concurrent pancreatic changes detected ultrasonographically (Marolf *et al.* 2012).

Definitive diagnosis of neutrophilic CCH requires a liver biopsy or biliary cytology and positive culture, obtained via a percutaneous ultrasound-guided gallbladder aspirate. If suppurative inflammation and bacteria are observed on bile cytology, a diagnosis of neutrophilic CCH can be confirmed (Twedt *et al.* 2014). Enteric bacteria, most often *Escherichia coli*, but also other species such as *Enterococcus sp., Bacteroides sp., Clostridia sp., Staphylococcus* and α-hemolytic *Streptococcus sp.* may be cultured from the bile or liver of cats with acute neutrophilic CCH. Most reported organisms are aerobic, but anaerobic organisms may also be found, therefore both aerobic and anaerobic cultures should be requested. Unfortunately, the rate of positive bile cultures tends to be low in neutrophilic CCH, even in untreated cats (Twedt *et al.* 2014). Using a florescence *in situ* hybridization (FISH) assay, a recent study observed intrahepatic bacteria in 33 % of cats with inflammatory liver disease examined (Twedt *et al.* 2013).

Cytologic examination of fine-needle aspirates from the liver showing neutrophilic or lymphoplasmacytic inflammation may help support the diagnosis. However, liver aspiration cytology has a poor correlation with histopathology, especially in inflammatory liver disease (Twedt *et al.* 2014). Fine-needle aspirates of cats with CCH may also reveal marked hepatocellular vacuolation if secondary hepatic lipidosis is present (Zoran 2012).

Definitive diagnosis of any form of CCH requires a liver biopsy with histopathology and identification of the cellular infiltrate (neutrophilic, mixed, or lymphocytic). Additional changes described with neutrophilic CCH include periportal hepatocellular necrosis and bile duct dilation and proliferation, while additional changes in lymphocytic CCH include periductal fibrosis, diminished bile duct number, and sclerosing cholangitis (Center 2009). In some cases, it may be difficult to differentiate lymphocytic CCH from lymphoma – in these cases additional diagnostic tests including polymerase chain reaction for T-cell receptor gene rearrangement may be helpful (Center 2009). Techniques for liver biopsy include ultrasound-guided needle biopsy and wedge biopsy via laparoscopy or laparotomy. The latter two techniques have the advantage that it allows examination of the extrahepatic bile system, pancreas, and other intra-abdominal structures (Twedt *et al.* 2014).

Treatment

Primary Treatment of Neutrophilic CCH

Antibiotic Therapy
- Should be based ideally on culture and sensitivity (Weiss *et al.* 1997)
- When cultures are negative or empiric selection is necessary:
  o Select antibiotic effective against most enteric gram-negative aerobes and has good penetration of the liver and bile such as cephalexin, cefadroxil, amoxicillin-clavulanate, amoxicillin, or enrofloxacin
  o Metronidazole can be added to extend the spectrum to anaerobes.
- Continue treatment for 4–6 weeks, even though most cats improve clinically within a week (Twedt *et al.* 2014)

Corticosteroid Therapy
- Considered in cats with neutrophilic CCH where liver biopsy sections contain relatively few neutrophils with a predominance of lymphocytes and plasma cells and where response to appropriate antibiotic therapy is poor or incomplete (Twedt *et al.* 2014).
- It may be difficult to ascertain if clinical improvement of these cases on corticosteroid therapy is attributable to resolution of the liver disease or perhaps due to improvement of the frequently concurrent IBD or pancreatitis.

Primary Treatment of Lymphocytic CCH

Corticosteroid Therapy
- Indicated to control the inflammatory component of the disease
- Prednisolone 1–2 mg/kg PO SID initially
  o Corticosteroid of choice, as it is well absorbed after oral administration in cats
- Monitor clinical signs and biochemical parameters for improvement
- Slowly taper the dose of prednisolone after 4–6 weeks if improvement is seen:
  o Reduce the dosage by 50 % every two weeks until 0.5 mg/kg PO SID is reached
  o If clinical and biochemical improvement is evident, a chronic dose of 0.5 mg/kg PO every second day can be administered for four weeks or long term, as needed to control clinical signs
- Treatment decisions should ideally be based on repeat liver biopsies, although this is not performed routinely in practice
- Long-term corticosteroid treatment is well tolerated by most cats, although cats should be carefully monitored for development of diabetes mellitus.
- Some anecdotal reports discuss the use of chlorambucil in conjunction with prednisolone in severe cases (Center 2009)
  o Chlorambucil 4 mg/m^2 PO every second day
- Other types of immunosuppressive therapy is sometimes advised for refractory cases, but no reported studies exist and severe side effects are commonly seen (Center 2009)
  o Cyclosporine: 3–5 mg/kg PO SID
  o Methotrexate: 0.13 mg PO TID for 3 doses at 7-day intervals
- It should be noted that corticosteroid therapy may not be contraindicated in cats with concurrent chronic pancreatitis or IBD – in fact, it may actually be beneficial (Twedt *et al.* 2014)

Acute Supportive Treatment of all Cases of CCH

Cats with CCH are frequently acutely ill and require intensive supportive care in conjunction with specific therapy.

- Intravenous fluids
  - A balanced polyionic crystalloid fluid is recommended.
- Correction of electrolyte abnormalities such as hypokalemia and hypophosphatemia
- Treat coagulation abnormalities (if present)
  - Vitamin K_1: 0.5–1.5 mg/kg SC BID for three injections or 5 mg PO SID
  - Allow adequate response interval after initiation of Vitamin K therapy before biopsies of the liver are obtained
- Ursodeoxycholic acid: 10–15 mg/kg PO SID
  - Beneficial effects include improvement of damage to cell membranes caused by retained toxic bile acids, improved biliary secretion of bile acids, improved bile flow (choleresis) and prevention of mitochondrial damage. It also has antifibrotic and immunomodulatory properties (Twedt *et al.* 2014)
- Nutritional support
  - Place a naso-esophageal feeding tube if voluntary food intake is inadequate
  - Feed a high-energy, high-protein diet such as Maximum Calorie (IAMS Veterinary Formula) and Prescription Diets a/d or m/d (Hill's Pet Nutrition), as protein is extremely important for liver repair and regeneration
  - Only restrict dietary protein if signs of hepatic encephalopathy are evident, and add lactulose (0.25–0.5 ml/kg TID PO) and neomycin (22 mg/kg TID PO) (Zoran 2012). It should be noted, however, that signs of hepatic encephalopathy are only rarely observed in cats with CCH (Twedt *et al.* 2014)
- Pain management is indicated in most cats with CCH, especially those with acute signs. Buprenorphine, hydromorphone, meperidine, or butorphanol can be used (Twedt *et al.* 2014). Fentanyl patch (25 μg/hr) can be used for longer-duration pain control. Effective blood levels are only reached after 3–12 hours in cats, therefore concurrent opioid administration will be needed initially.
- Control vomiting
  - Maropitant: 1 mg/kg SID IV, SC or PO is the drug of choice, however, as maropitant is metabolized by the liver a dosage of 0.5 mg/kg is sometimes used in cases with advanced hepatic dysfunction (Zoran 2012)
  - Ondansetron (0.1–1 mg/kg SID-BID IV/PO) or dolasetron (0.5–1 mg/kg SID-BID IV/PO) is advised if vomiting persists
  - Metoclopramide (0.2–0.5 mg/kg TID SC/PO) is a weak antiemetic in cats, but is commonly used for its prokinetic effects (Twedt *et al.* 2014)
- Surgery
  - Surgical therapy is uncommon, but may be required in some cases for gallbladder rupture, cholelith removal, or bile duct decompression if biliary obstruction is present (Weiss *et al.* 1997)

Quality of Life

Acute neutrophilic CCH may be a single curable event or it may recur (especially if antibiotic therapy is shortened), but the prognosis is generally good with timely diagnosis and appropriate treatment. Vigilant monitoring by the owner is important for early detection of anorexia, lethargy, vomiting, or abdominal discomfort, which could indicate recurrence of the condition. Lymphocytic CCH is a chronic condition but carries a fair to good prognosis with lifelong therapy. Owners should realize that compliance with medication administration might be a lifelong commitment.

Quality-of-life and end-of-life decisions will be influenced by the owner's ability to administer long-term treatment and the ease of handling the patient. The presence of concurrent diseases may also affect quality-of-life and treatment decisions; for example, corticosteroid treatment will negatively influence proper glucose control in patients with diabetes mellitus. Concurrent pancreatitis and/or IBD may also affect the long-term prognosis negatively.

References

Center SA. Diseases of the gallbladder and biliary tree. The Veterinary Clinics of North America: Small Animal Practice. 2009; 39: 543–598.

Gagne JM, Armstrong PJ, Weiss DJ, Lund EM, Feeney DA, King VL. Clinical features of inflammatory liver disease in cats: 41 cases (1983–1993). Journal of the American Veterinary Medical Association. 1999; 214(4): 513–516.

Marolf AJ, Gibbons DS, Bachand A, Twedt D, Leach L. Ultrasonographic findings of feline cholangitis. Journal of the American Animal Hospital Association. 2012; 48(1): 36–42.

Otte CMA, Penning LC, Rothuize J, Favier RP. Retrospective comparison of prednisolone and ursodeoxycholic acid for the treatment of feline lymphocytic cholangitis. Veterinary Journal. 2012; 195(2): 205–209.

Sherding RG. Feline jaundice. Journal of Feline Medicine and Surgery. 2000; 2: 165–169.

Twedt DC, Armstrong PJ, Simpson KW. Feline cholangitis. In: JD Bonagura and DC Twedt, Eds. Kirk's current veterinary therapy XV. Elsevier Saunders. 2014: 614–619.

Twedt DC, Cullen J, McCord K, Janeczko S, Dudak J, Simpson K. Evaluation of fluorescence in situ hybridization for the detection of bacteria in feline inflammatory liver disease. Journal of Feline Medicine and Surgery. 2013; 16: 395–406.

Weiss DJ, Armstrong PJ, Gagne J. Inflammatory liver disease. Seminars in Veterinary Medicine and Surgery (Small Animals). 1997; 12: 22–27.

Zoran D. Diseases of the liver. In: SE Little, Ed. The cat: clinical medicine and management. Elsevier Saunders. 2012: 533–536.

27

Chronic Kidney Disease
Gilad Segev

Introduction

Chronic kidney disease (CKD) is a common disease in companion animals. It may affect each part of the kidney, including glomeruli, tubules, interstitium, or blood vessels. Typically, the disease is characterized by structural changes and decreased kidney function, resulting in accumulation of uremic toxins and disruption of homeostasis. The disease is irreversible and tends to be progressive in nature, even if the underlying inciting cause is no longer present. Its clinical manifestation depends on the nature of the damage and its severity.

Diagnosis

The diagnosis of CKD is usually based on serum creatinine concentration (sCr), urine concentrating ability, presence of renal proteinuria, and imaging findings. sCr is the most commonly used screening marker, but it lacks sensitivity. It is commonly stated that at least a 75% reduction in glomerular filtration rate (GFR) occurs before an increase in sCr can be documented; however, it would be more accurate to state that for most animals, a 75% reduction in GFR is required for sCr to increase above the reference range (RR). One of the limitations of sCr is its variability between dog and, to a lesser extent, cat

breeds, despite a single RR for all breeds within each of the two species. Consequently, for some dog breeds (e.g., Yorkshire Terrier) a marked reduction in GFR occurs before sCr increases above the RR, while for others (e.g., Greyhound) only a mild decrease in GFR results in an increase of sCr above the RR. Establishing a normal range for the individual patient and assessing trends of sCr increase its sensitivity, and might indicate presence of CKD even before sCr exceeds the RR.

Management

Quality of medical care and the level of owner commitment are two major determinants of treatment success. Treatment goals include slowing down the disease progression rate, while providing a good quality of life. The former is achieved by feeding a designated diet, minimizing the pathophysiological consequences of the disease, and identifying and controlling known risk factors for rapid progression. Therapeutic targets should all be met even if clinical signs are absent.

There is good evidence that feeding a "kidney diet" is associated with slower progression rate and lower frequency of uremic crises (Jacob *et al.* 2002; Ross *et al.* 2006). Diets specifically designed for animals with CKD are modified from typical maintenance diets in several ways, therefore, diets only

Chronic Disease Management for Small Animals, First Edition. Edited by W. Dunbar Gram, Rowan J. Milner and Remo Lobetti.
© 2018 John Wiley & Sons, Inc. Published 2018 by John Wiley & Sons, Inc.

lower in protein content, are not satisfactory. Clinicians are advised to spend the time explaining the importance of consuming an appropriate diet, as an educated client is more likely to follow therapeutic recommendations. Transition to a new diet should be made gradually and only when clinical signs are controlled. Dogs and cats are often presented for medical care during an acute exacerbation of the disease, when they are unwilling to consume their regular diet, and are therefore even less likely to consume a therapeutic diet. An attempt to transition the animal to a therapeutic diet before clinical signs are controlled is more likely to fail and end up in food aversion.

Decreased appetite and weight loss are likely the most pronounced clinical signs of animals with advanced CKD. When animals are reluctant to eat, owners often replace the therapeutic diet by a more palatable diet; however, the latter might exacerbate the clinical manifestation of the disease (i.e., worsening azotemia, hyperphosphatemia and acid-base disorders), and consequently promote disease progression. When animals are reluctant to eat, owners often perceive quality of life as substantially deteriorated and might even elect euthanasia. In such instances, a variety of therapeutic diets, both dry and wet, should offered with concurrent use of medications such as anti-emetics (metoclopramide, maropitant, ondansetron), H_2 blockers (e.g., famotidine), proton pump inhibitors (e.g., omeprazole) and appetite stimulants (e.g., mirtazapine), so the animal will continue consuming the appropriate amount of a therapeutic diet. When these interventions are no longer effective, the use of feeding tubes should be considered.

Additional therapies are tailored for each patient according to the disease stage, the clinical signs and the presence and severity of secondary complications, such as hyperphosphatemia, hypertension, proteinuria, acid-based disorders, anemia, urinary tract infection, and dehydration. Each of these should be monitored regularly and treated

until predetermined therapeutic goals have been achieved (IRIS-website, 2017). When all therapeutic targets are met, quality of life is likely to improve and progression rate is likely to be slower. In this chapter, only a brief description of the management of CKD patients is provided. For a more detailed discussion, the reader is referred elsewhere (Polzin 2010).

Phosphorous control is achieved by prescribing a phosphorous restricted kidney diet and phosphorous binders, which should be mixed with food. The most common phosphorous binders are aluminum and calcium based. Lanthanum-based binders and Sevelamer are being used more frequently, but are also more costly. Recommended therapeutic goals are to maintain phosphorus concentration < 4.5 mg/dL in CKD stage II, < 5.0 mg/dL in stage III, and < 6.0 mg/dL in stage IV, but the accompanying risk of developing hypercalcemia or aluminum accumulation should not be overlooked.

Hypertension is another common complication of CKD and has been shown to be (directly or indirectly) associated with higher progression rates (Jacob *et al.* 2003; Syme *et al.* 2006). Thus, blood pressure should be monitored and controlled in any animal with CKD, but treatment should be initiated only when hypertension is documented persistently or when it is concurrent to documented damage to one of the end organs (e.g., eye). The most commonly used drugs to control systemic hypertension are angiotensin converting enzyme inhibitors (ACEi), angiotensin receptor blockers, and calcium channel blockers (e.g., amlodipine) with the goal of reducing systemic blood pressure to < 150/95 mmHg.

Renal proteinuria is more common in dogs compared to cats but is associated with progression of CKD in both species (Jacob *et al.* 2003; Syme *et al.* 2006). Renal proteinuria is managed using a low protein diet, omega 3 supplementation, ACEi, thromboxane inhibitors, angiotensin receptor blockers (e.g., telmisartan), and when indicated, immunosuppressant agents (Segev *et al.* 2013).

Metabolic acidosis is common in late Stage III and Stage IV CKD. The decision to institute alkalinization therapy is mostly based on serum pH and bicarbonate concentration. Treatment consists of sodium bicarbonate or potassium citrate administration.

Anemia is another sequel of advanced CKD, resulting from erythropoietin deficiency, blood loss (mostly to the gastrointestinal tract), reduced red blood cell lifespan, bone marrow toxicity, and nutritional (e.g., iron) deficiencies. Prior to erythropoietin treatment initiation, the clinician must be convinced that the main cause of anemia is erythropoietin deficiency. Premature treatment might result in antibody production and worsening of the anemia. When indicated (based on hematocrit level and presence of clinical signs), erythropoietin is administered together with iron supplementation.

Urinary tract infections (UTI) should be monitored on a regular basis to prevent pyelonephritis and acute exacerbation of CKD, as often UTIs are clinically silent and may not be diagnosed until they progressed to pyelonephritis and further decrease in kidney function. UTI should be treated based on culture and sensitivity results until clinical signs resolve and culture results are negative.

Subcutaneous (SQ) fluid administration is used to prevent dehydration. Although some veterinarians routinely administer SQ fluids to all CKD patients, it should not be considered as risk free. Adverse effects include sodium loading, overhydration, hypertension and an undesired interaction between owners and pets. Therefore, judicious amounts of SQ fluids should only be offered to patients with a risk of (or documented) dehydration. Cats, and animals with advanced CKD, appear to be more susceptible to chronic dehydration.

Managing Advanced CKD Patients

With further progression, clinical signs worsen and can no longer be controlled using conventional medical management. Some animals, however, (e.g., with congenital kidney disease) are more adapted or resilient than others to the consequences of uremia, and can therefore be managed successfully even when the disease is very advanced.

When clinical signs cannot be controlled using conventional management, owners might elect euthanasia or one of several other options, some of which might not be readily feasible. The first and most practical option is placing a feeding tube. The importance and utility of feeding tubes in animals with advanced CKD cannot be overemphasized. When the disease is very advanced, animals are not likely to consume enough food of the appropriate type. At this point owners also need to provide a myriad of medications to control clinical signs and clinicopathologic abnormalities. Placement of feeding tubes (esophagostomy or gastrostomy tubes) overcomes most of these obstacles. Feeding tubes are used to provide the amount of calories required (and not less importantly, of the appropriate diet), and to administer almost all the medication, some of which are being directly mixed with the food. Lastly, feeding tubes enable fluid administration in a more physiologic way, avoiding the undesired sodium load that is associated with SQ fluid administration, and the negative interaction between the owner and the pet. Unfortunately, many owners perceive an animal being fed with a feeding tube as having a poor quality of life, but the reality is that many CKD patients managed with a feeding tube have an excellent quality of life. When animals are being fed the appropriate type and amount of diet, and receive all the required medications and fluids, clinical signs often subside and consequently animals might even begin to re-consume the appropriate diet voluntarily. Nonetheless, before considering this option, owners need to be committed to this highly demanding type of care, as feeding 3–4 times a day (20–30 minutes each time) is required.

Chronic dialysis is performed successfully in dogs and cats and might provide an excellent quality of life for patients with advanced CKD that can no longer be medically managed. However, realistically speaking, this is not applicable for most owners due to financial constrains. Chronic dialysis is not only a financial commitment, but also a time commitment as the animal has to be presented for treatment twice or thrice weekly (for a whole day procedure), and the treatment does not replace the need for intense medical management. Nonetheless, if owners are willing to accept this commitment, animals can be successfully maintained on chronic dialysis even for years.

Kidney transplantation is another therapeutic intervention for animals with advanced CKD, but might be cost prohibitive. Kidney transplantation has been performed in both dogs and cats, but is substantially more successful in the latter. The perioperative mortality rate among cats undergoing kidney transplantation is 10–20%, with an additional 10–20% mortality during the 6 postoperative months due to various complications (Adin *et al.* 2001; Schmiedt *et al.* 2008). Nevertheless, those that survive may have an excellent quality of life for years with an overall 3-year survival rate of 40–50% (Adin *et al.* 2001; Schmiedt *et al.* 2008). In dogs, mortality rates are higher. In one study 15 and 100 days survival probability was 50% and 36%, respectively (Hopper *et al.* 2012).

Quality of Life

Before attempting to assess the long-term prognosis, one must ensure that the disease is irreversible and that the apparent kidney function tests represent a steady state rather than prerenal or postrenal complications, or acute decompensation (which may be reversible). In this regard, it is important to remember that compensatory hypertrophy and recovery after acute kidney insult might last up to 3 months.

Not all dogs and cats diagnosed with CKD will die from the disease (especially when diagnosed in Stage I or II). Particularly in cats, the progression rate might be very slow. For example, in one study of 211 cats with CKD and a sCr > 2.3 mg/dL, the overall median survival time was 771 days (Boyd *et al.* 2008). Cats with Stage III and IV CKD median survival time was 679 and 35 days, respectively. When communicating to owners about prognosis, however, clinicians should exercise realistic expectations and must always emphasize that there is a great deal of variability between animals and between circumstances.

A quality-of-life questionnaire has not been validated for veterinary CKD patients but a general quality-of-life assessment might be used (Lavan 2013), to improve the communication between clinicians and pet owners, to document changes in quality of life over time, to assess the response to treatment, and even to help guiding decisions regarding euthanasia.

Before electing euthanasia, owners need to consider the following questions:

- Does the pet have a poor quality of life?
- Is the current quality of life directly related to the presence of CKD, or do other reversible comorbidities contribute to the clinical signs, keeping in mind that CKD is typically well controlled until Stage IV, and in most patients until a certain (individual) point within stage IV?
- Is the current kidney function reversible (consider acute on chronic disease)
- What are the realistically available therapeutic options, and have they all been exhausted?

Weight loss and low body-condition score are markers of poor outcome (Elliott *et al.* 2003; Parker and Freeman 2011). When these are present, clinical signs cannot be controlled despite appropriate treatment, the disease is confirmed to be irreversible, and therapeutic options have been exhausted, euthanasia should indeed be considered.

References

Adin CA, Gregory CR, Kyles AE, Cowgill L. Diagnostic predictors of complications and survival after renal transplantation in cats. Veterinary Surgery. 2001; 30: 515–521.

Boyd LM, Langston C, Thompson K, Zivin K, Imanishi M. (Survival in cats with naturally occurring chronic kidney disease (2000–2002). Journal of Veterinary Internal Medicine. 2008; 22: 1111–1117.

Elliott J, Syme HM, Reubens E, Markwell PJ. Assessment of acid-base status of cats with naturally occurring chronic renal failure. Journal of Small Animal Practice. 2003; 44: 65–70.

Hopper K, Mehl ML, Kass PH, Kyles A, Gregory CR. Outcome after renal transplantation in 26 dogs. Veterinary Surgery. 2012; 41: 316–327.

IRIS-website. http://www.iris-kidney.com (accessed July, 2017).

Jacob F, Polzin DJ, Osborne CA, et al. Clinical evaluation of dietary modification for treatment of spontaneous chronic renal failure in dogs. Journal of the American Veterinary Medical Association. 2002; 220: 1163–1170.

Jacob F, Polzin DJ, Osborne CA, et al. Association between initial systolic blood pressure and risk of developing a uremic crisis or of dying in dogs with chronic renal failure. Journal of the American Veterinary Medical Association. 2003; 222: 322–329.

Lavan RP. Development and validation of a survey for quality of life assessment by owners of healthy dogs. The Veterinary Journal. 2013; 197: 578–582.

Parker VJ, Freeman LM. Association between body condition and survival in dogs with acquired chronic kidney disease. Journal of Veterinary Internal Medicine, 2011; 25: 1306–1311.

Polzin D. Chronic kidney disease. In: SJ Ettinger and EC Feldman, Eds. Textbook of Veterinary Internal Medicine, 7th ed. WB Saunders. 2010: 1990–2021.

Ross SJ, Osborne CA, Kirk CA, Lowry SR, Koehler LA, Polzin DJ. Clinical evaluation of dietary modification for treatment of spontaneous chronic kidney disease in cats. Journal of the American Veterinary Medical Association. 2006; 229: 949–957.

Schmiedt CW, Holzman G, Schwarz T, McAnulty JF. Survival, complications, and analysis of risk factors after renal transplantation in cats. Veteerinary Surgery. 2008; 37: 683–695.

Segev G, Cowgill LD, Heiene R, Labato MA, Polzin DJ. Consensus recommendations for immunosuppressive treatment of dogs with glomerular disease based on established pathology. Journal of Veterinary Internal Medicine. 2013; 27(Suppl 1): S44–S54.

Syme HM, Markwell PJ, Pfeiffer D, Elliott J. Survival of cats with naturally occurring chronic renal failure is related to severity of proteinuria. Journal of Veterinary Internal Medicine. 2006; 20: 528–535.

28

Chronic Urinary Tract Infection

Gilad Segev

Introduction

Urinary tract infection (UTI) is a common disease in companion animals. Bacterial infections are the most common cause of UTI, however fungal and viral infections may occasionally occur. The prevalence of UTI is higher in females compared to males, and in cats, it is substantially higher among the geriatric population. UTI usually results from an ascending migration of bacteria from the perineal urea into the urinary system. The infection might be confined to one anatomic area (e.g., urinary bladder) or involve multiple sites. The most commonly isolated urinary pathogen is *Escherichia coli*, accounting for approximately 50% of all isolates (Lees 1984; Ling 1984; Wooley and Blue 1976).

UTI occurs when the urinary system is overwhelmed with large quantities of virulent uropathogens, or due to temporary or permanent breach in host defense mechanisms, allowing virulent bacteria to adhere, multiply, and persist within the urinary tract. These include both local and systemic host defense mechanisms, but the former are more important.

UTI can be classified as uncomplicated (simple) or complicated. Uncomplicated UTI is defined as an infection in an otherwise healthy patient without abnormal urinary tract anatomy or function; whereas, complicated UTI is defined as an infection with a concurrent relevant comorbidity or when the infection is recurrent. Recurrent UTI is defined by the presence of ≥3 episodes of UTI during a 12-month period. Recurrent/ chronic UTI can be further classified as reinfection (i.e., multiple new infections), relapse (i.e., UTI caused by the same organism as the preceding infection that has occurred within 6 months), or persistent infection (i.e., bacteria isolated at any time point during an appropriate treatment course). Recurrent UTI might represent reinfections or relapses. The aforementioned classifications can only be made based on repeated urine cultures, before, during, and after treatment cessation.

The diagnosis of UTI is based on the presence of compatible clinical signs (pollakiuria, hematuria, dysuria, stranguria, or inappropriate urination) and is confirmed by urinalysis and a positive urine culture obtained by cystocentesis. While animals with upper urinary tract infection are often systemically ill, the absence of systemic clinical signs does not exclude upper UTI.

Management

Selection of antibiotics should rely primarily on urine culture and sensitivity (CandS) results, which are based on agar disk-diffusion or the minimum inhibitory concentration (MIC) method. In both methods, the results are interpreted as resistant, susceptible, or

Chronic Disease Management for Small Animals, First Edition. Edited by W. Dunbar Gram, Rowan J. Milner and Remo Lobetti.

intermediately susceptible. It is possible, however, that bacteria would be susceptible *in-vivo* despite *in-vitro* intermediate susceptibility or even resistance, provided the antibiotic is highly concentrated within the urine.

Renally excreted drugs and those being concentrated in the urine should be selected to manage chronic UTI, however, additional considerations include route and frequency of administration, adverse effects, cost, and the target organ (e.g. kidney, bladder, prostate). Ideally, antibiotic agents with high susceptibility should be used. The use of drugs with intermediate susceptibility might be appropriate when the other options are associated with a high prevalence of side-effects, are not easy to administer, should be reserved and used only as a last resort, or are cost prohibitive. In these scenarios, and when clinical signs are not life threatening, drugs with intermediate susceptibility can first be administered. In some instances, especially when more than one pathogen is involved, combination therapy might be indicated.

When UTI is recurrent it should not be regarded as an "antibiotic responsive disorder"; instead, predisposing factors should be sought and eliminated in addition to antibiotic therapy. Predisposing factors include anatomical abnormalities (e.g., ectopic ureters, abnormal vulvar conformation, urachal diverticulum), functional abnormalities (e.g., chronic kidney disease), metabolic disorders (e.g., diabetes mellitus, hyperadrenocorticism), neoplasia, urolithiasis, and causes for incomplete urinary bladder emptying. The diagnostic workup should be tailored for the individual patient. It always should include physical examination (including rectal examination to palpate the urethra) and may include a complete blood count, serum chemistry, survey and contrast radiography, ultrasonography, computed tomography, and cystourethroscopy.

Treatment of complicated or recurrent UTI should always be guided by culture and sensitivity testing due to relatively long treatment durations and the potential use of second- and third-line antibiotics. Misuse of antibiotics will promote resistance and when not based on culture and sensitivity results may also be ineffective. Whenever possible, the use of highly potent drugs (e.g., vancomycin, carbapenems) should be avoided and used only in rare instances of life-threatening or highly resistant infection. Treatment duration is determined by the nature of the infection and the organs involved. Evidence to support the treatment duration for complicated UTI is lacking, but administration of antimicrobials for a period of approximately 4 weeks is common practice. When pyelonephritis is suspected, treatment is indicated for an even longer period.

Monitoring

It is essential to monitor patients with complicated UTI to ensure eradication of the infection. Improvement of clinical signs cannot be used as proof of sterile urine. In complicated UTI, a urine culture is recommended before treatment initiation, during treatment (*in-vivo* susceptibility testing and ruling out super-infection) and 5–7 days following treatment cessation, to rule out relapse or early reinfection.

Treatment Failure and Chronic Management

UTI might be a frustrating disease to manage due to its high recurrence rate. Clinicians must always keep in mind that failure to identify and eliminate underlying causes is likely to result in failure to cure. If the UTI is recurrent, potential underlying causes should be revisited. Often the pathology is limited to the urethra and can therefore not be documented using routine diagnostic workup. In such instances, other diagnostic modalities (e.g., cystoscopy) should be considered.

In a subset of patients, where an underline disease either cannot be identified or eliminated, treatment is guided by culture and sensitivity testing. The selection of antibiotics might be challenging in some cases due the emergence of resistance (Couto *et al.* 2014; Delgado *et al.* 2007). When the isolated bacterium is resistant to all drugs available in the routine susceptibility panel, clinicians should communicate with the diagnostic laboratory to request an extended panel of antibiotics.

Both veterinarians and owners are often frustrated with the presence of repeated positive urine cultures despite a prolonged treatment using multiple medications. However, not every positive urine culture should be necessarily treated with the goal of achieving sterile urine. The results of a positive urine culture should be assessed in conjunction with the presence of clinical signs, presence of inflammation, and the risk for pyelonephritis. Asymptomatic bacteriuria is defined as the presence of bacteriuria (based on urine culture) in the absence of clinical signs or evidence of inflammation in the urine. Asymptomatic bacteriuria occurs commonly in human patients, and is documented in veterinary patients. Antimicrobial therapy in such patients is not indicated in the absence of clinical sings and inflammation, unless the risk of an ascending infection is considered high (e.g., given a previous history of pyelonephritis, predisposing anatomical abnormalities). One needs to consider, however, that in veterinary medicine it is more difficult to define asymptomatic bacteriuria, as animals may experience and even demonstrate symptoms but owners might not interpret those as clinical signs. Therefore, both the presence of clinical signs and urinary inflammation should be used in conjunction. A long-standing infection, even if not accompanied by clinical signs but associated with inflammation, might result in epithelial proliferation, and, in dogs, when urease positive bacteria are involved, also with struvite urolithiasis.

One of the common reasons for relapsing UTI and treatment failure is the presence of a deep-seated infection, in which the bacteria are not eliminated from tissues (e.g., bladder wall, kidney, prostate), despite their effective elimination from the urine, and therefore relapses occur days or weeks following cessation of antibiotic therapy. Deep-seated infections, infections in the upper urinary system, and those that involve the prostate, require longer treatment durations using antibiotics with good tissue penetration (e.g., fluoroquinolones).

In some cases, a long-standing infection induces epithelial proliferation in the urinary bladder or urethra, resulting in polypoid cystitis and proliferative urethritis, respectively (Crawford and Turk 1984; Martinez *et al.* 2003). These proliferations serve as a nidus for relapses and might intensify (or be the main cause of) clinical signs. Therefore, antibiotics should be used as described above for deep-seated infections, however, the addition of non-steroidal anti-inflammatory drugs should be considered in an attempt to relieve clinical signs and decrease epithelial proliferation. When only few urinary bladder polyps are present, resection using laser or a polypectomy snare under cystoscopic guidance can be attempted, but when diffuse and severe, surgical removal might be considered, depending on the nature of the polyps and their location.

A few ancillary therapies have been suggested in the management of recurrent and refractory UTI, including local instillation of antimicrobials and antiseptics into the urinary system, cranberry extracts, and urinary acidifiers. Currently, there is not enough evidence to support their use. However, side-effects using these therapies are uncommon and their use is not associated with emerging resistance. Such therapies can be considered in specific circumstances (see later), but should not replace proper use of antibiotics to treat an existing infection.

Instillation of antimicrobials and antiseptics directly into the lower urinary system has been suggested as treatment for refractory cases. One of the major disadvantages of this approach is the need to introduce a urinary catheter to deliver the treatment, which, in and of itself might introduce infection, and the fact that this treatment, in most cases, cannot be delivered by owners on a routine basis. However, if persistent urine diversion (e.g., a urine catheter or a cystostomy tube) is already in place, these therapies can be considered, as there is some evidence to suggest that the use of local antiseptics (e.g., chlorhexidine) decreases biofilm formation on urinary catheters (Segev *et al.* 2013).

Methenamine is a urinary antiseptic, which is converted in an acidic environment to formalin, and therefore interferes with bacterial growth (Lo *et al.* 2014). Concurrent administration of acidifying agents (ammonium chloride, vitamin C) is often required as the urine pH should acidic, however, caution should be used in animals that are already predisposed to metabolic acidosis (e.g., CKD).

Cranberry extract is known to inhibit attachment of particular uropathogens in people (Nowack 2007), but there is no solid evidence to suggest that these agents are effective in preventing UTI in dogs and cats. Cranberry extract should not be used to treat UTI. Rather, it might be considered as a preventative measure.

Prophylactic/Preventative Treatment

In some instances when an underlying cause cannot be identified or eliminated, but recurrent/persistent/reinfections are documented, prophylactic treatment should be considered. This practice involves the administration of long-term (i.e., months), once daily administration of first line antibiotics with minimal side effects, reaching high urine concentration (e.g., first generation β-lactam). Drugs should be administered at night after the pet has voided. The potential risk of emerging resistance resulting from this practice, however, should not be overlooked. Prophylactic treatment should never be applied before other options have been exhausted and only after the infection has been eliminated using the above guidelines. When performed, routine urine cultures should be carried out to document recurrence or super-infection, and if positive and associated with clinical signs or inflammation, it should be treated as a complicated UTI.

Quality of Life

It is uncommon that urinary tract infection, in the absence of an underlying morbidity, would substantially affect the quality of life of dogs and cats or be a reason for euthanasia, if appropriately treated. Treatment of recurrent UTI does require owner compliance, as prolonged treatment and monitoring are required. If severe clinical signs persist, despite appropriate use of antibiotics and good owner compliance, other comorbidities are likely to be present and should be looked for (e.g., polypoid cystitis and proliferative urethritis).

References

Couto N, Belas A, Couto I, Perreten V, Pomba C. Genetic relatedness, antimicrobial and biocide susceptibility comparative analysis of methicillin-resistant and -susceptible *Staphylococcus pseudintermedius* from Portugal. Microbial Drug Resistance. 2014; 20(4): 364–371.

Crawford MA, Turk MA. Ureteral obstruction associated with proliferative ureteritis in a dog. Journal of the American Veterinary Medical Association. 1984; 184: 586–588.

Delgado M, Neto I, Correia JH, Pomba C. Antimicrobial resistance and evaluation of susceptibility testing among pathogenic enterococci isolated from dogs and cats. International Journal of Antimicrobial Agents. 2007; 30: 98–100.

Lees GE. Epidemiology of naturally occurring feline bacterial urinary tract infections. The Veterinary Clinics of North America: Small Animal Practice. 1984; 14: 471–479.

Ling GV. Therapeutic strategies involving antimicrobial treatment of the canine urinary tract. Journal of the American Veterinary Medical Association. 1984; 185: 1162–1164.

Lo TS, Hammer KD, Zegarra M, Cho WC. Methenamine: a forgotten drug for preventing recurrent urinary tract infection in a multidrug resistance era. Expert Review of Anti-Infective Therapy. 2014; 12(5): 549–554.

Martinez I, Mattoon JS, Eaton KA, Chew DJ, DiBartola SP. Polypoid cystitis in 17 dogs (1978–2001). Journal of Veterinary Internal Medicine. 2003; 17: 499–509.

Nowack R. Cranberry juice: a well-characterized folk-remedy against bacterial urinary tract infection. Wiener Medizinische Wochenschrift. 2007; 157: 325–330.

Segev, G, Bankirer T, Steinberg D, Duvdevani M, Shapur NK, Friedman M, Lavy E. Evaluation of urinary catheters coated with sustained-release varnish of chlorhexidine in mitigating biofilm formation on urinary catheters in dogs. Journal of Veterinary Internal Medicine. 2013; 27: 39–46.

Wooley RE, Blue JL. Bacterial isolations from canine and feline urine. Modern Veterinary Practice. 1976; 57: 535–538.

29

Feline Interstitial Cystitis

Tanya Schoeman

Introduction

Feline lower urinary tract disease (FLUTD) is a common syndrome in small animal practice (Lund, Rimstad, and Eggertsdóttir 2012). Where appropriate investigations fail to identify a specific cause, a diagnosis of FIC is made. FIC accounts for between 55–73% of all cases seen for FLUTD (Buffington *et al.* 1997; Gerber *et al.* 2005). Although FIC is seen in all ages, cats 2–7 years old are at a higher risk (Lekcharoensuk, Osborne, and Lulich 2001). Certain risk factors have been identified for the development of FIC. Reported risk factors include male cats, long-haired cats, overweight, environmental stress, and feeding dry cat food (Buffington *et al.* 1997; Cameron *et al.* 2004; Defauw *et al.* 2011; Gerber *et al.* 2005).

Local bladder abnormalities and/or neuro-hormonal changes have been observed in a proportion of cats affected by FIC. Local bladder abnormalities identified in some affected cats include a decreased concentration of glycosaminoglycans (GAGs) in the urine (Buffington *et al.* 1996). It is thus possible that deficiencies in the mucopolysaccharide layer that overlies the bladder epithelium may contribute to damage, ulceration, and increased permeability of the underlying epithelium and also to submucosal haemorrhage (Lavelle *et al.* 2000). Similar to humans with interstitial cystitis, a number of neuro-hormonal abnormalities

have also been detected in cats with FIC that might play a role in the pathogenesis of the condition, including an increase in plasma norepinephrine (NE) and dihydroxyphenylalanine (DOPA) concentrations but without a concomitant increase in cortisol or adrenocorticotrophic hormone (ACTH) (Westropp, Kass, and Buffington 2006). These findings lend support to the fact that FIC appears to be associated with a stress response in many cats, but also suggests an uncoupling of the normal stress responses with increased sympathetic stimulation but suppressed adrenocortical responses (Westropp, Welk, and Buffington 2003).

Periuria (urinating in inappropriate locations), pollakiuria, stranguria, and gross hematuria are the most common clinical signs. Remarkably, these lower urinary tract signs subside within 1–7 days without therapy in up to 91% of cats with acute non-obstructive FIC. Signs recur after variable periods of time and again subside without treatment. Approximately 40–65% of cats with acute FIC will experience one or more recurrences of signs within 1 to 2 years (Defauw *et al.* 2011). A small subset of cats with FIC has also been described in which clinical signs persisted for weeks to months or are frequently recurrent. These cats are classified as having chronic FIC. Fortunately, less than 15% of cats evaluated because of acute FIC will develop chronic forms of the disease (Defauw *et al.* 2011).

Chronic Disease Management for Small Animals, First Edition. Edited by W. Dunbar Gram, Rowan J. Milner and Remo Lobetti.
© 2018 John Wiley & Sons, Inc. Published 2018 by John Wiley & Sons, Inc.

It is important to recognize that cats with FIC often have clinical problems outside the lower urinary tract. The comorbid conditions frequently encountered are related to the gastrointestinal tract, skin lesions (barbering of caudal abdomen), cardiovascular system, endocrine system (low adrenal cortical function), behavior problems (frightened, withdrawn, hiding, aggressive, overly attached) and obesity (Buffington 2004).

Diagnosis

A combination of findings from history (including details related to behavior, the environment, husbandry practices), physical examination (including all body systems in addition to the lower urinary tract), urinalysis, serum biochemistry, and quantitative urine culture are often needed to establish a definitive diagnosis for the causes of lower urinary tract disease (LUTD). Routine and advanced urinary tract imaging provide pivotal diagnostic anatomical information in cats with recurrent LUTD. Histopathology of urinary bladder or urethral tissue is rarely needed to make a diagnosis except in the instance of neoplasia. A diagnosis of FIC is only made once all other causes of LUTD have been ruled out; therefore, it is a diagnosis of exclusion.

A thorough diagnostic evaluation is indicated for all cats that fail to have spontaneous remission of clinical signs within one week or for those with recurrent episodes, urethral obstruction, a history or the presence of other health problems, or in older cats (>8 years of age).

In male and female cats with FIC, a varying degree of increased vessel number and tortuosity, oedema, and glomerulations (submucosal petechial haemorrhages) are often visualized in the urinary bladder during cystoscopy. An increase in the number and size of glomerulations often occurs in cats with FIC when higher bladder filling pressures (≥80 cm water) are used during cystoscopy. This finding does not occur in normal urinary bladders and can serve as a provocative test for FIC (Chew *et al.* 1996). Female cats with FIC rarely have lesions in the urethra whereas urethral lesions (erosions, hemorrhages, glomerulations) are observed in approximately 40% of male cats with FIC. It should be noted that lower urinary tract signs do not necessarily correlate with the degree or number of cystoscopic abnormalities identified in cats with FIC (Chew *et al.* 1996).

Reliable diagnostic markers for FIC are currently not yet clinically available. Urinary levels of antiproliferative factor, heparin-binding epidermal factor, and epidermal growth factor distinguish human patients with interstitial cystitis from healthy controls, but have not been investigated in cats with FIC.

Differential Diagnosis

- Bacterial cystitis
- Urolithiasis
- Urethral strictures
- Urethral plugs
- Urinary tract trauma
- Urinary tract neoplasia

Treatment

As there is currently no cure for cats with FIC, treatment options are aimed at keeping the clinical signs to a minimum and increasing the disease-free intervals. Because FIC can be a chronic condition in some cats, excellent client communication in conjunction with MEMO (multimodal environmental modifications) and dietary therapy and possibly pharmacologic agents, may be beneficial for managing FIC.

As environmental stressors can exacerbate clinical signs of FIC, MEMO therapy has been shown to be successful in most cats with FIC (Buffington *et al.* 2006). However, placebo controlled trials are difficult when evaluating cats with FIC due to the waxing and waning nature of the disease as well as the numerous variables that one encounters in a home environment. After the diagnosis of FIC is made, a thorough environmental history (including any inter-cat conflict), as well as notation of all other comorbidities present, needs to be obtained so the clinician can begin to tailor a plan to address all the needs of each individual cat. Helpful modifications can then be recommended to the client. Key resources to consider include water, food, litter boxes, interaction with humans and other animals, and hiding or resting areas (Herron and Buffington 2010).

Diet

Cats with FIC fed a canned diet tend to show a significant reduction in the clinical signs. (Markwell *et al.* 1999). Increasing water intake by feeding canned food — or other methods, such as broths or automatic water dispensers, may also be beneficial for cats with FIC. It is hypothesized that added water may help dilute the potential "noxious" stimulants in the urine such as urea and potassium chloride. One should also consider that for some cats, canned food or added dietary moisture in the forms described above may actually serve as a form of environmental enrichment (e.g., increased contact with humans who provide the food or differences in mouth feel/texture for the cat), which might have a positive impact on the cat's clinical signs (Westropp 2014). Recently is has been shown that feeding a commercially available multi-purpose urinary therapeutic food reduced the duration and episodes of FIC (Hill's Prescription Diet c/d Multicare).

Recent clinical studies have supported nutritional management with L-tryptophan and alpha-casozepine (Beata 2014). This may be especially as the daily administration of treatments can be potentially difficult or even stressful. As stated previously, stress may contribute to anxious behavior and it appears to play a key role in the pathogenesis of FIC. Use of dietary supplements or therapeutic foods may therefore be helpful to decrease anxiety and stress, however, clinical studies are needed with the final product showing that the expected efficacy is present.

Pheromones

Feliway® is the synthetic F3 fraction of the naturally occurring feline facial pheromone. Treatment with this pheromone has been reported to reduce the amount of anxiety experienced by cats in unfamiliar circumstances, a response that may potentially be helpful for FIC cats (Westropp 2014). In a pilot study evaluating Feliway® in cats with FIC, a decrease in the number of days they exhibited clinical signs was reported, although this finding was not significant (Gunn-Moore and Cameron 2004).

Drug Therapy

A variety of drugs has been used in cats with FIC, including amitriptyline and glycosaminoglycans. Unfortunately, prospective, randomized, properly masked, placebo-controlled studies are lacking to confirm their clinical efficacy (Westropp 2014). If MEMO and dietary (and possibly pheromone) therapy fails to control signs, these medications can be considered. It must be emphasized that these drugs should not be used for cats on initial presentation for care of FIC; they should be considered only for cats after their environmental and dietary needs have been addressed, and should not be discontinued abruptly.

Amitriptyline (2.5–7.5 mg/cat PO SID), a tricyclic antidepressant appears to help clinical signs in some cats with severe, refractory FIC (Chew *et al.* 1998). This drug, or possibly clomipramine, (0.25–0.5 mg/kg PO SID), may need to be administered for at least one week or longer before a beneficial effect may be noted. If there is no improvement or medicating the cat is too stressful (for owner or cat), these drugs should be gradually discontinued over 1–2 weeks.

Pentosan polysulfate sodium is a semi-synthetic carbohydrate derivative similar to glycosaminoglycans that are approved for humans with IC. A multi-centered, placebo-controlled, masked study in cats with FIC reported no significant differences when comparing pentosan polysulfate sodium with placebo (Chew *et al.* 2009). However, all groups had clinical benefit, suggesting a strong "placebo" effect. All medication was provided to the cat in a food treat; the authors of this study hypothesized that improving the interaction and environmental needs of the cat may inadvertently have contributed to the positive outcomes noted in all groups. Similar findings were reported in two other studies evaluating GAG replacers in cats with FIC (Westropp 2014).

Analgesics to reduce pain during acute episodes are advocated, although studies evaluating their use have not been reported. Current management includes opioid analgesics (butorphanol or buprenorphine) and/or NSAIDS.

Glycosaminoglycans, pheromones, serotonin modulating drugs, or salt supplementation have been shown to be no better than a placebo but can be considered in difficult, highly recurrent or chronic cases of FIC.

Quality of Life

Although FIC is not a life-threatening disease, a cat with chronic or recurrent FIC can have a significantly reduced quality of life due to chronic pain and discomfort. Owner compliance is essential with feeding and environmental modifications. End-of-life decisions may become unavoidable in refractory chronic cases of confirmed FIC that do not seem to respond to any type of modifications or medications.

References

Beata C. L-tryptophan and alpha-casozepine: What is the evidence? Scientific Proceedings Hill's Global Symposium on Feline Lower Urinary Tract Health, Prague. 2014: 37–41.

Buffington CA. Comorbidity of interstitial cystitis with other unexplained clinical conditions. Journal of Urology. 2004; 172: 1242–1248.

Buffington CA, Blaisdell JL, Binns SP, Woodforth BE. Decreased urine glycosaminoglycan excretion in cats with interstitial cystitis. Journal of Urology. 1996; 155: 1801–1804.

Buffington CA, Chew DJ, Kendall MS, et al. Clinical evaluation of cats with non-obstructive urinary tract diseases. Journal of the American Veterinary Medical Association. 1997; 210: 46–50.

Buffington CA, Westropp JL, Chew DJ, Bolus RR. Clinical evaluation of multimodal environmental modification (MEMO) in the management of cats with idiopathic cystitis. Journal of Feline Medicine and Surgery. 2006; 8: 261–268.

Cameron ME, Casey RA, Bradshaw JWS, Waran NK, Gunn-Moore DA. A study of environmental and behavioural factors that may be associated with feline idiopathic cystitis. Journal of Small Animal Practice. 2004; 45: 144–147.

Chew DJ, Buffington CA, Kendall MS, DiBartola SP, Woodworth BE. Amitriptyline treatment for severe recurrent idiopathic cystitis in cats. Journal of the American Veterinary Medical Association. 1998; 213: 1282–1286.

Chew DJ, Buffington CA, Kendall MS, Osborn SD, Woodworth BE. Urethroscopy, cystoscopy, and biopsy of the feline lower urinary tract. Veterinary Clinics of North America: Small Animal Practice. 1996: 26: 441–462.

Chew DJ, et al. Randomized, placebo-controlled clinical trial of pentosan polysulfate sodium for treatment of feline interstitial (idiopathic) cystitis. Journal of Veterinary Internal Medicine. 2009; 23: 690.

Defauw PA, Van de Maele I, Duchateau L, Polis IE, Saunders JH, Daminet S. Risk factors and clinical presentation of cats with feline idiopathic cystitis. Journal of Feline Medicine and Surgery. 2011; 13: 967–975.

Gerber B, Boretti FS, Kley S, et al. Evaluation of clinical signs and causes of lower urinary tract disease in European cats.

Journal of Small Animal Practice. 2005; 46: 571–577.

Gunn-Moore DA, Cameron ME. A pilot study using feline facial pheromone for the management of feline idiopathic cystitis. Journal of Feline Medicine and Surgery. 2004; 6(3): 133–138.

Herron ME, Buffington CA. Environmental enrichment for indoor cats. Compendium of Continuing Education for Veterinarians. 2010; 32: E4.

Lavelle JP, Meyers SA, Ruiz WG, Buffington CAT, Zeidel ML, Apodaca G. Urothelial pathophysiological changes in feline interstitial cystitis: a human model. American Journal of Renal Physiology. 2000; 278: F540–F553.

Lekcharoensuk C, Osborne CA, Lulich JP. Epidemiologic study of risk factors for lower urinary tract diseases in cats. Journal of the American Veterinary Medical Association. 2001; 218: 1429–1435.

Lund HS, Rimstad E, Eggertsdóttir AV. Prevalence of viral infections in Norwegian cats with and without feline lower urinary tract disease. Journal of Feline Medicine and Surgery. 2012; 14: 895–899.

Markwell PJ, Buffington CA, Chew DJ, Kendall MS, Harte JG, DiBartola SP. Clinical evaluation of commercially available urinary acidification diets in the management of idiopathic cystitis in cats. Journal of the American Veterinary Medical Association. 1999; 214: 361–365.

Westropp JL. Feline idiopathic cystitis: evidence-based management. Scientific Proceedings Hill's Global Symposium on Feline Lower Urinary Tract Health, Prague. 2014: 31–36.

Westropp JL, Kass PH, Buffington CA. Evaluation of the effects of stress in cats with idiopathic cystitis. American Journal of Veterinary Research. 2006; 67: 731–736.

Westropp JL, Welk KA, Buffington CA. Small adrenal glands in cats with feline interstitial cystitis. Journal of Urology. 2003; 170: 2494–2497.

30

Canine Chronic Bronchitis

Richard K. Burchell

Introduction

Canine chronic bronchitis (CCB) is often a difficult condition to diagnose, manage, and to append an accurate prognosis. This is partly due to the fact that CCB has a poorly understood etiopathogenesis, making pathophysiologically rationalized treatment difficult to tailor, and also due to the fact patients are often older, overweight small breed dogs with comorbid conditions such as canine myxomatous mitral valve disease, and canine hyperadrenocorticism, which may obfuscate an accurate diagnosis and complicate therapeutic interventions. Notwithstanding this disagreeable situation, a careful stepwise systematic approach will permit the optimal management of each case and ensure that clients are given accurate feedback. Traditionally CCB is defined as a chronic inflammatory lower airway disease, fulminating as a harsh dry cough, which has persisted for at least two months. Corticosteroids and antitussives are the mainstay of therapy. Many patients can be maintained on inhaled glucocorticoids, which are associated with fewer side effects.

Etiology

CCB is purportedly a chronic indolent, slowly progressive inflammatory response, which results in airway inflammation and goblet cell hypertrophy (Rozanski 2014).

Proposed pathogenesis of the condition has been environmental pollutants (dust and cigarette smoke) (Rozanski 2014; Yamaya, Sugiya, and Watari 2015) and allergies (Yamaya and Watari 2015). Further work has demonstrated that cigarette smoke exposure results in damage to DNA in the lungs of dogs with CCB, suggesting that smoke inhalation may induce inflammatory changes in the airways of dogs with CCB (Yamaya *et al.* 2015).

Diagnosis

A definitive diagnosis of CCB is premised on radiographs and bronchoscopy with cytology/culture (Rozanski 2014; Ristic and Herrtage 2001). The typical signalment of dogs with CCB is older small breed dogs, who are also at risk for a number of other diseases such as tracheal collapse, myxomatous mitral valve disease (MMVD), and canine hyperadrenocorticism; which may complicate the diagnosis and treatment. It is not uncommon that a patient is presented with a cough and the veterinarian detects a heart murmur during a physical examination with possible scenarios being primary respiratory disease with an incidental cardiac murmur; or primary respiratory disease and pulmonary hypertension, resulting in right sided heart disease; or MMVD with cardiomegaly and a cardiac cough. The presence of a slow

Chronic Disease Management for Small Animals, First Edition. Edited by W. Dunbar Gram, Rowan J. Milner and Remo Lobetti.
© 2018 John Wiley & Sons, Inc. Published 2018 by John Wiley & Sons, Inc.

heart rate with a sinus rhythm tends to negate heart disease as a possible cause for the cough. In addition, it has been demonstrated that congestive heart failure (CHF) is not a common cause of coughing in MMVD, while left atrial enlargement is. Resultantly, a cardiac cough, is most likely due to pressure on the left main stem bronchus, due to increased atrial pressure. Thus it may be possible from a thorough physical examination and radiographs to differentiate between MMVD and CCB. Alternatively, pro-BNP is a useful biomarker to exclude cardiac disease as a cause of coughing and dyspnea (Oyama 2015; Prosek *et al.* 2007). Furthermore, since glucocorticoids are often the mainstay of therapy, it must be remembered that these patients are also at risk for developing hyperadrenocorticism, given the age and breeds normally affected by CCB. Therefore, along with the fact that patients require anesthesia if a definitive diagnosis is to be reached, a complete blood count, urinalysis, fecal flotation (for lung worm), heart worm antigen (if indicated), and serum biochemistry should be performed. Echocardiography is useful to screen for pulmonary hypertension, which can cause, or contribute to coughing. This will allow a comprehensive stratification of the individual patient with regards to possible comorbid diseases, ensuring that the management is most successful. Furthermore, the clinician should remember that steroid therapy may alter the outcome of diagnostic tests (such as liver enzymes, platelets, and cytology) and therefore, once started may obscure the diagnosis of diseases such as liver disease, hyperadrenocorticism, and may mask cytological typical lesions on bronchioalveolar lavage (BAL) fluid analysis.

Therapy and Monitoring

Given the paucity of therapeutic trials in patients with CCB, firm evidence-based recommendations are not possible, and the following section is based on the limited evidence and the opinion of the author. Data obtained from well-structured trials will supersede that of the opinion of experts.

The reality confronting most practicing veterinarians is that many owners have a limited budget, which does not necessarily preclude the successful management of CCB. Owners with limited funds should not be denigrated and excluded from compassionate and dedicated care. Indeed, it is often more challenging (and possibly rewarding) to successfully manage a chronic disease based on clinical data and limited diagnostics.

In cases where funds are limited and in the absence of a cytological confirmed diagnosis, a trial of doxycycline or fluoroquinolones (typically 10–14 days) can be considered to exclude bacterial diseases such as *Bordetella* and *Mycoplasma*. The combination of antimicrobials and glucocorticoids should be avoided, as this may obscure the interpretation of a therapeutic trial. It is this author's opinion that antimicrobial cover should be reserved for patients that have cytological/bacterial culture or clinic-pathological evidence of bacterial infection. Neutrophilia on blood smear, fever, productive cough, exposure to other coughing dogs, an elevated respiratory rate and systemic illness are compelling reasons to treat with antibiotics. Existing and emerging antimicrobial resistance is a concerning global phenomenon, threatening the health of human and animal patients (Weese *et al.* 2015). Therefore, clinicians should carefully consider the probability of bacterial infection before instituting a therapeutic antibiotic trial. Glucocorticoids (GC) is currently the recommended therapy in CCB. The response to GC is variable, and owners should be warned of this at the beginning of therapy. Recent work has demonstrated the utility of inhaled GC in the management with CCB, which has the added advantage of having fewer unwanted GC side effects, and endocrine perturbations. The response to inhaled GC is variable, and doses required to control clinical signs vary from patient to patient; therefore, the author treats with oral GC first to assess whether the coughing is GC responsive. Inhaled GCs tend to be expensive, and some capital outlay for the spacers and mask is needed. Oral doses are typically initially high (e.g., prednisone 1.5–2 mg/kg/d) for 7–10 days, and are tapered once a reduction in the clinical signs is documented. Worsening of clinical signs, or failure to respond should prompt a reassessment of the case, and possibly cessation of therapy. In cases where the response is encouraging; the dose is tapered gradually over 1–2 months, in an attempt to determine the minimal dose required to control clinical signs. If the dog tolerates an inhaler, the owner is shown how to use an inhaler with the spacer. If an inhaler is used, an inhaled bronchodilator such as salbutamol can also be used for symptomatic relief. If the patient tolerates the inhaler, oral GC is slowly withdrawn and the patient is maintained on inhaled GC. The author sometimes finds that pulse therapy of oral GC is needed to "buy back" control occasionally, but inhaled GC seems to reduce the requirement of oral GC and is associated with fewer side effects. This author prefers budesonide, given its negligible interference with the hypothalamic-pituitary-adrenal axis compared to fluticasone, but either of these drugs appear to be effective (Melamies *et al.*, 2012). Owners who cannot afford inhaled GCs would need to titrate the oral GC dose to the minimum effective dose long term.

In addition to GC therapy, weight-loss is important in overweight patients as it greatly improves comfort and ease of breathing. Where possible avoidance of cigarette smoke, dust, and environmental pollutants is advisable and if possible owners should humidify the air in very dry environments. In addition, in cases where the coughing is causing distress, and is unproductive, antitussives can be used for symptomatic relief, but should be reserved for patients that have worrisome coughing, as cough suppression will reduce the clearance of mucous and pathogens.

Quality of Life

The poorly understood etiology and that CCB is probably better described as a syndrome, as opposed to a disease as a finite entity, makes prognostication difficult, because not all patients experience the same response. In addition, long-standing cases, may have experienced damage to the respiratory tract, that may be irreversible, and therefore therapy is less likely to be successful. Owners need to understand that CCB is not normally cured but merely managed. Owners are encouraged to keep a diary of coughing, which serves to document if a change in frequency occurs. In addition, owners are asked to occasionally record sleeping respiratory rates, to track possible worsening lung function, or development of parenchymal lung lesions such as pneumonia. Documenting the incidence and severity of coughing to some extend gives an indication of how often the dog is affected by CCB. Other markers of quality of life, such as appetite, tolerance of exercise, and long periods of uninterrupted sleep usually help to decide whether CCB is progressively worsening.

In refractory cases, where coughing is severe, and/or dyspnea ensues, and particularly if pulmonary hypertension is documented, euthanasia should be considered. In owners without budget constraints repeat radiographs, echocardiography, and possibly repeating endoscopy BAL may provide additional data, such as pulmonary hypertension or an infection, which may improve quality of life if managed. The most common reasons for owners to seek euthanasia are the presence of dyspnea, exercise intolerance, and bouts of severe coughing.

References

Melamies M, Vainio O, Spillmann T, Junnila J, Rajamäki MM. Endocrine effects of inhaled budesonide compared with inhaled fluticasone propionate and oral prednisolone in healthy Beagle dogs. The Veterinary Journal. 2012; 194: 349–353.

Oyama MA. Using cardiac biomarkers in veterinary practice. Clinics in Laboratory Medicine. 2015; 35: 555–566.

Prosek R, Sisson DD, Oyama MA, Solter PF. Distinguishing cardiac and noncardiac dyspnea in 48 dogs using plasma atrial natriuretic factor, B-type natriuretic factor, endothelin, and cardiac troponin-I. Journal of Veterinary Internal Medicine. 2007; 21: 238–242.

Ristic J, Herrtage M. Chronic bronchitis in dogs. The Veterinary Record. 2001;148: 320.

Rozanski E. Canine chronic bronchitis. The Veterinary Clinics of North America: Small Animal Practice. 2014; 44: 107–116.

Weese JS, Giguère S, Guardabassi L, et al. ACVIM consensus statement on therapeutic antimicrobial use in animals and antimicrobial resistance. Journal of Veterinary Internal Medicine, 2015; 29: 487–498.

Yamaya Y, Sugiya H, Watari T. Methylation of free-floating deoxyribonucleic acid fragments in the bronchoalveolar lavage fluid of dogs with chronic bronchitis exposed to environmental tobacco smoke. Irish Veterinary Journal. 2015; 68: 7.

Yamaya Y, Watari T. Increased proportions of CCR4(+) cells among peripheral blood CD4(+) cells and serum levels of allergen-specific IgE antibody in canine chronic rhinitis and bronchitis. The Journal of Veterinary Medical Science. 2015; 77, 421–425.

31

Bronchiectasis

Richard K. Burchell

Introduction

Bronchiectasis (BE) is a permanent dilation of the bronchi, with resultant fluid accumulation that occurs secondary to chronic inflammation, and damage to the elastic layers of the airways. BE has been described secondary to a number of etiologies, but is most commonly observed secondary to chronic bronchitis. Diagnosis is based on radiography/computed tomography and bronchoscopy. Bacterial culture and sensitivity testing are strongly advocated to ensure that antibiotic therapy is appropriate. Therapy is typically tailored to contr infection, and if possible man the underlying cause to prevent further damage to the airways. Long-term antibiotic therapy may be required and adjunctive mucolytic therapy, and nebulization may be of benefit in some cases. The prognosis is typically guarded, given the irreversible nature of the lesion, and is aimed at amelioration of clinical signs and prevention of secondary infection.

Etiology and Classification

As with many chronic inflammatory diseases the etiology of bronchiectasis (BE) is enigmatic and poorly understood. Simply stated, BE purportedly occurs secondary to indolent chronic inflammatory process in the bronchi and is insidious, culminating in destruction of the elastic layers of the airways, leading to secondary dilation thereof (Cannon *et al.* 2013; Marolf, Blaik, and Specht 2007; Meler *et al.* 2010). A number of primary etiologies have been described in association with BE, namely, chronic bronchitis, eosinophilic bronchopneumopathy (Meler *et al.* 2010), primary ciliary dyskinesia, tracheal collapse, and bronchomalacia (Marolf *et al.* 2007). The overarching theory of BE is inflammatory damage, however, it is unclear as to why only certain patients with chronic airway inflammation develop BE while others do not. In addition, causality has not been proven in the case of BE and it is possible that the diseases implicated in the genesis of BE are associated with and not the cause of BE per se.

Diagnosis

Radiographically, BE is classified as cylindrical or saccular (Cannon *et al.* 2013). In cylindrical BE there is tapering of the bronchi peripherally, whereas in saccular BE there is not. There is currently no evidence as to the clinical significance of this finding. In some cases with radiographically ambiguous lesions, computed tomography (CT) may be a more sensitive imaging modality. Bronchoscopy is commonly used as the gold standard for diagnosis of BE (Figure 31.1),

Chronic Disease Management for Small Animals, First Edition. Edited by W. Dunbar Gram, Rowan J. Milner and Remo Lobetti.

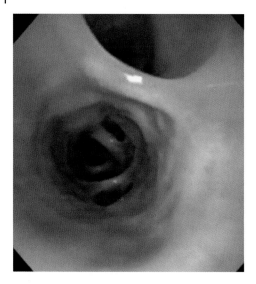

Figure 31.1 Bronchoscopy from a dog with bronchiectasis.

however; it should be noted that there is an aspect of subjectivity in the interpretation of bronchoscopy. Bronchoscopy can show thinning of the bifurcations and dilation of the walls of the bronchi, which are often filled with mucus plugs. Ideally cases with BE should have samples collected for cytology, culture, and antibiogram.

Patients with BE are typically older and often smaller breed dogs. Consequently, there may be a number of comorbid diseases that may complicate the management of BE. Resultantly, the author will usually advise a complete blood count, serum biochemistry, and urinalysis to screen for any concurrent medical conditions that may require management. Fecal analysis is also normally advised, and depending on the geographical location, it may be worthwhile to screen for specific lung parasites.

Treatment

Treatment of BE can be quite challenging, given the fact that these patients have impaired ability to eliminate bronchial secretions from the lower respiratory tract. Most cases of BE are associated with persistent coughing and

refractory chronic bacterial lung infections. Many patients with BE will require prolonged courses of antibiotics but given the rising incidence of antibiotic resistance; it is incumbent to use antibiotics judiciously. Thus, antibiotic selection in the case of a chronic disease like BE, that requires prolonged antibiotic cover, should always be based on culture and sensitivity. Ideally, first-line antibiotics such as amoxicillin, first-generation cephalosporins and sulphonamides should be used. The main challenge of antibiotic therapy is monitoring therapy and titrating treatment according to the severity of the disease. Repeat sampling of lung fluid is not routinely performed, and thus there are currently no objective parameters to measure the progress of patients with BE. Resultantly, the monitoring is typically clinical, and thus demonstrating improved level of comfort and reduction in the frequency of coughing, if present is typically the way in which progress is monitored. Follow up radiographs/CT can be performed, especially where deterioration is observed, and serve to assess the development of complications such as worsening bronchopneumonia or development of inspissated areas of infection or abscesses that may require surgical removal. In general, surgery is not indicated and the majority of cases are managed medically. Adjunctive therapies such as nebulization, humidification of air, reduction of aero-pollutants (such as cigarette smoke) coupage, and mucolytic therapy are often also prescribed in order to improve clearance of mucus from the airways. Currently there are no evidence-based recommendations supporting the use of any particular therapeutic interventions, however, the use of these treatment methodologies is intuitively reasonable.

Wherever possible the underlying disease process should be managed. In the case of allergic/immune mediated inflammatory diseases this may include circumspect use of glucocorticoids (GCs) but needs to be carefully considered and the risk/benefit ratio needs to be discussed with the client. In the case of a florid bacterial pneumonia, the use of GCs particularly higher doses may be contraindicated, and thus are probably best reserved for when the patient is more stable, and the infection is under control. In cases where the underlying etiology is likely due to chronic inflammatory diseases such as chronic bronchitis a short course of steroids may be of benefit. A sensible approach may be to start with a dose of 0.5–1 mg/kg once daily for 5–7 days, and if an improvement is noted the dose can be tapered to effect over a number of weeks, and reduced to the lowest effective dose. Alternatively, the author has found that inhaled GCs (fluticasone, budesonide) are also sometimes effective, and in some cases can be used alone, or may reduce the required amount of oral prednisolone required to control the clinical signs. Inhaled GCs are particularly helpful in cases were systemic GCs are inappropriate such as in patients with diabetes mellitus or hyperadrenocorticism. The author will normally advise that the owner obtains a humidifier and if possible a nebulizer. Humidifiers are helpful in dry and dusty climates, and can be placed near to where the pet sleeps, and anecdotally seem to improve the comfort level of the patient. Coupage also appears to be of some benefit. Certain owners can be shown how to perform this, or alternatively some clinics provide a service, where physiotherapy and general physical therapy can be performed.

Quality of Life

Given the paucity of literature pertaining to BE no firm prognostic factors are available, and each case needs to be assessed individually. The presence of comorbid diseases such as congestive heart failure, chronic renal failure, diabetes mellitus, and hyperadrenocorticism generally complicate the management of BE, and if present need to be discussed with the owners, in order to align their expectations with a realistic outcome in such cases. In addition, recurrent pneumonia, development of pulmonary abscesses, worsening dyspnea, or coughing in spite of treatment would be considered negative prognostic factors. Most importantly, the patient's quality of life should be assessed, and euthanasia should only be considered when this has deteriorated, regardless of the radiographic or bronchoscopy findings.

References

Cannon MS, Johnson LR, Pesavento PA, Kass PH, Wisner ER. Quantitative and qualitative computed tomographic characteristics of bronchiectasis in 12 dogs. Veterinary Radiology and Ultrasound. 2013; 54: 351–357.

Marolf A, Blaik M, Specht A. A retrospective study of the relationship between tracheal collapse and bronchiectasis in dogs. Veterinary Radiology and Ultrasound. 2007; 48: 199–203.

Meler E, Pressler BM, Heng HG, Baird DK. Diffuse cylindrical bronchiectasis due to eosinophilic bronchopneumopathy in a dog. Canadian Veterinary Journal. 2010; 51: 753–756.

32

Interstitial Lung Diseases
Richard K. Burchell

Introduction

Interstitial lung diseases (ILDs) are a diverse group of conditions of various etiologies that result in inflammatory degenerative changes within the pulmonary parenchyma that usually does not communicate directly with the airways. Possible etiologies include inflammatory or infectious causes, toxins (paraquat), neoplasia, immune-mediated, and idiopathic. Resultantly, the outcomes may vary from complete resolution to death or euthanasia. ILDs can be challenging to diagnose, due to difficulty in obtaining representative samples non-invasively. Definitive diagnosis is based on radiographs, computed tomography, endoscopy, fine–needle lung aspirate, and lung biopsy. Adjunctive tests such as fecal flotation, heartworm antigen, echocardiography, and NT-ProBNP may also be of use in some cases. Unfortunately, many ILDs are frustrating to manage and markedly affect quality of life, often necessitating euthanasia.

Etiology and Classification

The classification of ILDs is somewhat hampered by the plethora of pathologies that can manifest as an ILD pattern on radiographs (Reinero and Cohn 2007). Furthermore, ILDs can be described as diffuse or nodular. Generally, nodular patterns are more consistent with neoplastic diseases with fungal disease, eosinophilic lung diseases and cardiogenic lung edema in cats serving as other possible differential diagnoses. Finding a nodular lung pattern on a radiograph typically necessitates the exclusion of neoplasia, and ultrasound guided fine-needle aspirates are useful to achieve this. Diffuse ILDs can result from a number of pathophysiological processes such as immune mediated/allergic, infectious, toxicological, parasitic, idiopathic, and, more rarely, neoplastic disease.

Diagnosis

Radiographic signs of ILD may be fairly subtle in the face of advanced and severe clinical signs, and often the clinical signs correlate poorly with radiographic severity. In addition, many dogs with ILD are older, and there may be some overlap in lesions from ILDs and age-related changes within the lungs. Where lesions are readily radiographically demonstrable (Figure 32.1, Figure 32.2); endoscopy and broncho-alveolar lavage (BAL) will likely elucidate the etiology of the lesions. However, it is not uncommon that a patient is fulminant dyspneic with seemingly mild radiographic lesions. In these cases,

Chronic Disease Management for Small Animals, First Edition. Edited by W. Dunbar Gram, Rowan J. Milner and Remo Lobetti.
© 2018 John Wiley & Sons, Inc. Published 2018 by John Wiley & Sons, Inc.

pulmonary hypertension and pulmonary thromboembolism should be considered. In order to differentiate between these conditions, echocardiography, clotting tests such as thromboelastography and D-dimers, and computed tomography (CT) or CT angiography may be required. In the case of ILDs with subtle radiographic signs, CT may be of great use in diagnosing conditions such as interstitial pulmonary fibrosis (IPF) (Heikkilä-Laurila and Rajamäki 2014). Biomarkers such as serum endothelin 1 and procollagen type III aminoterminal propeptide in BAL fluid have demonstrated some utility in differentiating between IPF and chronic bronchitis (Krafft *et al.* 2011; Heikkilä-Laurila and Rajamäki 2014), but to the author's knowledge, these assays are not yet commercially available. A typical diagnostic clinical conundrum is when to recommend a lung biopsy, when an ILD is suspected. Although incontrovertible recommendations cannot be made, a lung biopsy should only be performed once all other reasonable non-invasive options have been exhausted. The author finds it useful to pursue a lung biopsy in cases where immunosuppression is sought as a therapeutic intervention. Given the generally poor response of IPF to immunosuppression, the author would counsel the client against treating IPF aggressively for long periods of time, in the interests of the patient's quality of life, and this discussion is often best guided when informed by a sound histological report.

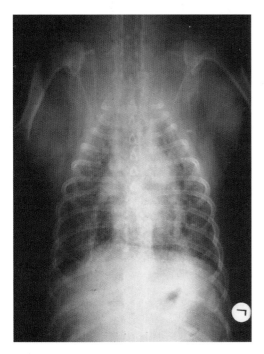

Figure 32.1 Ventro-dorsal thoracic radiograph of 6-year-old dog with pulmonary fibrosis showing advanced interstitial pattern involving all the lung lobes.

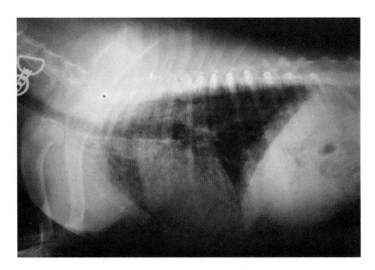

Figure 32.2 Lateral thoracic radiograph of 6-year-old dog with pulmonary fibrosis showing advanced interstitial pattern tending to be bronchial to nodule and involving all the lung fields.

Treatment

Therapy based on a definitive diagnosis is always preferable, and most likely to ensure the best outcome. However, in many cases owners do not have the financial resources to fund all the tests needed to reach a definitive diagnosis. In cases like these, the author explains to owners that manageable ILDs generally respond to antibiotics/antiparasitics or corticosteroids. In rare cases, the author has diagnosed indolent bacterial infections fulminating as ILDs, especially in cats, but it bears mention that irrevocable pulmonary damage had been sustained in these cases. In some cases, especially in cats, if there is heart disease, it may be difficult to exclude cardiac causes of dyspnea without echocardiography, in which case a short trial of diuretics (furosemide) can be tried. Depending on the geographical location, parasitic migration (*Dirofilariasis, Spirocerca lupi, Angiostrongylus vasorum, Paragonimus, Ancylostoma*) may result in interstitial lung disease, and if there is a sufficient index of suspicion, it may be worthwhile treating with an appropriate therapeutic program for each of the aforementioned parasites. Treatment with either a macrocyclic lactone or febendazole may also be warranted as intestinal verminosis may have resulted in pulmonary parasitic migration. Infectious causes of ILDs include viruses (parainfluenza, distemper, adenovirus, influenza), and the vaccination status of the patient should be checked. Bacterial causes of ILD are probably rare, with *Bordetella* and *Mycoplasma* possibly being able to cause ILD. Bacteria may complicate ILDs, especially in cases of viral ILD, and therefore a judicious trial of antibiotics can be considered, if there is a clinical suspicion. In light of growing antibiotic resistance, the use of antibiotics should be carefully considered, and should be reserved for cases in which a reasonable possibility of a bacterial infection exists.

Some cases of ILD, such as eosinophilic bronchopneumopathy (EB), may be exquisitely responsive to corticosteroids. The management of EB is beyond the scope of this chapter and the reader is referred elsewhere for a comprehensive review of the topic (Bexfield *et al.* 2006; Clercx and Peeters 2007; Mesquita *et al.* 2015).

ILDs are commonly associated with pulmonary hypertension (PH), which negatively impacts on the patient's quality of life (Heikkilä-Laurila and Rajamäki 2014). A right-sided heart murmur and exercise intolerance should alert the clinician to the possibility of PH. Radiographic evidence of right heart enlargement, supports the diagnosis of PH, which is usually confirmed with echocardiography. Abrogation or attenuation of PH often significantly improves the patient's quality of life, even though it may not improve overall longevity. Based on the current evidence (which is scant) sildenafil is the drug of choice in managing PH, if the underlying cause cannot be addressed (Brown, Davison, and Sleeper 2010; Wung 2013). Another option is pimobendan, which has phosphodiesterase III inhibitory action. The author has used both of these drugs to manage PH. In the case of ILD such as pulmonary fibrosis the clinician should specifically screen for PH where possible, because it is commonly associated with this condition.

ILDs are typically monitored clinically, as there is limited value in serial evaluation of radiographs, BAL findings, or tissue sampling. Monitoring of the respiratory rate is a particularly useful appraisal of the respiratory system. In addition, reduction in the frequency of coughing (if present) or an improved tolerance of exercise, are also useful clinical indicators of improvement. Ultimately quality of life is the most important factor in the management of ILDs. Clinicians need to guide owners in the assessment of quality of life, as many owners do not have the medical background to appreciate the signs of suffering in their pets, and even compassionate owners may not appreciate the severity of a condition in pets that are still eating, or wag their tail when spoken to. The author finds that getting owners to keep a respiratory rate diary, and if present keeping a record of coughing and exercise tolerance, allows owners to visually track the progress of their pets, and provides objective data, rather than a subjective assessment of quality of life. In the case of PH, the author typically performs a repeat echocardiogram 2 weeks after instituting therapy. However, studies to date have failed to demonstrate the efficacy of drug therapy in reducing the echocardiographic severity of PH, but have shown an improvement in the quality of life, which re-emphasizes the importance of objectively assessing patient comfort as an overarching clinical assessment paradigm.

Quality of Life

The prognosis of ILDs depends very much on the cause and varies from good (in the case of EB and some parasitic ILDs) to dismal (in the case of certain neoplasia and IPF). As the understanding of the pathogenesis of ILDs improves, novel therapies may be developed, but currently the array of drugs available to clinicians is frustratingly limited. Notwithstanding this scenario, careful and systematic management of the clinical consequences of ILDs, such as managing PH and environmental modification can vastly improve the patient's quality of life.

References

Bexfield NH, Foale RD, Davison LJ, Watson PJ, Skelly BJ, Herrtage ME. Management of 13 cases of canine respiratory disease using inhaled corticosteroids. The Journal of Small Animal Practice 2006; 47: 377–382.

Brown AJ, Davison E, Sleeper MM. Clinical efficacy of sildenafil in treatment of pulmonary arterial hypertension in dogs. Journal of Veterinary Internal Medicine. 2010; 24: 850–854.

Clercx C, Peeters D. Canine eosinophilic bronchopneumopathy. Veterinary Clinics of North America: Small Animal Practice. 2007; 37: 917–935, vi.

Heikkilä-Laurila HP, Rajamäki MM. Idiopathic pulmonary fibrosis in West Highland white terriers. Veterinary Clinics of North America: Small Animal Practice. 2014; 44: 129–142.

Krafft E, Heikkilä HP, Jespers P, *et al.* Serum and bronchoalveolar lavage fluid endothelin-1 concentrations as diagnostic biomarkers of canine idiopathic pulmonary fibrosis. Journal of Veterinary Internal Medicine. 2011; 25: 990–996.

Mesquita L, Lam R, Lamb CR, McConnell JF. Computed tomographic findings in 15 dogs with eosinophilic bronchopneumopathy. Veterinary Radiology and Ultrasound. 2015; 56: 33–39.

Reinero C, Cohn L. 2007. Interstitial lung diseases. Veterinary Clinics of North America: Small Animal Practice. 2007; 37: 937–947.

Wung D. Treatment of canine pulmonary arterial hypertension: is tadalafil an appropriate alternative to sildenafil? International Journal of Pharmaceutical Compounding. 2013; 17: 24–27.

33

Feline Asthma

Frank Kettner

Introduction

Feline asthma is a common chronic inflammatory airway disease of the lower respiratory tract and may account for more than 60 % of feline lower respiratory tract diseases (Dye *et al.* 1996; Johnson and Drazenovich 2007; Padrid 2014; Trzil and Reinero 2014). It is estimated to affect between 1–5% of cats of all breeds, ages, and genders, with the Siamese breed reported to have a higher prevalence. The underlying pathogenesis is increased airway mucus production, together with intermittent bronchiolar smooth muscle contraction and bronchoconstriction in response to inhaled aeroallergens or irritants (Reinero 2011; Trzil and Reinero 2014). With time irreversible airway remodeling occurs.

Diagnosis

The single most common (and frequently the only) clinical sign reported by caregivers is chronic coughing (Moise *et al.* 1989; Dye *et al.* 1996; Johnson and Vernau 2011; Lin *et al.* 2015). Wheezing, increased respiratory rate and effort, with or without respiratory distress, may be noted by astute caregivers. Clinical signs have often been present for a prolonged period prior to presentation. Clinical signs may occur sporadically and

show temporary improvement with corticosteroid treatment.

In the mildly affected patient physical examination findings may be unremarkable. In more severely affected cats non-specific findings include respiratory distress, abnormal lung sounds (wheezing, crackles), tachypnea, and increased expiratory effort (Padrid 2014; Trzil and Reinero 2014).

In most instances, the diagnosis is usually a clinical one (i.e., there is no single confirmatory test). A diagnosis is made by combining patient signalment, history, physical examination, and diagnostic findings to complete a clinical picture (Reinero 2011; Lin *et al.* 2015). Excluding differentials is vital in the workup of the asthmatic patient. A full blood count may demonstrate eosinophilia in some cases, but this is neither specific nor sensitive for asthma. Fecal analysis is performed to look for parasites (*Toxocara cati, Aelurostrongylus abtrusus*) that may be associated with eosinophilic airway inflammation (Conboy 2009), and heartworm needs to be excluded in endemic areas. Thoracic radiographs remain the most readily available diagnostic tool; but is neither sensitive (up to 23% of cases may lack radiographic abnormalities) nor specific. It does, however, assist in ruling out differentials (Adamama-Moraitou *et al.* 2004). Thoracic ultrasound in the emergency setting is useful in excluding differentials causing

Chronic Disease Management for Small Animals, First Edition. Edited by W. Dunbar Gram, Rowan J. Milner and Remo Lobetti.
© 2018 John Wiley & Sons, Inc. Published 2018 by John Wiley & Sons, Inc.

respiratory distress and N-terminal pro-BNP can help distinguish congestive heart failure from primary respiratory disease. Bronchoscopy with broncho-alveolar lavage (BAL) for cytological evaluation, polymerase chain reaction (PCR) and culture is performed to exclude other airway diseases (e.g., bacterial bronchopneumonia, parasitic lung disease) (Johnson and Drazenovich 2007; Johnson and Vernau 2011).

Comorbid Conditions, Diagnostic Conundrums, and Differential Diagnoses

Hairballs and reverse sneezing might be mistaken for coughing by caregivers. Taking a thorough history and requesting video footage of the cough should clarify uncertain cases. Investigating respiratory disease involves looking at the entire airway, including the upper respiratory tract.

Asthmatic airway inflammation is typically eosinophilic (with eosinophils >17% on BAL cytology), however a neutrophilic (neutrophils >7%) and mixed inflammatory reaction (eosinophils >17% and neutrophils >7%) may be observed (Johnson and Vernau 2011; Lin *et al.* 2015). Eosinophilic inflammation may be found in other respiratory diseases (e.g., parasitic) as well as with bromide therapy, so this finding is not specific for feline asthma. Additionally, airway inflammation may be non-uniform between varying lung areas and collecting more than one BAL sample is advisable (Johnson and Vernau 2011; Ybarra *et al.* 2012).

Chronic bronchitis differs from feline asthma in that it is primarily a non-degenerative neutrophilic airway inflammatory reaction, which causes airway remodeling and fixed irreversible changes in airway resistance. Differentiating feline asthma from feline chronic bronchitis is challenging (Nafe *et al.* 2010; Reinero 2011; Allerton *et al.* 2013; Trzil and Reinero 2014; Lin *et al.* 2015). Unlike feline asthma, sporadic bronchoconstriction does not occur in chronic bronchitis and bronchodilators are ineffective in resolving respiratory distress (Nafe *et al.* 2010). This differentiates asthma from chronic bronchitis (Trzil and Reinero 2014; Lin *et al.* 2015). There is, however, significant overlap between these two conditions. The history, physical examination, and radiographic features may be similar between the two entities. While differentiating between chronic bronchitis and feline asthma is ideal, it is often difficult in the clinical setting and also probably of limited value until targeted therapies become available for clinical use and are proven to affect outcome. Of clinical significance is the sporadic bronchoconstriction seen in feline asthma, which must be managed as a respiratory emergency. Definitive diagnosis of asthma allows pre-emptive measures to be put in place, such as training caregivers for home emergency treatment. Fortunately, in most cases collecting a good history will provide enough information to discriminate between the two clinical entities. Biomarkers, as a tool of differentiating between various inflammatory lung diseases, remain research tools (Nafe *et al.* 2010; Reinero, Liu, and Chang 2012).

Bacterial pneumonia mimics the respiratory signs seen in asthma. Even the absence of visible intracellular bacteria on BAL cytology does not exclude bacterial pneumonia, necessitating treatment trials in selected cases (Johnson and Vernau 2011). In one study, cats with bacterial pneumonia did not have a BAL eosinophil count >21% (Johnson and Vernau 2011). The role of *Mycoplasma* in feline asthma is uncertain and diagnosing mycoplasma lower respiratory infections is difficult. A 42-day treatment with doxycycline may be appropriate to eliminate this bacterium as a contributing factor, especially in cases that do not undergo lung sampling (Foster and Martin 2011).

Comorbid conditions and complications associated with feline inflammatory lower airway disease include tracheal and bronchial collapse, bronchiectasis, pneumonia, lung lobe torsion, dynamic upper airway obstruction, pulmonary hypertension, and pneumothorax. Further differentials that cause respiratory distress and a change in breathing pattern include pleural effusions, cardiogenic and non-cardiogenic causes of pulmonary edema, and pulmonary fibrosis.

In cases where a complete and thorough workup cannot be undertaken (e.g., caregivers cannot afford or are unwilling to undergo a complete or even a partial investigation, unco-operative patients) a practical approach would include treating for parasites and attempting a therapeutic trial with corticosteroids after the patient's clinical picture has been critically considered. If at all possible, a minimum data-base (blood, urine, and fecal analyses) together with thoracic radiographs should be done. If the clinical picture is consistent with asthma, invasive diagnostics (bronchoscopy with BAL) may not be necessary at initial presentation due to the risks involved (Padrid 2014). A good history and physical examination can go a long way to clinically excluding differentials. The longer the history of coughing, in an oth-erwise healthy cat with a negative examina-tion finding, the greater the probably it has inflammatory lower airway disease; especially considering that feline asthma is one of most common respiratory disorders. A history that is short (days to weeks) in an ill cat is likely to have another diagnosis (e.g., pneumonia) and caregivers should be convinced to undertake some form of diagnostic investigation. Needless to say, this approach is a compro-mise and caregivers must clearly understand the advantages and risks.

Therapeutics

Treatment options are summarized below and have been reviewed in more detail else-where (Hawkins and Papich 2014; Padrid 2014; Trzil and Reinero 2014; Reinero 2015).

Supportive Measures

- Weight loss
- Environmental temperature control
- Avoiding airway irritants
- Regular anthelmintic treatment, heartworm prophylactics in endemic areas, ecto- and endoparasite control.

Medical Therapy

- Oxygen
- Anxiolytics
- Bronchodilators – administrated via inha-lation (metered dose inhaler with face mask or nebulization), parenteral or oral formulations.
- Corticosteroids remain the mainstay of medication used to modulate airway inflam-mation and are considered the primary treatment after emergency stabilization.
- Novel, alternative, or ancillary therapies, which may be beneficial, but with good clinical veterinary evidence lacking:
  - Inhaled lidocaine (Nafe *et al.* 2013)
  - Tyrosine kinase inhibitors (Bellamy *et al.* 2009; Lee-Fowler *et al.* 2012)
  - Omega-3 polyunsaturated fatty acids
  - Stem cell therapy (Trzil *et al.* 2014; Trzil *et al.* 2015)
  - Cyclosporine has been used with success where corticosteroids were not tolerated (Nafe and Leach 2014).
- Allergen specific immunotherapy
- Antibiotics – have no role in either acute or chronic cases of feline inflammatory airway disease, which is primarily a non-infectious disorder. Secondary bacterial infections do on occasion complicate cases, requiring appropriate anti-microbial therapy.
- Heartworm diagnostics and treatment in endemic areas
- Ineffective therapies (Schooley *et al.* 2007; Trzil and Reinero 2014; Grobman *et al.* 2015a, 2015b):
  - Leukotriene inhibitors
  - Cyproheptadine
  - Antihistamines (cetirizine)
  - Inhaled N-acetylcysteine
  - Neurokinin-1 receptor antagonist – maropitant

Approach to the Acute Patient in Crisis

Acute therapy usually refers to treatment of patients presenting with acute respiratory distress or *status asthmaticus*. Emergency therapy includes supplying oxygen and administrating anxiolytics and corticosteroids. Bronchodilators are critical to successful emergency management and asthmatic crises are best treated by using injectable formulations. Antitussives in the acute setting are generally not required as coughing is a marker of the underlying asthmatic disease. Treatments must be administered without excessive physical restraint or exacerbating anxiety, both of which increase oxygen demand and breathing effort in an often extremely compromised and hypoxic patient.

Approach to Chronic Management

Chronic treatment goals are to control the airway inflammation and decrease airway remodeling. Corticosteroids are currently still considered the primary treatment for management of feline asthma, despite their side effects. Oral, injectable, and inhaled formulations have all been used successfully. Inhaled formulations for chronic management carry the least risk of systemic side effects and remain first choice. Not all cats can be controlled with inhaled formulations alone; others will not tolerate this administration route. Bronchodilators are rarely required as an ongoing therapy, but held in reserve for acute episodes of bronchoconstriction. They play no role in managing airway inflammation and should not be used as monotherapy.

Patients have traditionally been started on a high dose of glucocorticoids with treatment being tapered to the lowest effective dose based on resolution of clinical signs (wheezing, increased inspiratory rate and effort, coughing, etc.) together with improvement of radiographic changes. This practice is, however, less than ideal. In cats with controlled clinical signs, up to 70% had persistent sub-clinical airway inflammation based on repeat BAL cytology (Cocayne *et al.* 2011). Additionally, asthma waxes and wanes in severity, making assessment of treatment responses difficult and thoracic radiographs may be normal in a good proportion of asthmatic cats. Best-practice recommendations may develop over time to monitoring treatment success objectively by means of repeat BAL cytology.

Quality of Life

Unless the disease trigger is identified and removed, patient management will, in many cases, be lifelong. The overall prognosis is dependent on how well the airway inflammation and remodeling can be controlled. Patients that fail to improve after 1 month of aggressive appropriate treatment are unlikely to benefit further from extending the same treatment plan. In these cases, the diagnosis should be reconsidered; the therapeutic plan changed (by adding or changing medications); and concurrent morbidities and or complications should be investigated (e.g., is heart disease now present?). Up to a third of cats diagnosed with feline asthma will have some persistent clinical signs despite appropriate treatment. This may be acceptable provided activity levels and breathing are unaffected.

From the caregiver's perspective, coughing, exercise intolerance, weight loss, and respiratory distress are the signs perceived to be affecting patient quality of life. Rarely does coughing affect the patient's quality of life directly and cough suppressants are generally not needed, especially after corticosteroid use has been initiated. *Status asthmaticus* is life threatening and severely distressing to both patient and caregiver. Caregiver anxiety is best addressed by training and helping clients become comfortable with emergency home treatment measures (e.g., bronchodilator therapy).

Managing feline asthma is a lifelong commitment. Treatment options are stressful in some cats which may affect the human-animal bond. Treatment formulations should be discussed and tailored to the individual patient and client needs and abilities. Although least ideal, depot formulations of glucocorticoids remain a practical solution in those cats that cannot be pilled or where the owner is unwilling to invest the time and effort required for effective management.

Cats that have persistent respiratory distress or hypoxia will show weight loss, decreased appetite, and become withdrawn and inactive. Individuals with treatment failure will be poorly responsive to treatment (glucocorticoids and bronchodilators) and respiratory difficulty/hypoxia will persist despite appropriate medications, increasing dosages, rescue therapies, and treatment duration. Severely affected cats (or those that cannot be treated) in treatment failure, where even mild activity induces respiratory distress, should be considered for euthanasia.

References

Adamama-Moraitou KK, Patsikas MN, Koutinas AF. Feline lower airway disease: a retrospective study of 22 naturally occurring cases from Greece. Journal of Feline Medicine and Surgery. 2004; 6: 227–233.

Allerton FJW, Leemans J, Tual C, Bernaerts F, Kirschvink N, Clercx C. Correlation of bronchoalveolar eosinophilic percentage with airway responsiveness in cats with chronic bronchial disease. Journal of Small Animal Practice. 2013; 54: 258–264.

Bellamy F, Bader T, Moussy A, Hermine O. Pharmacokinetics of masitinib in cats. Veterinary Research Communications. 2009; 33: 831–837.

Cocayne CG, Reinero CR, Declue AE. Subclinical airway inflammation despite high-dose oral corticosteroid therapy in cats with lower airway disease. Journal of Feline Medicine and Surgery. 2011; 13: 558–563.

Conboy G. Helminth parasites of the canine and feline respiratory tract. Veterinary Clinics of North America: Small Animal Practice. 2009; 39: 1109–1126.

Dye JA, Mckiernan BC, Rozanski EA, et al. Bronchopulmonary disease in the cat: historical, physical, radiographic, clinicopathologic, and pulmonary functional evaluation of 24 affected and 15 healthy cats. Journal of Veterinary Internal Medicine. 1996; 10: 385–400.

Foster SF, Martin P. Lower respiratory tract infections in cats: reaching beyond empirical therapy. Journal of Feline Medicine and Surgery. 2011; 13: 313–332.

Grobman M, Graham A, Outi H, Dodam JR, Reinero CR. Chronic neurokinin-1 receptor antagonism fails to ameliorate clinical signs, airway hyper-responsiveness or airway eosinophilia in an experimental model of feline asthma. Journal of Feline Medicine and Surgery. 2015a; 18(4): 273–279.

Grobman M, Krumme S, Outi H, Dodam JR, Reinero C R. Acute neurokinin-1 receptor antagonism fails to dampen airflow limitation or airway eosinophilia in an experimental model of feline asthma. Journal of Feline Medicine and Surgery. (2015b) 18(2) 176–181.

Hawkins EC, Papich MG. Respiratory drug therapy. In: J Bonagura and D Twedt, Eds. Kirk's Current Veterinary Therapy XV. Saunders Elsevier. 2014: 622–628.

Johnson LR, Drazenovich TL. Flexible bronchoscopy and bronchoalveolar lavage in 68 cats (2001–2006). Journal of Veterinary Internal Medicine. 2007; 21: 219–225.

Johnson LR, Vernau W. Bronchoscopic findings in 48 cats with spontaneous lower respiratory tract disease (2002–2009). Journal of Veterinary Internal Medicine. 2011; 25: 236–243.

Lee-Fowler TM, Guntur V, Dodam J, Cohn LA, Declue AE, Reinero CR. The tyrosine kinase inhibitor masitinib blunts airway inflammation and improves associated lung mechanics in a feline model of chronic allergic asthma. International Archives of Allergy and Immunology. 2012; 158: 369–374.

Lin CH, Wu HD, Lee JJ, Liu CH. Functional phenotype and its correlation with therapeutic response and inflammatory type of bronchoalveolar lavage fluid in feline lower airway disease. Journal of Veterinary Internal Medicine. 2015; 29: 88–96.

Moise NS, Wiedenkeller D, Yeager AE, Blue JT, Scarlett J. Clinical, radiographic, and bronchial cytologic features of cats with bronchial disease: 65 cases (1980–1986). Journal of the American Veterinary Medical Association. 1989; 194: 1467–1473.

Nafe LA, Leach SB. Treatment of feline asthma with ciclosporin in a cat with diabetes mellitus and congestive heart failure. Journal of Feline Medicine and Surgery. 2014; 17(12): 1073–1076.

Nafe LA, Declue AE, Lee-Fowler TM, Eberhardt JM, Reinero CR. Evaluation of biomarkers in bronchoalveolar lavage fluid for discrimination between asthma and chronic bronchitis in cats. American Journal of Veterinary Research. 2010; 71: 583–591.

Nafe LA, Guntur VP, Dodam JR, Lee-Fowler TM, Cohn LA, Reinero CR. Nebulized lidocaine blunts airway hyper-responsiveness in experimental feline asthma. Journal of Feline Medicine and Surgery. 2013; 15: 712–716.

Padrid PA. Chronic bronchitis and asthma in cats. In: J Bonagura and D Twedt, Eds. Kirk's Current Veterinary Therapy XV. Saunders Elsevier. 2014: 673–680.

Reinero C. Management of feline inflammatory airway diseases. ACVIM Forum, 2015.

Reinero CR. Advances in the understanding of pathogenesis, and diagnostics and therapeutics for feline allergic asthma. The Veterinary Journal. 2011; 190: 28–33.

Reinero CR, Liu H, Chang CH. Flow cytometric determination of allergen-specific T lymphocyte proliferation from whole blood in experimentally asthmatic cats. Veterinary Immunology and Immunopathology. 2012; 149: 1–5.

Schooley EK, Turner JB, Jiji RD, Spinka CM, Reinero CR. Effects of cyproheptadine and cetirizine on eosinophilic airway inflammation in cats with experimentally induced asthma. American Journal of Veterinary Research. 2007; 68: 1265–1271.

Trzil JE, Reinero CR. Update on feline asthma. Veterinary Clinics of North America: Small Animal Practice. 2014; 44: 91–105.

Trzil JE, Masseau I, Webb TL, et al. Long-term evaluation of mesenchymal stem cell therapy in a feline model of chronic allergic asthma. Clinical and Experimental Allergy. 2014; 44: 1546–1557.

Trzil JE, Masseau I, Webb TL, et al. Intravenous adipose-derived mesenchymal stem cell therapy for the treatment of feline asthma: a pilot study. Journal of Feline Medicine and Surgery 2015; 18(12): 981–990.

Ybarra WL, Johnson LR, DrazenovichTL, Johnson EG, Vernau W. Interpretation of multisegment bronchoalveolar lavage in cats (1/2001–1/2011). Journal of Veterinary Internal Medicine. 2012; 26: 1281–1287.

34

Collapsing Trachea

Frank Kettner

Introduction

Tracheal collapse is a common respiratory condition in which progressive dorso-ventral flattening of the trachea occurs with consequential collapse of the airway lumen. A part of or the whole trachea may be involved. The exact cause is unknown, and is most likely multifactorial, but chondromalacia of the tracheal rings has been documented as a mechanism (Herrtage 2009; Maggiore 2013). Bronchomalacia or bronchial collapse may occur concurrently or in isolation and airway collapse in dogs is frequently associated with non-infectious inflammatory airway disease (e.g., eosinophilic bronchopneumopathy). The exact relationship between tracheal and bronchial collapse is unclear. Airway collapse induces and perpetuates secondary changes such as airway inflammation, mucus secretion, and decreased mucociliary clearance, all of which complicates overall management (Sun *et al.* 2008; Maggiore 2013). In mild cases, tracheal collapse may be asymptomatic. As the condition progresses, or an inciting trigger factor is encountered; it is associated with coughing, loss of airway function, and respiratory distress. Tracheal collapse rarely affects cats, but when present it is typically associated with inflammatory airway disease (Johnson and Vernau 2011).

Diagnosis

The typical patient is a middle aged to elderly small or toy breed dog presenting with a classical goose honking cough as the primary complaint. A prolonged history (months to years) is common and useful in distinguishing tracheal collapse from differentials. Caregivers may observe exercise intolerance, respiratory distress, and/or cyanosis with or without syncope in more severely affected animals.

A nonspecific harsh honking cough is frequently elicited by tracheal palpation. Respiration and lung sounds may be normal or abnormal, especially if concomitant lung disease is present. In some patients, the tracheal collapse may be palpable in the neck region. Increased airway noises are potentially audible in severely collapsed tracheas and increased respiratory effort may be observed. Hepatomegaly may be palpated.

Tracheoscopy remains the gold standard diagnostic modality (Johnson, Singh, and Pollard 2015). Figure 34.1 shows a tracheoscopy from a dog with tracheal collapse. While most practitioners have access to thoracic radiographs; falsely diagnosing or excluding the condition with this diagnostic modality is not uncommon (Johnson and Pollard 2010; Johnson *et al.* 2015; Lindl Bylicki, Johnson, and Pollard 2015). When available, fluoroscopy may show the dynamic

Chronic Disease Management for Small Animals, First Edition. Edited by W. Dunbar Gram, Rowan J. Milner and Remo Lobetti.

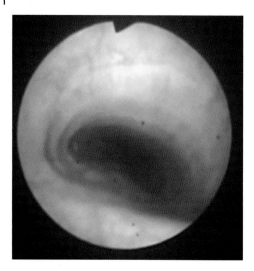

Figure 34.1 Tracheoscopy from a dog with tracheal collapse.

changes of the tracheal diameter during the respiratory cycle, aiding diagnosis with a greater accuracy than radiography. The use of ultrasound has also been reported, but remains an ancillary diagnostic tool that is surpassed by the other modalities (Rudorf, Herrtage, and White 1997; Eom *et al.* 2008). Computed tomography and tidal breathing flow-volume loop analysis have also been able to document tracheal collapse but remain largely available only in referral practices. Echocardiography and broncho-alveolar lavage are not useful in the diagnosis of tracheal collapse *per se*, but are frequently performed as part of a holistic cardio-respiratory system investigation, especially considering the association between inflammatory airway disease and tracheal/airway collapse (Singh *et al.* 2012; Zhu, Johnson, and Vernau 2015).

Comorbid Conditions, Diagnostic Conundrums, and Differential Diagnoses

Comorbid conditions include concurrent bronchial collapse, laryngeal paralysis, and bronchiectasis (Bottero *et al.* 2013, Johnson and Pollard 2010; Chisnell and Pardo 2015). Airway inflammatory changes as determined by BAL cytology is seen in a large proportion of dogs with airway collapse (Johnson and Pollard 2010; Singh *et al.* 2012), but whether there is a causal relation, or whether it represents a concurrent, but independent condition, requires further investigation. Ideally, all patients investigated for collapsing airway disease should also be investigated for chronic bronchitis or inflammatory airway disease.

Patients with tracheal and bronchial collapse potentially have decreased mucociliary clearance mechanisms, leading to increased risk for secondary bacterial bronchitis and bronchopneumonia; although concurrent airway infections in newly diagnosed cases of tracheal collapse is not a common finding (Johnson and Pollard 2010). Acute infectious tracheobronchitis may be mistaken for tracheal collapse and patients with tracheal collapse can become infected with *Bordetella bronchiseptica*.

Mitral valve regurgitation caused by myxomatous degeneration may result in coughing as a result of left atrial enlargement with compression of the left main stem bronchi without the dog being in congestive heart failure. The collapsing trachea patient in congestive heart failure is expected to have an increased sleeping respiratory rate; and increased serum NT-proBNP concentrations help differentiate cardiac causes of respiratory signs from respiratory diseases (Oyama *et al.* 2009; Schober *et al.* 2010; Rishniw *et al.* 2012; Ferasin *et al.* 2013). Respiratory sinus arrhythmia is not expected in a patient with congestive heart failure, but may be present in a dog with tracheal collapse and mitral valve regurgitation not in heart failure. Pulmonary hypertension may complicate airway collapse (Bottero *et al.* 2013) and would need to be addressed as a comorbid condition.

Up to 55 % of dogs may have a co-associated condition at the onset of clinical signs (White and Williams 1994).

Therapeutics

Treatment is aimed at relieving immediate respiratory distress, managing acute and persistent coughing, and addressing underlying co-existing or exacerbating factors (e.g., concurrent congestive heart failure or laryngeal paralysis). These have been reviewed in more detail elsewhere (Sun *et al.* 2008 ; Herrtage 2009; Maggiore 2013; Hawkins and Papich 2014; Scansen and Weisse 2014).

Supportive Measures

- Avoiding collars
- Weight loss
- Environmental temperature control and humidification
- Avoiding airway irritants
- Minimizing anxiety
- Controlled exercise – provided it is does not cause coughing or respiratory distress
- Management of concurrent diseases.

Medical Treatments

- Oxygen therapy
- Anxiolytics (opioids, acepromazine, trazodone, or others)
- Antitussives
  - Opioids (butorphanol, hydrocodone, and others)
  - Nebulized lignocaine and furosemide (reported in human medicine but very little literature in veterinary medicine)
- Corticosteroids (Parental, oral, and inhaled)
- Bronchodilators – no proven benefits, but have traditionally been used and are recommended in texts. A therapeutic trial can be attempted.
- Antibiotics. Tracheal collapse is a non-infectious disorder thus no need for antibiotics unless bacterial infections complicate the case.
- Experimental treatment
  - Stanozolol (Adamama-Moraitou *et al.* 2011)

- Unproved/ineffective/low evidence based therapies (although often used in practice)
  - Doxycycline (unless susceptible infectious airway disease is present)
  - Polysulfated glycosaminoglycan
  - Neurokinin-1 receptor antagonist – maropitant (Grobman *et al.* 2015a; Grobman *et al.* 2015b)

Surgical Options (Sun *et al.* 2008; Chisnell and Pardo 2015)

- External tracheal ring prostheses
- Intraluminal stent.
- Procedures largely replaced by the above
  - Dorsal tracheal ligament plication
  - Tracheal ring chondrotomy
  - Prosthetic polypropylene mesh reconstruction

The Asymptomatic Patient

When tracheal collapse is identified incidentally, or as asymptomatic disease (those with only the occasional spontaneous cough and without respiratory compromise) treatment is usually not required. Emphasis is placed on addressing concurrent co-associated disorders (e.g., chronic bronchitis) and supportive measures. Confirming the diagnosis in this group of patients by tracheoscopy is unlikely to change the treatment.

The Coughing Patient Without Respiratory Compromise

Medical management as an outpatient is usually sufficient. The diagnostic and therapeutic approach is aimed at diagnosing collapsing trachea; identifying associated disorders; and addressing and applying supportive measures, including antitussives. Glucocorticoids, preferably inhaled formulations, remain central to controlling secondary airway inflammation and coughing, especially with the evidence that bronchomalacia is associated with chronic inflammatory airway disease. Corticosteroids are titrated to the lowest effective dose. Initial clinical improvement with medical therapy can be expected in over two-thirds of patients (White and Williams 1994).

The (Coughing or Noncoughing) Patient with Respiratory Compromise

Generally, these patients have been previously diagnosed and are already on treatment. Medical and supportive management has been applied, but is no longer effective. Respiratory distress may be episodic, resolving spontaneously, or severe and persistent with the patient presenting as a respiratory emergency, severely compromised. Immediate treatment goals are aimed at decreasing the breathing rate and effort by supportive measures, such as cooling, and medical treatment. These include oxygen therapy, decreasing anxiety (i.e., decreasing hyperventilation), antitussive therapy (coughing exacerbates airway collapse), short-acting glucocorticoids, bronchodilators when bronchoconstriction is a comorbid problem, and providing ventilator support when *in extremis* by means of intubation with positive pressure ventilation (PPV). It is important to note that supplying oxygen by facemask or oxygen chambers may have limited success in patients with severe tracheal collapse as these animals are unable to ventilate and move oxygen enriched air into the lungs.

Patients that require PPV will mostly require a surgical solution. If PPV is not available, then endotracheal intubation will be necessary. Placing an oxygen delivering feeding tube through an endotracheal tube to the level of the carina will bypass tracheal (but not bronchial) collapse. Unless a stent is readily available for placement or the precipitating factor that induced ventilation failure can be rapidly corrected (e.g., severe panting due to heat stroke), intubation and ventilation will not aid long-term survival and euthanasia should be considered. While PPV is not ideal; it may provide a sufficient bridge in those dogs that have an acute reversible exacerbating factor.

In patients with episodic airway compromise, managing the *whole* airway is crucial. Diagnosing and correcting problems that increase airway resistance (such a chronic rhinitis, narrow nares, elongated soft palate, laryngeal collapse, everted laryngeal ventricles, and chronic lower airway inflammatory disease) will alleviate airway collapse by decreasing the effort required to breathe, without directly affecting the underlying tracheal collapse, and hopefully delaying the need for surgical intervention.

When respiratory compromise progresses or becomes refractory, surgical options remain the only means of providing relief in cases of airway collapse (Sun *et al.* 2008). Failure to administer medication is not a valid reason to seek surgical solutions, as most animals will require additional medical management afterwards.

Quality of Life

Respiratory distress and coughing are the two main signs that affect patient quality of life (QOL) in animals with tracheal collapse. Persistent coughing is likely to cause tracheal pain or discomfort in addition to the irritation. Additionally, obstructive airway episodes may be trigged by coughing. Controlling coughing should be a primary treatment goal in addressing QOL. Severe intractable coughing is a trigger for end-of-life discussions.

Airway obstruction is an extremely distressing experience and with time becomes progressively more frequent and severe, eventually resulting in hypoxic syncope episodes, which may be fatal. Between obstructive episodes patient QOL may be reasonable; however, obstructive episodes may be episodic and unpredictable. In early stages, obstruction may be mild, such that patient distress is minimal and short lived. At this point treatment options not yet addressed, or poorly implemented, must be explored and optimized. Once respiratory distress is severe and cannot be controlled (due to financial reasons or otherwise) end of life should be discussed with the caregiver.

Many caregivers experience helplessness when they are unable to provide relief to their pets' coughing attacks or respiratory distress. Alternatively, clients may be willing, but unable to provide treatment for various reasons, such as cost. Intraluminal tracheal stents cost in the excess of $1000, excluding placement, and caregivers may feel guilt at not being able to afford treatment. The unpredictable nature of coughing or airway obstruction can elevate the anxiety of the caregiver. Some caregivers will request euthanasia due to intractable coughing.

Euthanasia should be advised whenever respiratory distress cannot be controlled or relieved by the combination of supportive, medical and surgical treatment options. When airway obstruction is severe, prolonged or frequent; quality of life is poor and should prompt euthanasia.

References

Adamama-Moraitou KK, Pardali D, Athanasiou LV, Prassinos NN, Kritsepi M, Rallis TS. Conservative management of canine tracheal collapse with stanozolol: a double blinded, placebo control clinical trial. International Journal of Immunopathology and Pharmacology. 2011; 24: 111–118.

Bottero E, Bellino C, Lorenzi D, Ruggiero P, Tarducci A, D'angelo A, Gianella P. Clinical evaluation and endoscopic classification of bronchomalacia in dogs. Journal of Veterinary Internal Medicine. 2013; 27: 840–846.

Chisnell HK, Pardo AD. Long-term outcome, complications and disease progression in 23 dogs after placement of tracheal ring prostheses for treatment of extrathoracic tracheal collapse. Veterinary Surgery. 2015; 44: 103–113.

Eom K, Moon K, Seong Y, et al. Ultrasonographic evaluation of tracheal collapse in dogs. Journal of Veterinary Science. 2008; 9: 401–405.

Ferasin L, Crews L, Biller DS, Lamb KE, Borgarelli M. Risk factors for coughing in dogs with naturally acquired myxomatous mitral valve disease. Journal of Veterinary Internal Medicine. 2013; 27: 286–292.

Grobman M, Graham A, Outi H, Dodam JR, Reinero CR. Chronic neurokinin-1 receptor antagonism fails to ameliorate clinical signs, airway hyper-responsiveness or airway eosinophilia in an experimental model of feline asthma. Journal of Feline Medicine and Surgery. 2015a; 18(4): 273–279.

Grobman M, Krumme S, Outi H, Dodam JR, Reinero C R. Acute neurokinin-1 receptor antagonism fails to dampen airflow limitation or airway eosinophilia in an experimental model of feline asthma. Journal of Feline Medicine and Surgery. 2015b; 18(2): 176–181.

Hawkins EC, Papich MG. Respiratory drug therapy. In: J. Bonagura and D. Twedt, Eds. Kirk's current veterinary therapy XV. Saunders Elsevier. 2014: 622–628.

Herrtage ME. Medical management of tracheal collapse. In: J Bonagura and D Twedt, Eds. Kirk's current veterinary therapy XIV. Elsevier. 2009: 630–635.

Johnson LR, Pollard RE. Tracheal collapse and bronchomalacia in dogs: 58 cases (7/2001–1/2008). Journal of Veterinary Internal Medicine. 2010; 24: 298–305.

Johnson LR, Vernau W. Bronchoscopic findings in 48 cats with spontaneous lower respiratory tract disease (2002–2009). Journal of Veterinary Internal Medicine. 2011; 25: 236–243.

Johnson LR, Singh MK, Pollard RE. Agreement among radiographs, fluoroscopy and bronchoscopy in documentation of airway collapse in dogs. Journal of Veterinary Internal Medicine. 2015; 29: 1619–1626.

Lindl Bylicki BJ, Johnson LR, Pollard RE. Comparison of the radiographic and tracheoscopic appearance of the dorsal tracheal membrane in large and small breed dogs. Veterinary Radiology and Ultrasound. 2015; 56(6):602–608.

Maggiore A. Tracheal and airway collapse in dogs. Veterinary Clinics of North America: Small Animal Practice. 2013; 44: 117–127.

Oyama MA, Rush JE, Rozanski EA, et al. Assessment of serum N-terminal pro-B-type natriuretic peptide concentration for differentiation of congestive heart failure from primary respiratory tract disease as the cause of respiratory signs in dogs. Journal of the American Veterinary Medical Association. 2009; 235: 1319–1325.

Rishniw M, Ljungvall I, Porciello F, Haggstrom J, Ohad DG. Sleeping respiratory rates in apparently healthy adult dogs. Research in Veterinary Science. 2012; 93: 965–969.

Rudorf H, Herrtage ME, White RA. Use of ultrasonography in the diagnosis of tracheal collapse. Journal of Small Animal Practice. 1997; 38: 513–518.

Scansen BA, Weisse C. Tracheal collapse. In: J Bonagura and D Twedt, Eds. Kirk's current veterinary therapy XV. Saunders Elsevier. 2014: 663–668

Schober KE, Hart TM, Stern JA, et al. Detection of congestive heart failure in dogs by Doppler echocardiography. Journal of Veterinary Internal Medicine. 2010: 24: 1358–1368.

Singh MK, Johnson LR, Kittleson MD, Pollard RE. Bronchomalacia in dogs with myxomatous mitral valve degeneration. Journal of Veterinary Internal Medicine. 2012; 26: 312–319.

Sun F, Uson J, Ezquerra J, Crisostomo V, Luis L, Maynar M. Endotracheal stenting therapy in dogs with tracheal collapse. The Veterinary Journal. 2008; 175: 186–193.

White RAS, Williams JM. Tracheal collapse in the dog – is there really a role for surgery? A survey of 100 cases. Journal of Small Animal Practice. 1994; 35: 191–196.

Zhu BY, Johnson LR, Vernau W. Tracheobronchial brush cytology and bronchoalveolar lavage in dogs and cats with chronic cough: 45 ases (2012–2014). Journal of Veterinary Internal Medicine. 2015; 29: 526–532.

35

Allergic Rhinitis
Remo Lobetti

Introduction

Chronic nasal disease can be a common problem in dogs, with clinical signs being a combination of sneezing, nasal discharge, epistaxis, nasal stertor, paroxysmal reverse sneezing, coughing, halitosis, open-mouth breathing, facial deformities, facial pain, discoloration of the nares, and exophthalmos (Burgener, Slocombe, and Zerbe 1987; Tasker *et al.* 1999). Various diseases of the nasal cavity present with similar clinical signs, with no one-sign being pathognomonic for any particular disease (Davidson, Mathews, and Koblik 2000), rendering clinical diagnosis difficult.

Common causes of chronic nasal disease in dogs are neoplasia, fungal rhinitis, and idiopathic lympho-plasmacytic rhinitis (LPR), the latter also referred to as inflammatory rhinitis (Bolln *et al.* 2003; Davidson *et al.* 2000; Meler, Dunn, and Lecuyer 2000; Tasker *et al.* 1999; Windsor and Johnson; 2006). Other less common causes include nasal foreign body, rhinitis secondary to dental disease, parasitic rhinitis (*Pneumonyssoides caninum*), and primary ciliary dyskinesia (Pownder, Rose, and Crawford 2006).

In dogs, idiopathic LPR is frequently presented with clinical signs typical of other chronic nasal diseases (Lobetti 2014; Windsor *et al.* 2004). Idiopathic LPR is characterized microscopically by the infiltration of lymphocytes and plasma cells within the nasal mucosa; although variable numbers of neutrophils and eosinophils may also be present (Mackin 2004; Windsor *et al.* 2004). Histologically, idiopathic LPR closely resembles the human non-polyploid chronic rhinosinusitis (CRS), where nasal tissue infiltration is dominated by lymphocytes and neutrophils, with eosinophilic inflammation being of minor importance (Rudack, Sachse, and Alberty 2004). The definitive cause of idiopathic LPR is unknown, with speculated hypotheses being chronic inflammatory response to infectious agents, high microbial load, inhaled irritant, pollutant, immune dysregulation, or aeroallergens (Burgener *et al.* 1987; Mackin 2004; Windsor *et al.* 2004; Windsor and Johnson 2006).

Idiopathic LPR is an important and common cause of chronic nasal disease in dogs with clinical signs similar to those of other chronic nasal disorders. In one study, idiopathic LPR was diagnosed in 30% of cases (Lobetti 2014).

Diagnosis

Idiopathic LPR is generally a disease of middle-aged to older dogs (Lobetti 2014; Burgener *et al.* 1987; Windsor *et al.* 2004) with a predilection for the Dachshund, Yorkshire Terrier, and German shepherd dog (Lobetti 2014; Windsor *et al.* 2004). Common clinical findings are mucoid nasal

Chronic Disease Management for Small Animals, First Edition. Edited by W. Dunbar Gram, Rowan J. Milner and Remo Lobetti.

discharge and stertor and occasionally epistaxis. (Lobetti 2014; Tasker *et al.* 1999; Windsor *et al.* 2004). Typical radiographic changes are opacification of the nasal passages with nasal turbinate destruction being uncommon (Lobetti 2014; Burgener *et al.* 1987; Tasker *et al.* 1999). Contrast-enhanced CT and MRI show a patchy inflammatory response with either no or mild conchal destruction.

Rhinoscopy often shows hyperemic and swollen nasal mucous membranes (Figure 35.1a and Figure 35.1b) and the accumulation of mucoid material within the nasal passages (Lobetti 2014; Tasker *et al.* 1999); with plaque-like lesions (Lent and Hawkins 1992) and mass-like lesions (Willard and Radlinksy 1999) also reported.

The diagnosis of idiopathic LPR is made on finding a lymphoplasmacytic infiltration within the nasal mucosa on histopathology, absence of fungi and pathogenic bacteria on culture, and resolution of the rhinitis with systemic corticosteroids and/or cyclosporine therapy, and/or topical corticosteroid therapy, and/or desensitization therapy; without the use of any antibiotic therapy.

Therapy

Long-term administration of antibiotics (doxycycline) together with glucocorticoids (oral or topical) and/or non-steroidal anti-inflammatory agents usually control the condition, but recurrence following cessation of medication is common. Generally speaking the best response to therapy is seen in the dogs that undergo desensitization therapy (complete resolution), followed by corticosteroids and cyclosporine (marked reduction and duration of response). Doses for cortisone and cyclosporine are 1 mg/kg SID and 3–5 mg/kg SID, respectively. If the dog will tolerate a spray, intra-nasal cortisone spray would be the best for long-term treatment. In dogs where only corticosteroids are used, clinical signs are merely controlled and tend to return once the corticosteroids are discontinued. The use of antibiotics appears to be neither effective nor sustained in eliminating clinical signs but helps to reduce the

(a) (b)

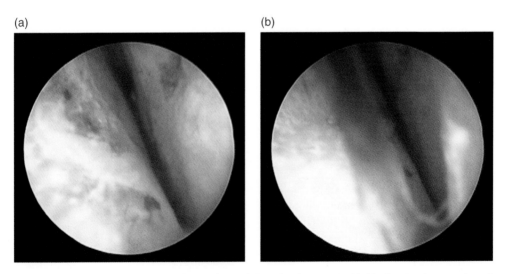

Figure 35.1(a, b) Rhinoscopy image from a dog with lymphoplasmacytic rhinitis showing hyperemic and swollen nasal mucous membranes.

nasal discharge and the type in some dogs – from a muco-purulent to serous. Thus, it is most likely that antibiotics merely reduce secondary bacterial colonization without diminishing the nasal discharge caused by idiopathic LPR (Windsor *et al.* 2004). In people with CRS and allergic rhinitis the use of topical corticosteroids is more beneficial than antihistamines and antibiotics for achieving symptomatic improvement both in children and adults, with systemic corticosteroids indicated in severe cases (Mori *et al.* 2010).

Idiopathic LPR needs to be managed with long-term corticosteroids and cyclosporine therapy if the underlying triggers are not identified and suppressed with desensitization therapy.

Quality of Life

The perceived changes are often best observed from the owner and not from the dog as with idiopathic LPR pain and/or discomfort is not obvious, there is no loss of function, and there are no overt cosmetic changes. It is important that the owner is fully educated in the disease and that treatment at best is aimed at some form of control rather that cure and that clinical signs may well be life-long for the dog. Despite the poor long-term response, idiopathic LPR is unlikely to result in the death of the dog.

References

Bolln G, Wölk U, Bausch M, Kresken JG, Höptner C. Retrospective study of 143 cases (1997–2001) of chronic nasal discharge in the dog and cat. Praktische Tierarzt. 2003; 84: 742–751.

Burgener DC, Slocombe RF, Zerbe CA. Lymphoplasmacytic rhinitis in five dogs. Journal of the American Animal Hospital Association. 1987; 23: 565–568.

Davidson AP, Mathews KG, Koblik PD. Diseases of the nose and nasal sinuses. In: SJ Ettinger, Ed. Textbook of veterinary internal medicine, 5th edn. WB Saunders. 2000: 1003–1025.

Lent SE, Hawkins EC. Evaluation of rhinoscopy and rhinoscopy-associated mucosal biopsy in diagnosis of nasal disease in dogs: 119 cases (1985–1989). Journal of the American Veterinary Medical Association 1992; 201: 1425–1429.

Lobetti RG. Idiopathic lymphoplasmacytic rhinitis in 33 dogs. Journal of the South African Veterinary Association. 2014; 85(1): 1–5.

Mackin A. Lymphoplasmacytic rhinitis. In: LG King, Ed. Respiratory diseases in dogs and cats. WB Saunders. 2004: 305–310.

Meler E, Dunn M, Lecuyer M. A retrospective study of canine persistent nasal disease: 80 cases (1998-2003). Canadian Veterinary Journal. 2000; 49: 71–76.

Mori F, Barni S, Pucci N, Rossi ME. Orsi Battaglini C, Novembre E. Upper airway disease: role of corticosteroids. International Journal of Immunopathology and Pharmacology. 2010; 23, 61–66.

Powder S, Rose M, Crawford R. Radiographic techniques of the nasal cavity and sinuses. Clinical Techniques in Small Animal Practice. 2006; 21: 46–54.

Willard MD, Radlinksy MA. Endoscopic examination of the choanae in dogs and cats: 118 cases (1988–1998). Journal of the American Veterinary Medical Association. 1999; 215: 1301–1305.

Rudack C, Sachse F, Alberty J. Chronic rhinosinusitis – need for further classification? Inflammatory Research. 2004; 53: 111–117.

Tasker S, Knottenbelt CM, Munro EAC, Stonehewer J, Simpson JW, Mackin AJ.

Aetiology and diagnosis of persistent nasal disease in the dog: a retrospective study of 42 cases. Journal Small Animal Practice. 1999; 40: 473–478.

Windsor RC, Johnson LR, Herrgesell EJ, De Cock, HE, Idiopathic lymphoplasmacytic rhinitis in dogs: 37 cases (1997–2002). Journal of the American Veterinary Medical Association. 2004; 224: 1952–1957.

Windsor RC, Johnson LC. Canine chronic inflammatory rhinitis. Clinical Techniques in Small Animal Practice. 2006; 21: 76–81.

Further Reading

Willemse A. Canine atopic disease: investigations of eosinophils and the nasal mucosa. American Journal of Veterinary Research. 1984; 45: 1867–1869.

Part Three

End of Life

36

Hospice Care and End of Life

Mary Gardner

Hospice Care

As hard as we may try to thwart the progression of disease and the aging process, there comes a time when we simply need to care for the pet (and the owner) and provide the best quality of life possible regardless of the quantity of time left. This is when veterinary hospice services are best utilized. The term hospice has a Latin derivative stemming word *hospitium*, which means to host. Hospice for humans has been around for centuries as a place of hospitality for the sick, wounded, or dying. The more modern concept of hospice is a type of care that focuses on the palliation of pain and symptoms of a terminally or chronically ill patient which could occur in the hospital, nursing home, or in the patient's home (Figure 36.1) or in the home of family members. Within the veterinary world, hospice is still very much misunderstood.

Some define veterinary hospice as a medically supervised service dedicated to providing comfort and quality of life for the pet (and the owners) until euthanasia is elected or natural death occurs. It is important to understand that hospice is not prolonging suffering nor is it intended to preclude euthanasia. The AVMA has established guidelines for Veterinary Hospice Care and states that if the practice is consistent with veterinary practice acts, veterinary hospice gives clients time to make decisions regarding a companion animal with a terminal illness or condition and to prepare for the pending death of the animal (AVMA 2017).

Hospice does not mean you stop treatment for the pet or even possible curable options. Take the case of Romeo. Romeo was a male, neutered, 12-year-old domestic short hair, cat with a 2-month history of vomiting and diarrhea also exhibiting signs of decreased appetite and dehydration; Romeo was just not "himself." After being diagnosed with intestinal lymphoma by the primary care veterinarian, the caregiver was told that not much could be done for Romeo besides supportive care and steroids which they had already started. Romeo's caregiver Anthony reached out to me for hospice care and advice on quality-of-life assessment. After examination of Romeo (Figure 36.2) and a long conversation with Anthony, I suggested a consultation with an oncologist since the owner was willing to do anything for Romeo. I felt that minimally we could get a better idea of length of time left and to give Anthony the opportunity for other treatment options from an expert. He followed my suggestion and took Romeo to the oncologist the next day and Romeo was started on chemotherapy right away. Anthony however knew that chemotherapy may not work so he wanted to continue hospice care. I worked in tandem with the oncologist, providing updates from

Chronic Disease Management for Small Animals, First Edition. Edited by W. Dunbar Gram, Rowan J. Milner and Remo Lobetti.
© 2018 John Wiley & Sons, Inc. Published 2018 by John Wiley & Sons, Inc.

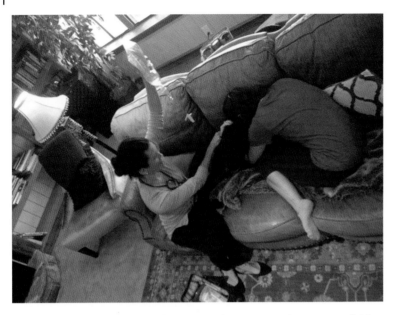

Figure 36.1 Dr. Dani McVety teaching owners how to give sub-cutaneous fluids to a terminally ill patient. (Courtesy of Dr. Dani McVety.)

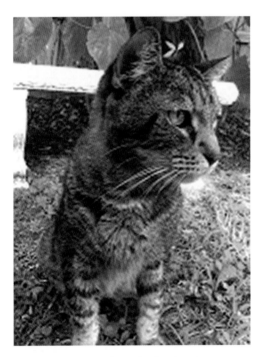

Figure 36.2 Romeo during his first hospice appointment.

the home visits, changing supportive care protocols when needed and helping Anthony with quality-of-life assessments and preparing him for the eventual euthanasia.

Four months later, Romeo was doing really well and his quality of life was actually great. He was the first hospice patient that I happily suspended from hospice care. Almost 30 months later, Anthony reached out to us again and this time it was to help say goodbye to Romeo. We provided a peaceful passing in his home with no regrets. The reason I tell you about this case is to exemplify that Romeo's family was prepared to say goodbye during his first struggle but they still wanted to try curative measures. Hospice does not mean we have to give up all hope and treatment – but it can be used in conjunction with treatment in order to afford owners a better sense of control over the entire process.

What qualifies a pet for hospice treatment? Much of the answer is based on the evaluation of the pet, the beliefs of the family, and the goals for care.

Here are a few scenario's in which pets can benefit from veterinary hospice care:

- Advanced aged and dealing with symptoms that limit their quality of life
- Struggling with symptoms from a chronic disease

- Diagnosed with a terminal illness with no treatment options or treatments have failed
- Diagnosed with an illness but treatment is not pursued by the family
- Struggling with life limiting disease but still attempting curative options
- Family's ability to care for the sick pet is not conducive to quality of life

Hospice can be a part of any life stage. In veterinary medicine, there are the three well known stages of life; puppy, adult, and senior. I encourage us to consider geriatrics as the fourth life stage. A pet can be within any one of these life stages but circumstances present themselves such that hospice is warranted. It could be a kitten with FIP, a 5-year-old Great Dane with osteosarcoma or a 17-year-old Chihuahua in heart failure. All could greatly benefit from hospice care and the caregivers would value the support your team provides.

Many families wish to keep their pets alive for as long as possible while maintaining a good quality of life but simply don't know how, which leads to feelings of helplessness. With the advancement of treatment options, we have never been in a more powerful position to provide comfort care to pets and help owners face the struggles of dealing with a dying pet.

While much of veterinary hospice is ideally done in the home (one can garner a lot of information in the home environment that may be missed at the clinic) where the pet is most comfortable, foundational discussions and treatments should be started at the clinic with their primary veterinarian who has enjoyed a long-term relationship with the pet parent.

Hospice veterinarian Tamara Shearer uses a Five Step strategy for hospice care including:

- Evaluation of the pet owner's needs, beliefs, and goals for the pet
- Education about the disease process
- Development of a personalized plan for the pet and pet owner
- Application of palliative or hospice care techniques

- Emotional support during the care process and after the death of the pet (Shearer 2011, p. 508).

By using the word "hospice" with your clients, it redirects their thoughts from curing their pet to caring for their pet and preparing themselves for death and grieving. This, then allows you to tailor your medical management appropriately to make sure the pet is kept comfortable and safe.

Every veterinary practice should provide a Hospice Package (similar to "puppy/kitten" packages) to families with pets in hospice care. Included in the package is disease information, quality of life assessment information and scales, ways to tell if a pet is in pain or discomfort, information on local adjunctive services (mobile pet grooming, acupuncture, etc), information on euthanasia (what to expect, how to make the appointment, and local in-home euthanasia services), information on aftercare (plus crematory contact information in case the pet passes on its own and they need assistance), and pet loss information.

In addition to the Hospice Package, clinics can offer the following services to their clients:

Consultations: Dedicating 30–60 minutes with the veterinarian to discuss the disease or ailment the pet is facing, the progression or trajectory of the symptoms, and creating a plan can be of tremendous benefit to the care giver. When a client calls us for euthanasia but says, "It's not time yet – but I want to be in your system" – to me, this signifies a call for help. Their pet is bad but not quite ready for euthanasia. This is the perfect opportunity to offer a consultation (Figure 36.3).

Pain and Anxiety Management: Providing adequate pain medication is vital and evaluating its effectiveness is just as important. I also equip the owner with an "emergency intervention" they can do themselves. For example, a dog with osteosarcoma should leave your clinic with a dose of injectable pain medication and the client should have knowledge of how to administer it in case

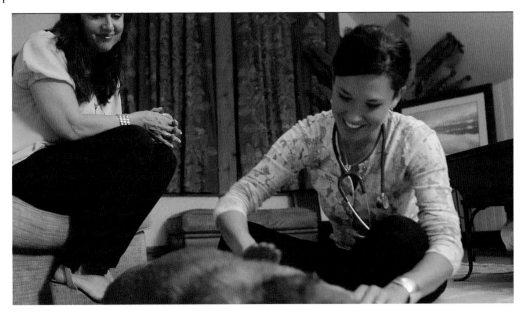

Figure 36.3 Dr. Dani McVety during a hospice visit with patient Fiona.

of a pathologic fracture. This allows the pet some relief while the next steps are organized.

Anxiety Control: Many dogs are up all night panting and pacing. Providing medications that help the pet sleep through the night helps the anxiety level and can be appreciated by everyone in the house. In addition, anxiety and distress change pain perception and pain threshold which can exacerbate the pet's level of pain and making management even more difficult.

Hygiene Maintenance and Infection Control: Urinary and fecal incontinence is usually an ailment geriatric pets succumb to. Although incontinence may not affect quality of life too drastically – some pets do become anxious when they have accidents in the house. Let unmanaged infection and urine scalding can occur. It's important to keep the pet clean with sanitary grooming/shaving, baby-wipes, diapers, waterproof bedding, low litter boxes, and frequent walks. A pet that has inappropriate urination can also lead to the human–animal bond being tested as well as internal disputes among family members.

Nutritional Support: Some diseases will lead to a decrease in appetite. While appetite stimulants are useful at times, often their effectiveness decreases quickly (Figure 36.4). Many owners are willing to cook for their pets, so providing nutritious recipes with alternating protein sources can be helpful.

Nausea Control: Often pets dealing with certain illnesses or those on medications can become nauseous. It's best to control nausea proactively so that the pet doesn't stop eating which can lead to even more issues.

In Home Technician Visits and Care: Seeing the pets in their own environment is important since they can act differently in familiar surroundings. More importantly, modifications can be made that may have been overlooked and treatments can be done in the home without a potentially distressing trip to your clinic.

Visiting Hours: If an aging pet is in your hospital for treatment or boarding for more than a day – encourage visiting hours. The joy both the pet and owner receive is priceless.

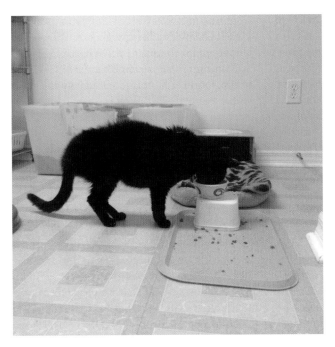

Figure 36.4 Hospice patient Lance who's food bowl needed to be elevated.

Specialized Boarding: Create a special boarding program for geriatric or hospice pets including specialized cage/kennel set up, visiting hours (Figure 36.5), twice daily pictures, and updates.

While offering veterinary hospice may not provide the largest avenue of revenue – the immeasurable benefits are great. The satisfaction your clients will have with the full circle of veterinary care at your clinic will be priceless. This can lead to positive word of mouth, referrals, and repeat business with other pets from that client when necessary and most importantly – it's what's best for the pet. A study in 2010 looked at patients that received palliative care early in their treatment of metastatic lung cancer. It was found that those patients had better quality of life at the end as well as an increased survival time (Temel *et al*. 2010). One could extrapolate that this may also occur with our companion animals – that not only can they live longer but the time they live is better.

With more and more people having positive experiences with human hospice, I believe veterinary hospice will continue to become a requested service and the future of the field looks promising. Textbooks are being written on this topic, national groups have been formed with annual conferences (www.IAAHPC.org), there has even been an increase in pet loss counseling certifications and possibly in the works is an AVMA approved board certification.

Client Needs

According to a study published in the *Journal of Palliative Medicine*, a lack of preparedness when a person was dying resulted in a prolonged grieving period. It showed that caregivers whose loved ones were in a hospice program for as little as 4 days had a significantly reduced amount of depression and grieving than those who did not have hospice services (Hebert *et al*. 2006). The benefits of caregiver well-being with human hospice

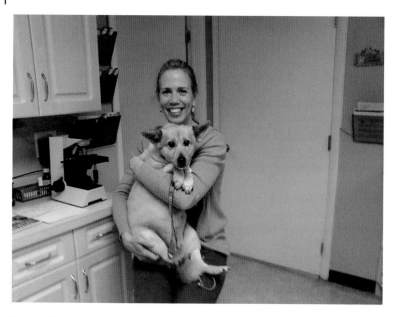

Figure 36.5 Dr. Mary Gardner and hospice patient Cali. Cali needed to be boarded for IV fluids and her owner was allowed to come in the morning and evening for visits and the clinic would send texts with pictures to the mom during the day.

may be carried over to pets in hospice. The more caregivers are able to cope with their decisions, feel confident in their ability to care for their pets, and are properly prepared for the death of their pet, grief and depression may be less – as seen with human hospice.

With all the diagnostic tools and treatment options, we sometimes fail to recognize the other half of the equation – the family and their budgets – what I call 'The 4 Family Budgets":

- *Time*: Caring for a chronically, terminally ill, or advanced-aged, pet requires more time than most realize. Owners must dedicate time to be at home, come home frequently, or make sure someone can care for the pet multiple times throughout the day and in many cases, give medications at an increased frequency. Many families don't have enough time for a healthy pet, let alone one that requires, in many cases, double the amount of time. Often caregivers will not take vacations or postpone work responsibilities just so they can care for their pet during this stage.

- *Emotional*: The stress of caring for a sick pet can tax the human system to a point where the owner becomes anxious, stressed, sick, and even angry. I have helped families that struggle emotionally since this was not the first pet they had with a particular disease and they felt guilt for the way they handled their other pet. Or they simply have many personal, emotional issues to deal with (divorce, sick relative, themselves sick, bankruptcy, moving, etc.) and this can greatly compound the responsibility of a sick pet making it almost too much to bear.

- *Physical*: (Particularly larger dogs with mobility issues.) Physically handling a pet with decreased abilities can be a challenge for many care givers or the home is not ideal when trying to care for particular ailments pets may face.

- *Financial*: The financial budget can be one of the most central of all four budgets however, in my experience, it's not the one that stresses the family the most. Care givers are often willing to pay for their pet's comfort and in most cases, hospice treatment is not an exorbitant amount of money – it's the other three budgets that make caring difficult.

A family may have any component of the budgets strained during the care of their pet – however, if one of the four budgets is exhausted, then humane intervention is not only acceptable, often encouraged. For example, if a pet requires medications every 6 hours as well as to be let out to go to the bathroom and the care giver works an 8 hour shift with an hour commute and has no one to assist them, quality of life for the pet is not sustainable.

Learning what the family most values, the boundaries surrounding their pet's daily life, where their "stop point" is in relation to the pet's disease condition, and what their idea of a "good death" is for their pet is key in helping address the client's needs. Using open-ended questions during the consultation will give the clinician a better understanding of their client's needs.

Below are some example questions to ask owners:

1) Have you ever been through the loss of a pet before? If so, what was your experience (good or bad, and why)?
2) What do you hope the life expectancy of your pet will be? What do you think it will be?
3) What is the ideal situation you wish for your pet's end of life experience? (at home, pass away in her sleep, etc.)
4) Do you hold any stress or anxiety about any of these issues? (This section is meant to help identify the main concerns the family has.)
   - Pet suffering
   - Desire to perform nursing care for pet
   - Ability to perform nursing care for pet
   - Pet dying alone
   - Not knowing the right time to euthanize
   - Coping with loss
   - Concern for other household animals
   - Concern for other members of the family (i.e., children).

Ideally, every family's budgets and boundaries align with the disease process at hand. It's vital to avoid having owners feel guilty about any of the budgets that they can't afford or if their values and boundaries are not what you would do for your pet in your situation.

Pet Needs

One of the most important components in veterinary hospice is obviously the needs of the pet. In the role of "veterinarian," we do our best to manage pain and anxiety, keep nutrition at the highest levels possible, attempt to slow the progression of terminal diseases or manage chronic ones, while at the same time trying to stay within the financial budget of the family. Those are the subjective aspects for the pet's care but the more objective needs of the pet is usually managed by the family. Is the pet happy? That may be an anthropomorphic concept – but one that most of us could agree is used when describing the pet's condition and what's important to the family. In my practice, when I ask owners what is most important for them in terms of their pet's needs, invariably they all say 'I don't want him in pain and I want him to be happy.' This can be challenging because how do you know if the pet is happy or what makes them happy? It usually comes down to the family and their profound knowledge of their pet's personality, daily activities, simply put – their favorite things (Figure 36.6).

As a hospice veterinarian, I attempt to ensure pets are as free from pain and anxiety as possible, that they are kept clean, have a support system to care for them, are properly nourished and hydrated and that they still receive love and care from the family. Often, older or sick pets are demanding to manage, they may smell horrible, urine soaked, pant and whine at night, and so on and this leads to them being banished to another section of the home or outside. In those cases, the pet's needs are not being met and the fine line of doing what's best for the pet while maintaining

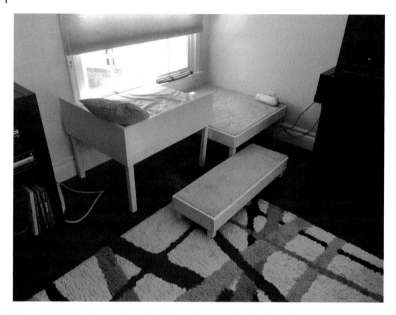

Figure 36.6 Hospice patient Andy loved to sit on his bed by the window but it was too high for him to jump into anymore. Owners build him a modified bed so he could easily enjoy his favorite pastime.

a non-judgmental attitude towards the family becomes a difficult one to assess.

The two most common symptoms to manage in a hospice case are pain and anxiety. Both of which, when left unmanaged, can escalate to the pet suffering. It's a common perception that "animals hide their pain." However, there are many professionals who believe that carnivorous animals, such as cats and dogs, do not "hide" their pain, rather pain simply does not bother them the same way it bothers humans. Animals do not have an emotional attachment to their pain like we do. Humans react to the diagnosis of cancer much differently than Fluffy does. Fluffy doesn't know she has a terminal illness, it bothers us more than it bothers her. With that said, this is vastly different when compared to prey animals like rabbits or guinea pigs, who must hide their pain to prevent carnivorous attacks. Chapter 5 in Temple Grandin and Catherine Johnson's book *Animals in Translation* goes into great detail on this topic (Grandin and Johnson 2005).

If you consider that most pain scales ask owners to perform visual assessments of their pets – then one has to hope that the pet is not "hiding" the pain that is being evaluated. We talk about cat's whiskers or ear positioning when looking for signs of pain. The shear fact that we are looking for these signs is counter intuitive to the thought that they are hiding it. The drawback is that once in pain, animals cannot sense an ending to their hurt. As humans, we can take a pill knowing that the headache will eventually subside but animals have no perception of their suffering ending. Robin Downing, once said in a lecture "Pets do not fear or anticipate death – but they do fear and anticipate pain." I use that often in hospice consultations as well as euthanasia appointments and it really helps owners understand the importance of managing their pet's pain.

Anxiety is not often brought up by the owner unless they actively see it or feel the pain of it occurring during the night when they are trying to sleep. We should be just as concerned about anxiety in our pet as we are about pain. Let's look at dyspnea – in human medicine it is correlated to the unpleasant sensory experience – not just defining the act of labored breathing. Research shows that dyspnea should to be considered as sufferable as chronic pain. My dog rarely looks as distraught when she's in pain as she does when she's anxious. It's the same for animals that are dying. End-stage arthritis patients begin panting, pacing, whining, and crying, especially at night time. Anti-anxiety medications can sometimes work for a time but for pets that are at this stage, the end is certainly near. Cognition also plays a role in the increased anxiety levels. Circling back to the client's needs – an anxious pet, particularly one that does not sleep well – inhibits the family from sleeping well and thus effects their quality of life too.

The best way to manage the pet's needs during the end-of-life stage is to work with the family using a quality-of-life assessment tool as described later in this chapter. The family can be your biggest ally in figuring out what makes the pet "themselves," what makes them happy and what their needs are and how we can work as a team to make sure those are being met.

Expectations on how painful or dramatic the death may depend on the pet's disease. It is most important to help the family understand the disease process their pet is facing. Although we cannot predict exactly what will happen in the future, we can use our medical training and experience to give each family facing an end-of-life experience with their pet, a possible and probable progression of their pet's disease process. As doctors, this is the most important piece of information we can communicate to families as well as a valuable tool they can use in the decision-making process. We must explain to the best of our abilities the most likely "natural" method of death if the pet is left unattended. This educated approach to the physicality of death is essential to veterinary hospice care; by providing the family with knowledge and expectations, we give them the ability to make an informed decision based on their personal wishes for their pet with the gentle guidance by their veterinarian.

When there is a disease present, I will categorize them based on the trajectory of progression and quickness of death (or likelihood of emergency situation occurring in the end). The three categories are Imminent, Intermediate, and Non-Imminent.

- *Imminent diseases* are the ones that have a quick progression and a high likelihood of an emergent situation at the end. Examples might be heart disease, uncontrolled seizers, osteosarcoma, laryngeal paralysis, collapsing trachea, and hemangiosarcoma. The decline resulting from these diseases, in many cases, will happen quickly and most likely not allow for planning or arranging a relaxed and peaceful euthanasia.
- *Intermediate diseases* are ones that may have a longer trajectory and give a bit more time to plan for euthanasia services. Example diseases might be lymphoma, mast cell cancer, nasal tumors, and liver failure.
- *Non-imminent diseases* tend to have the longest trajectory as decline will most likely be slow, allowing families to plan ahead. Example diseases might be chronic renal failure, mobility issues, and cognitive dysfunction. Due to the longer decline period as well as the lack of appearance of active suffering in these pets, it can be difficult for families to make the decision. In those cases, they need to be assured that they are making the right decisions and often the use of quality-of-life scales can be a huge benefit to families. They tend to have the time to track the pet's progression and see the patterns change.

I am able and willing to help extend life as long as pain and anxiety are controlled, but this is always preceded by a lengthy discussion on the progression of the disease process present and a clear "stop point" which we agree is the ending of a good quality of life. Communication, preparation, and more communication is the hallmark of a successful end-of-life case.

Quality of Life

One of the most common questions care givers will ask their veterinarian is "How will I know when it's time?" This question comes with a heavy heart and is not one that can be quickly answered or given a stock answer such as "you will know" or "when they stop eating" – often the answer can be more convoluted than that. Although, at times, those stock answers can be good indications of it being time, often, they are not. The 13-year-old Labrador with osteoarthritis may still be eating and looking excited when his owner comes home, yet he can barely get up, falls down the stairs and is sitting in his own feces half the day. Assessing quality of life is an important part of helping families navigate the end of life stage.

There are three core components to evaluating quality of life: the pet's disease or ailments, the pet's personality, and the owner's abilities, beliefs, and wishes

The Pet's Disease or Ailments

Each disease or ailment a pet faces will carry a different set of struggles, pain, anxiety, or even suffering. A thorough discussion of the symptoms the pet is currently facing, what they will face in the short term and maybe what they will face during the dying process is needed. The quality of life for the German Shepard with hip dysplasia may be within an acceptable level if they are still maintaining nutrition, hydration, pain control, and interaction with family. However, the cat in heart failure that struggles with respiratory distress everyday may have an unacceptable quality of life and intervention may be needed sooner than later.

When discussing the pet's disease, one must cover what the disease process means in terms of how it feels to the pet. Often owners with cats in kidney failure are told it is not painful, however, dehydration, toxin buildup, ulcers, nausea are not without discomfort. Outlining the most common future problems, time frame, and expectations can help a family navigate through the assessment process and also create a "stop point" for when they should consider intervention.

The Pet's Personality

One must consider how the pet deals with different situations such as pain, anxiety, medications, equipment, and the like and, just like humans, every pet will handle things a little differently. So much so that where one pet may easily tolerate a harness, the next pet will do everything in its power to get out of it. Giving medications to some pets can be very difficult whether it be orally, sub-lingually, or sub-cutaneously. It may be easy for the veterinary team to administer but to the family it can be a struggle which can cause a pet to grow weary of their family consequently straining/compromising the human–animal bond.

What the pet enjoys in life is also important. If a dog enjoys laying around being a couch potato, then a disease that limits mobility may not be as quality crushing as a herding dog whose "job" in life is to heard the flock or family. The very quality that we love in pets – individuality – can be a limiting factor when trying to manage a chronic disease.

Owner's Abilities, Beliefs and Wishes

The ability and desire to care for an aging or terminally ill pet can impact the quality of life for the pet as well as the owner. Some owners may seek treatment until all options have been exhausted, while others will opt for a simpler approach to keep them as comfortable for as long as possible without going to the medical "extremes." Since pets are unfortunately seen as property, we cannot force a caregiver to partake in medical treatment for the pet. We can step in as the pet's advocate but in chronic cases, that would typically mean euthanasia vs forcing treatment.

As discussed earlier, regarding the family's budget, the quality of life of a pet can be altered by the family's ability to care for the pet, their beliefs of what is right, and what they wish for the pet near the end (Figure 36.7). What one person considers good "quality" can differ from the others.

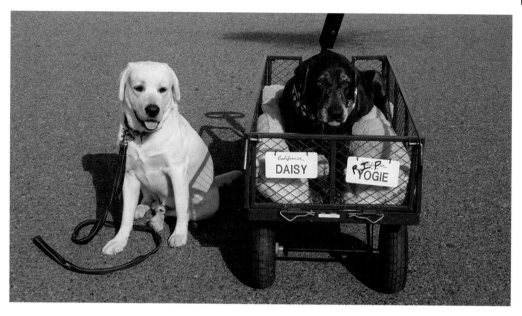

Figure 36.7 Hospice patient Daisy in a cart used for walks. Daisy's owner was willing to do whatever it took to allow Daisy to enjoy her final days.

Luckily most people will agree on one thing – that they don't want their pet to suffer but suffering can still be subjective. This is where assessing quality of life quantitatively can help. But what do you measure? The most commonly used objective measurements for quality of life by veterinarians are mobility, appetite, pain, and proper voiding. I certainly do not disagree with any of these but the presence of quality of life based on these items should not be answered with a "yes or no," but rather "if/then."

Quality-of-Life Assessment Tools

There are many tools available that can assist owners and the veterinary team with evaluating quality of life; some are very simple and others are complex. Selecting the right tool for the family will enable them to monitor the quality progression. There is no perfect tool for all situations, pets, and families but finding a tool that covers the most significant concerns is best. Below are some commonly used tools.

Basic Quality of Life Assessment Tools

- *Rule of 5*: A common suggestion the veterinary team or friends of the family will tell an owner is to pick the pet's five most favorite things to do (Figure 36.8). When the pet no longer does three or more of those, then it's time to consider intervention. This may be eating, going for walks, interacting with family, toys, and so on. The one drawback to this is that the pet may actually still be doing those five favorite things yet their quality of life is clearly not well. For example, cognition issues. While a pet is "alert" they may act, eat, play normally – but when they are in a cognitive state, they are pacing uncontrollably or staring frozen into space until they become physically exhausted. I've witnessed pets that are in a "trance" like state for up to 18 hours a day and the rest of the time they are eating, playing or sleeping comfortably. If this method of evaluation is used, I also suggest including something a pet does NOT like. If they have passion for hating something and they lose that passion – they may not be well. So if the

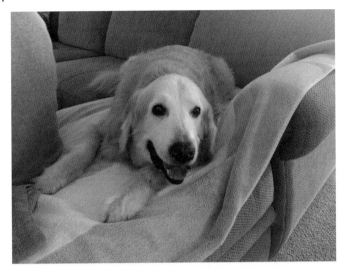

Figure 36.8 Bogey on his favorite couch. It was important to the family that Bogey was still able to get on his couch – even with assistance. And they wanted this final moments to be on the couch.

dog hates the doorbell and eventually doesn't have enough energy to make the smallest bark when it is rung, then the quality of life may be poor.

- *Good Days Vs Bad*: Ensuring that the good days outweigh the bad may seem like a logical way to evaluate quality however most people don't actually record the number of good days. A suggestion I make with all my clients who want to use this method of evaluation is to simply use a calendar to mark and track the bad days. Actually seeing the bad days accumulate helps owners visualize the severity of the situation. It also prevents them from inadvertently forgetting how bad previous days or weeks were when the cherished "good" day comes around. This calendar was developed by Lap of Love for owners to use (http://lapoflove.com/Pet_QoL_Calendar.pdf).

- *Pennies in a Jar*: Another uncomplicated way to track quality of life is to get two jars – one labeled "good day" and the other "bad day." Have the owner put a penny in the appropriate day jar based on the pet's behavior, habits, daily functions, and so on. After a few weeks – you can see if the pet is having more bad days than

good and can signal an appropriate time to recommend euthanasia.

Advanced Quality of Life Assessment Tools

- *HHHHHMM Scale*: Developed by Dr. Alice Villalobos, the HHHHHMM Scale (http://pawspice.com/clients/17611/documents/QualityofLifeScale.pdf) was one of the first tools that veterinarians could instruct a client to use to evaluate clinical signs with a more objective lens. This scale takes into consideration hurt, hunger, hydration, hygiene, happiness, mobility, and more good days than bad. Owners score those symptoms with a 1–10 (one being worst and 10 being best) and add the values up to create a grand total. If the pet is above or below a certain mark, then they may be in an acceptable state or in need of intervention.

- *Lap of Love Quality of Life Scale and Daily Diary*: This scale (http://www.lapoflove.com/Pet_Quality_of_Life_Scale.pdf) is similar to the HHHHHMM scale in terms of scoring and meeting an acceptable threshold but has six criteria (mobility, nutrition, hydration, interaction/attitude, elimination, and favorite things). It also has space dedicated to daily notes so that the owners can jot down any significant changes in their pet that day.

- *Lap of Love Pet's Quality of Life and Family Concerns*: This scale is a tool that also has questions for the family to make sure their needs are addressed. You can download this tool from http://lapoflove.com/Pet_Quality_of_Life_Scale_DrMcVety.pdf. The scale is produced here.

Pet's Quality of Life

Score each subsection on a scale of 0–2:

- 0 = agree with statement (describes my pet)
- 1 = some changes seen
- 2 = disagree with statement (does not describe my pet)

1) Social Functions
   a) Desire to be with the family has not changed.
   b) Interacts normally with family or other pets (i.e., no increased aggression or other changes).
2) Natural Functions
   a) Appetite has stayed the same.
   b) Drinking has stayed the same.
   c) Normal urination habits.
   d) Normal bowel movement habits.
   e) Ability to ambulate (walk around) has stayed the same.
3) Mental Health
   a) Enjoys normal play activities.
   b) Still dislikes the same things. (i.e., still hates the mailman = 0, or doesn't bark at the mailman anymore = 2)
   c) No outward signs of stress or anxiety.
   d) Does not seem confused or apathetic.
   e) Nighttime activity is normal, no changes seen.
4) Physical Health
   a) No changes in breathing or panting patterns.
   b) No outward signs of pain. (See Resources Below)
   c) No pacing around the house.
   d) My pet's overall condition has not changed recently.

Results:

0–8 = Quality of life is most likely adequate. No medical intervention required yet, but guidance from your veterinarian may help you identify signs to look for in the future.

9–16 = Quality of life is questionable and medical intervention is suggested. Your pet would certainly benefit from veterinary oversight and guidance to evaluate the disease process he/she is experiencing.

17–36 = Quality of life is a definite concern. Changes will likely become more progressive and more severe in the near future. Veterinary guidance will help you better understand the end stages of your pet's disease process in order to make a more informed decision of whether to continue hospice care or elect peaceful euthanasia.

Family's Concerns

Score each section on a scale of 0–2:

- 0 = I am not concerned at this time.
- 1 = There is some concern.
- 2 = I am concerned about this.

I am concerned about the following things:
1) Pet suffering
2) Desire to perform nursing care for your pet
3) Ability to perform nursing care for your pet
4) Pet dying alone
5) Not knowing the right time to euthanize
6) Coping with loss
7) Concern for other household animals
8) Concern for other members of the family (i.e., children)

Results:

0–4 = Your concerns are minimal at this time. You have either accepted the inevitable loss of your pet and understand what lies ahead, or have not yet given it much thought. If you have not considered these things, now is the time to begin evaluating your own concerns and limitations.

5–9 = Your concerns are mounting. Begin your search for information by educating yourself on your pet's condition; it's the best way to ensure you are prepared for the emotional changes ahead.

10–16 = Although you may not place much value on your own quality of life, your concerns about the changes in your pet are valid. Now is the time to prepare yourself and to build a support system around you. Veterinary guidance will help you prepare for the medical changes in your pet while counselors and other health professionals can begin helping you with anticipatory grief.

Interactive Quality of Life Assessments

Pet Hospice Journal

This online quality-of-life scale is the first interactive assessment tool that was developed by Lap of Love. The biggest concern with most quality-of-life scales is that they do not take into consideration the disease the pet has and what symptoms they will experience with that particular disease. The dog with arthritis may score a "0" for mobility but their eating gets a "3" as does their favorite things. This will falsely elevate the Quality-of-Life score. The Pet Hospice Journal was developed so that a caregiver could create a profile for their pet and based on the disease they selected, the criteria for assessment would change as well as the "weight" each answer earned. This tool is free for vets and pet owners and can be found at www.pethospicejournal.com.

Suggestions when using any quality-of-life scale:

1) Complete the scale at different times of the day, note circadian fluctuations in well-being. (We find most pets tend to do worse at night and better during the day.)
2) Request multiple members of the family complete the scale; compare observations.
3) Take periodic photos of the pet to help remember their physical appearance.
4) Keep detailed notes.
5) Create a stop point of when intervention will be sought.
6) Don't get frustrated – this is not an easy time and there is no black and white answer.
7) Pick the tool that best fits the pet's ailment and family's personality. Not everyone is willing to do the interactive tool, yet some people want more than a jar of pennies.

Using any method to help evaluate quality of life of the pet in conjunction with the family's quality of life has helped many owners feel empowered over their decisions – whether to continue with treatment/care or euthanize their pets.

How I wish the answer to the question of "when is it time" was simple and clear cut. I believe that it is our duty to assist owners with end-of-life decisions and to help end and prevent suffering of animals. There are many ways to help families explore quality-of-life questions but the one way that is an injustice to our profession is if you simply say, "Call me when it's time." Owners need more than this and animals deserve more.

Cultural Sensitivities

There are many religions or cultures that do not believe in euthanasia which makes providing hospice even more important. It is the veterinary team's role to educate, care, and support the pet and the owner during this time. Equally important is to avoid judging a pet owner's beliefs and wishes. At that time, focusing on comfort care is paramount.

Even for those families that elect euthanasia, the decision might be conflicting with their core religious beliefs and they may be struggling with the decision. I've often been asked if I am a Christian. After I answer that I was born and raised a Roman Catholic, inevitably they ask me how I justify taking a life. I usually answer that I was blessed with the ability to help end suffering and that is what I am doing. Refocusing back to the pet's needs and undesirable situation is usually all that it takes, but often people lament on this decision.

As far as aftercare, some families may carry their personal "human" beliefs/rituals over to their pets. Table 36.1 presents some ritual differences that one should know and respect if a client requests a particular process.

Developing an awareness and appreciation for the variations among rituals, feelings of death, attitudes towards animals, and the mourning practices surrounding death in different cultures provides a meaningful context and can help you lead families through the death process with more dignity and empathy.

Dying Naturally

Faced with a terminal illness or a geriatric pet in a declining state, pet owners have to eventually come to terms with their pet's passing and make the decision between a "natural death" and humane euthanasia. Many owners fear their pet "passing alone" while others do not. I imagine just about everyone would like their pet to comfortably crawl into their bed one night, drift off to sleep, and pass away peacefully while sleeping. I hope that I personally pass that way as well and I believe this is what many people think "natural death" is. However, more often than not, this is not how a pet dies naturally and a "natural" death does not necessarily mean a peaceful death.

Table 36.1 Variations between religious rituals and beliefs.

Religion	Cremation	Funeral Details	Mourning
Catholic	Cremation is allowed but body present for the funeral is preferred	Funerals do not occur on certain holy days	No specific mourning period or memorial events
Baptist	Cremation is allowed	Burial should take place within three to five days of the death	No specific mourning period or memorial events
Buddhist	Cremation is acceptable in Buddhism	Traditionally held on the third, seventh, forty-ninth, and one-hundredth day after the death.	In Tibet the day of death is thought of as highly important. It is believed that as soon as the death of the body has taken place, the personality goes into a state of trance for four days. Some Buddhists will keep the body out for this period of time.
Jewish	Depending on the degree of orthodoxy of the deceased, the rituals around cremation may vary. For Orthodox Jews, cremation and embalming is not acceptable.	There is no generally no viewing, visitation, or wake in Jewish tradition.	The first mourning period ('Shiva') is 7 days following the funeral, the second mourning period ('shloshim") lasts 30 days. On the first year anniversary, a memorial event called the "Yahrzeit" is held.
Muslim	Cremation is forbidden for Muslims.	According to Islamic law the body should be buried as soon as possible from the time of death.	It is acceptable in Islam to express grief over a death. Crying and weeping at the time of death, at the funeral, and at the burial are all acceptable forms of expression. However, wailing and shrieking, tearing of clothing and breaking of objects, and expressing a lack of faith in Allah are all prohibited.

Source: Data from Everplans.com.

Occasionally I am asked to help families through the natural dying process with their pet. For different reasons, these families are against euthanasia. I explain everything I possibly can, from how a natural death may look to how long it may take, and what their pet may experience.

I also educate the family that they may be present for the death and that can be difficult to watch, especially for non-medically oriented people. Most people can watch a human family member in pain much more easily than they can their pet. To an extent, we can talk other humans through physical pain or discomfort.

To begin with, one has to understand how an animal actually dies. Unfortunately, this is not fully understood in many cases as it is dependent on the disease or issue the pet is suffering from. Many "end stage" diseases can be extremely painful or full of anxiety for the pet.

When I consult with clients who desire a "natural passing" for their pet – I explain what their pet may experience during that process depending on their ailment. I also ask why they want a natural passing for their pet. More often than not, I receive two answers.

1) They do not want to make the decision (or make the decision too early) which is understandable. However, death will occur eventually but it is up to us to help relieve pain, anxiety, and suffering for our furry family members by electing humane euthanasia which is the gentlest, most caring thing one can do for an ailing pet.

2) The second most common answer I hear is that they think euthanasia hurts and entails giving a poison to their pet or giving them a heart attack. None of which are true.

Another thing to keep in mind about a "natural" passing is that it doesn't always happen at night while they are in bed. It can happen when the owner runs to the store, when they are at work, when they are outside getting the mail, and so on. More often than not, death doesn't occur while they are asleep but instead the pet eventually does fall unconscious which people then perceive as having occurred while they were asleep.

A natural passing doesn't always happen very quickly either. I have had many frantic phone calls from people wanting me to rush to their home because they wanted a natural passing for their pet but the process is taking too long or not very peaceful. The pet might start having a seizure, they may start to choke or they may have difficulty breathing. This is not easy to watch or let your pet go through and people need to be prepared for this. I wouldn't want to be alone during my final moments, so families with pets that are near the end should have someone with them at all times to make sure they are not suffering.

Points to cover with families during the dying process:

- It can happen at any time – day or night
- The dying process can take hours
- The pet may stretch, put their head back, yawn, seize, and even vocalize
- Afterwards, they will first have a period of muscle relaxation (including the release of urine and feces) followed by rigor mortis
- Plan for aftercare – provide the family with information on how to handle the body after including information on burial, crematory information, or a local emergency clinic that will arrange cremation.

A family should know that it is never too late to call a veterinarian if the natural route is not going as they had planned. The owner should give themselves permission to choose humane euthanasia if their plan for natural death is not what they had envisioned for their pet's end-of-life experience.

Dying with Assistance – Euthanasia

The euthanasia appointment is unparalleled in emotion and sentiment. What you say, how you say it, and what you don't say during the euthanasia becomes a delicate dance that should be carefully choreographed and continually improved upon.

Making the decision to euthanize a pet can feel gut-wrenching, murderous, and immoral. Yes, those are strong words, but that is what our pet families' experience. They feel they are letting their pet down or that they are the cause of their friend's death (which is why so many say "I'm sorry" to their pet as they are passing). They forget that euthanasia is a gift, something that, when used appropriately and timely, prevents further physical suffering for the pet and emotional suffering of the family.

If there is one thing to keep in the forefront of the team's approach to the euthanasia appointment, it's this: "What would I do for my own family's pet?" This goes for the environment, the medicine, and even how they are handled afterwards. When you consider what you would do for you own pet – that becomes the minimum of how you treat your patients and their caregivers. The entire euthanasia process can be broken down into three major sections. Before, during, and after the appointment.

Before

The most difficult phone call an owner has to make about their pet is the euthanasia appointment. The moment the receptionist knows the call is for a euthanasia, they should immediately show empathy and focus entirely on the conversation. Owners should never be put on hold – particularly if the hold music is advertisements for care of pets. Prices for services should be memorized or cheat sheets available to enable a quick response to any questions. It's best if all services are priced as a group instead of itemized which can be difficult for a receptionist to list and even more upsetting for a client to hear. For example – the price for the euthanasia should automatically include sedation and catheter placement and so on.

The most concerning trend I have encountered is when clinics will charge more if the client wants to be present. Although I understand the rationale behind this – receptionists dislike talking about that and owners will

wonder what a clinic does to their pet (or services not provided) when they are not around to witness. This doubt instantly puts a shadow on the already emotionally fragile appointment.

During

When a family is on the schedule for a euthanasia, appoint someone on the team to manage that appointment including watching out for the family as they pull up. Assist them with their pet getting out of the car, open the door for them and direct them to the exam room as quickly as possible. If there is one message I would give, it is to never break the human–animal bond – particularly during the last appointment. I would never want my pet separated from me at the end nor would I want them to experience even the slightest bit of anxiety. This is why I feel that all pets should be allowed to stay in the room with their family while all preparations are made. Ideally, pets should be sedated before any type of catheter (indwelling or butterfly) is placed. I cannot tell you how many owners will comment on how nice it is to see their pet calmly resting one last time (Figure 36.9). It gives the owners a sense of peace and is a nice transitional step before the final medication is given. I've also seen that it helps the entire staff to see this peaceful resting period. All too often pets are not sedated (or they struggle for an indwelling catheter first) and it is putting emotional pressure on the staff when most feel a struggle with this type of appointment already.

Communication is paramount during this time. Everything should be explained especially how the euthanasia medication works (Figure 36.10). Too often owners think the medication stops the heart and think it's painful, or they do not realize how fast the process can be. Explaining every possible side-effect is not necessary but the two key ones are relaxing the bladder and the eyelid muscles relaxing and not tightly closing.

Offering time alone before or after the euthanasia is suggested in case the family

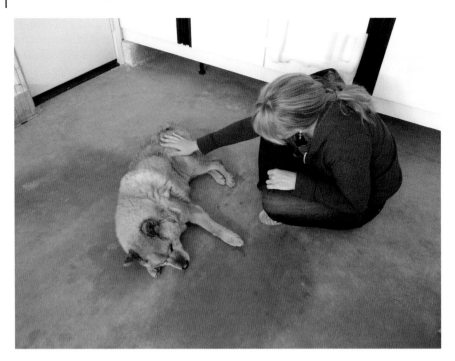

Figure 36.9 Dr. Mary Gardner and Jindu. The patient had a difficult night and the owners called at 6am asking for Dr. Gardner to get there as soon as she could. (After giving the sedation, the owners wanted to take a picture of him so peaceful as they had not seen him resting that well in weeks.)

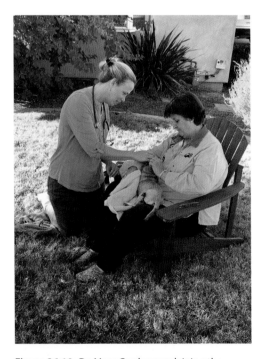

Figure 36.10 Dr. Mary Gardner explaining the euthanasia process to a client.

needs time to prepare or grieve. They should never feel rushed or awkward for their wishes.

After

After the appointment, follow up with the family to make sure they don't have any questions or are in need of support. It is recommended to call the family the following day to simply offer your condolences and let them know you are there if they need anything. The power behind that small gesture is priceless. Sympathy cards personalized by the entire staff show the owners that everyone at the clinic cared for their pet as well as the family and that the bond they shared is recognized and honored. Creating a good experience and memorial has a positive effect on many people dealing with loss and allows them to appreciate the life and memory of the lost one.

Although everyone knows the exam room contains the "cold sterile table" – the sterility of the appointment comes from multiple facets – not just the steel table. The feeling of support during the illness and decision process, how the receptionist warmly communicates to the family, the service and caring nature the entire team handling the appointment, to the follow up – all can turn a difficult moment for a family, into something a little better than expected.

Dying Well

Whether a family elects euthanasia or a natural passing, it is paramount that the pet remains in as little discomfort as possible. I believe that it is our responsibility as veterinary professionals and advocates for the pets to ensure the comfort of the pets and educate the owners on the disease they are facing and setting expectations.

There will be some families that want to wait for as long as possible before they decide on euthanasia and that may be more important to them then a peaceful passing. They are fearful of doing it too soon and giving up without a good fight. With that said, pain and anxiety medication is typically required to support the pet through the final weeks and days. I also have a frank conversation with the owners about what to expect in the end and where the emergency clinic is in case it occurs during off hours. Often, just hearing about the side-effects and possibility of emergency clinics will gently guide an owner to euthanasia sooner.

It is often easier for families to decide on euthanasia if they actually see their pet in pain, anxiety, or suffering – it reduces the guilt they feel. This of course is not always fair for the pet and I encourage families to say goodbye on a "good day." Make it an experience that they can remember as a positive one. Do their favorite things the day before (or day of), provide whatever they want to eat (even chocolate!), take pictures/videos, and so on. Usually regret happens when they wait too long – but it requires that to occur before they realize that. An interesting trend that I did not expect when starting my hospice practice is that the more times families experience the loss of a pet, the sooner they make the decision to euthanize. With the first passing, they tend to reflect back on the past days, weeks, or months, and feel guilty for putting their pet through those numerous trips to the vet or uncomfortable medical procedures that did not improve their pet's quality of life. The next time they witness the decline of a pet, they are much more likely to make the decision at the beginning of the decline instead of the end.

Encouraging and supporting a "good death" on a "good day" can help mitigate feelings of guilt as well as the suffering of the pets. I've been to euthanasia parties for the pet and as odd as that may sound – it is actually quite lovely. The entire family is supported and the pet feels how loved they are (Figure 36.11). There is no better way to say goodbye.

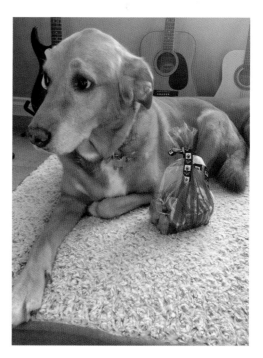

Figure 36.11 12-year-old Dixie was diagnosed with Osteosarcoma and the family wanted to say goodbye to Dixie on a good day – before she ever struggled with the disease. This picture was taken the morning of her euthanasia when she was given treats and love by the entire family.

Death and Aftercare of the Body

Technically, death is the termination of the biological functions that sustain a living organism. Human medicine differentiates "brain death" from "biological death" from "legal death." Clearly this is problematic and not well defined.

Whether a family chooses euthanasia or the pet passes on their own, it is important to know and at times, educate the families to set expectations appropriately.

Events associated with natural death:

1) Cardiac arrest
2) Muscle spasms or convulsions – cells lose connections
3) Agonal breath – up to hours after (humans), usually no more than 10 minutes at most in vet med; spasmodic open mouth with contraction of the diaphragm and retraction of the hyoid apparatus which occurs at death (mechanism not fully known)
4) Fluid from nostrils or mouth – if fluid back up in lungs (i.e., CHF, neoplasia)

Events associated with injection of barbiturates (euthanasia):

1) Cerebral death
2) Respiratory arrest
3) Cardiac arrest
4) Agonal breath
5) Fluid from nostrils or mouth

Occasionally caregivers will question what happens after the pet dies or questions why the pet still feels warm, why the eyes are open or even why they may see slight muscle twitching. Typically one does not need to go into much details but it is good to understand the process to give a summarized answer if asked.

Five stages of decompensation

Stage 1 – Fresh
  a) Pallor mortis – paleness, 15–120 minutes after death
  b) Livor mortis – settling of the blood in the lower portion of the body
  c) Algor mortis – reduction in body temperature.
    • Each hour the body temperature falls about 1.5 degrees.
  d) Rigor mortis – limbs stiffen due to lack of ATP
    • 30 minutes to 2 hours
    • onset is faster at higher temperatures and with a lot of muscular activity immediately prior to death, which depletes glycogen stores and ATP in the muscle

Stage 2 – Bloat
  a) Anaerobic metabolism continues leading to the accumulation of gases, such as hydrogen sulphide, carbon dioxide, and methane. This causes the distention of the abdomen and gives a cadaver its overall bloated appearance.
  b) Intestinal anaerobic bacteria transform hemoglobin into sulfhemoglobin and other colored pigments. Gases aid in the transport of sulfhemoglobin throughout the body giving the body an overall marbled appearance.

Stage 3 – Active Decay
  a) Period of greatest mass loss. This loss occurs as a result of both maggots and the purging of decomposition fluids into the surrounding environment. Liquefaction of tissues and disintegration become apparent during this time and strong odors persist. The end of active decay is signaled by the migration of maggots away from the body to pupate.

Stage 4 – Advanced Decay
  a) Decomposition and insect activity are reduced. When the carcass is located on soil, the area surrounding it will show evidence of vegetation death.

Stage 5 – Dry Remains
  a) All that remains of the cadaver is dry skin, cartilage, and bones, which will become dry and bleached if exposed to the elements. (Forbes 2008; Everplans. com 2017)

Aftercare varies based on situation and family wishes. Often in general practices, cremation is elected. With that said, many people would like to bury their pets at home and are not often given that option. It is important to offer that option but let the owner's know that it is their responsibility to learn about local ordinances as well as proper burying techniques.

The crematory you use is the most important pet loss partner for your clinic. Before selecting a crematory, one should tour the facility to observe how they handle the pets, how the procedure is done (mainly regarding identification) and learning the differences between a private, individual, and communal cremation.

Anticipatory Grief and Honoring the Pet

Our society in general is a "death avoidance" society. We try to move away from the pain of death and tend to not want to acknowledge its existence. The death of a pet is, for many, the worst personal loss they have ever experienced. Complicate the event with the possibility of euthanasia and the emotions can be too much for some pet parents to bear. How, when, and why veterinary professionals can make a difference at such an important time is essential to maintaining not only the human–animal bond, but the doctor–client bond as well. There is no better time to show your clients you care than by helping through the difficult journey of pet loss.

Many people experience what is referred to as "Anticipatory Grief." This is when emotions such as grief, despair, anger occur before the impending loss of a pet. Once an owner learns of a terminal illness or sees the long-term decline of their geriatric pet, their grief emotions can start to manifest and can even make some physically sick. The five stages of grief, listed below, can also be present in anticipatory grief. However, this period can also allow pet owners time to do things with their pet that they may have put off in the past and for some, it prompts a conscious closure before the loss.

With the lack of social acceptance of grief over a pet that has passed, it is even more compounded when someone is facing anticipatory grief. A caregiver may feel that no one understands them or they may even feel "silly" that they are getting so emotional over "just an animal." But most pet owners that love their pets do understand and it is important that this period of grief is recognized, and us as pet professionals assist our clients during this difficult time.

This period of anticipatory grief doesn't usually take the place of post-loss grief. There will typically still be a degree of grief after the pet has passed.

Regardless if the pet is old or young, if death is sudden or expected, grief is a natural reaction to the loss of that pet. Similar to when a person passes away, many people can experience what is commonly called the five states of grief – although not everyone experiences all of these emotions and there is no set pattern that people follow when grieving.

1) Denial
2) Anger
3) Bargaining (i.e., trying to find an activity or action that either could have helped avoid the loss or that will take it away)
4) Depression
5) Acceptance

Pet loss grief is a real and sometimes crippling emotion. As pet professionals we need to recognize, embrace, and help (within limits) our clients through this time. Your clinic should have available information on local pet loss groups and even counselors for clients not only dealing with pet loss but also the upcoming loss of their pet to help with anticipatory grief. A recommended source for pet loss information as well as companion certification is at Two Hearts Pet Loss Center (http://twoheartspetlosscenter.com).

Honoring their Memory

Honoring a lost pet is an important part of both the grieving and healing process. Some don't want any remembrance of their pet as the emotional pain is too intense while others need many ways to remember and honor their pet. In the clinic, the most common memorial item we provide is the paw impression in clay. I encourage all doctors to make the paw impression personally and after every euthanasia. This simple act can provide so much peace and happiness to the client – often rubbing off on the veterinary team.

Below are some ideas we can provide owners to help them to honor their pet once their time together has come to an end:

1) Start a scrapbook with photos, drawings and/or stories.
2) Plant a tree in the backyard – choose one as a family that "reminds" you of the pet. For example, a snowball bush for a white, fluffy dog/cat or a big, oak tree for a working breed dog.
3) Plant flowers yearly in a flower bed and take that time to reminisce and remember the pet.
4) Make a tribute table with items that remind the family of the pet; pictures, toys, a collar or leash, favorite stick or mementos from various trips together (Figure 36.12). This can be a particularly useful when small children are in involved in the grieving process.
5) Have all family members wear something that reminds them of the pet. For example, get all shirts to match the same color as the pet's favorite collar, get a picture of your pet on a nightshirt, a ring with the pet's birthstone or engrave the pet's name in a locket.
6) Make each family member a small pillow out of the pet's favorite blanket or bandana.
7) Hold a memorial service – let children take part in the planning as much as possible (older children can do the planning/ inviting independently).
8) Make a donation in the pet's name and let children choose the charity.

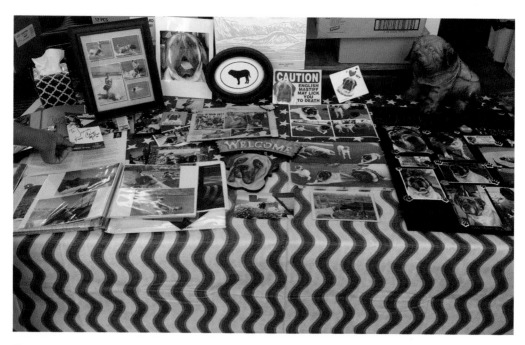

Figure 36.12 Jupiter's Memorial Table. This was created the day of the euthanasia and left out for the family to look at for a week.

9) Write a letter or a "will" from the pet – this will serve as a nice family activity to share and a forum for memories and stories.

10) Have all family members write (or if they are too young, you can do it for them) a letter to the pet to express their feelings or perhaps things they wish they could say to the pet.

11) Keep a list of all the things the pet did that brought about a smile or laugh. The family can experience the joy the pet brought to their lives now and for years to come.

12) Keepsakes: There are many companies that specialize in creating personalized treasures like stone markers, sculptures, paintings, jewelry, even diamonds that can all incorporate the cremains of your pet.

Resources for Coping with Pet Loss

- Good resources for pet loss help can be found through the "Association for Death Education and Counseling" and the "Association for Pet Loss and Bereavement".
- Dr. Alan Wolfelt, Pet Loss expert, has created the 'Pet Lover's Code' which helps owners with the loss of a pet
- Petlosspartners.org

Pet Loss Books for Children

- *When a Pet Dies* ~ F. Rogers

- *Dog Heaven* ~ C. Rylant
- *Cat Heaven* ~ C. Rylant

Pet Loss Books for Adults
- *Grieving The Death of a Pet* ~ Betty Carmack
- *Sorrow on the Loss of Your Pet* ~ M. Anderson
- *Pet Loss and Human Bereavement* ~ W. Kay
- *Animals as Teachers and Healers* ~ S. McElroy
- *A Final Act of Caring: Ending the Life of an Animal Friend* ~ M. Montgomery
- *Pet Loss: A Thoughtful Guide for Adults and Children* ~ H. Neiburg.
- *It's Okay To Cry* ~ M.L. Quintana

Summary

The end of life stage can be an emotionally fragile time for caregivers but it is also one of the most precious times. As veterinary professionals it is our duty to assist the families through this time with education, support, sound medical decisions, and thoughtful preparations.

By honoring the human–animal bond in everything we do can not only help owners and pets but the entire veterinary team. Developing an End-of-Life program in your clinic including hospice services, quality-of-life consultations and best practices in euthanasia will ensure you are doing everything possible to help caregivers give the best care for their pets.

References

AVMA Guidelines for Veterinary Hospice Care. Online at: https://www.avma.org/KB/Policies/Pages/Guidelines-for-Veterinary-Hospice-Care.aspx (accessed June 5, 2017).

Everplans.com. Health and medical. Online at: https://www.everplans.com/health-medical (accessed June 5, 2017).

Forbes SL. Decomposition chemistry in a burial environment. In: M Tibbett and DO Carter, Eds. Soil analysis in forensic taphonomy. CRC Press. 2008: 203–223.

Grandin T, Johnson C. Animals in translation. Bloomsbury. 2005.

Hebert RS, Prigerson HG, Schulz R, Arnold RM. Preparing caregivers for the death of a loved one: a theoretical framework and suggestions for future research.

Journal of Palliative Medicine. 2006; 9(5): 1164–1171.

Janaway RC, Percival SL, Wilson AS. Decomposition of human remains. In: SL Percival, Ed. Microbiology and aging. Springer Science + Business. 2009: 13–334.

Shearer T. Palliative medicine and hospice care, an issue of veterinary clinics. Elsevier Health Sciences. 2011.

Temel JS1, Greer JA, Muzikansky A. et al. Early palliative care for patients with metastatic non-small-cell lung cancer. New England Journal of Medicine. 2010; 363(8): 733–734.

Index

Chronic Disease Management for Small Animals, First Edition. Edited by W. Dunbar Gram,
Rowan J. Milner and Remo Lobetti.
© 2018 John Wiley & Sons, Inc. Published 2018 by John Wiley & Sons, Inc.